SHARING THE
BURDEN OF
SICKNESS

SHARING THE BURDEN OF SICKNESS

A History of Healing and Medicine in Accra

—⁓—

Jonathan Roberts

INDIANA UNIVERSITY PRESS

This book is a publication of

Indiana University Press
Office of Scholarly Publishing
Herman B Wells Library 350
1320 East 10th Street
Bloomington, Indiana 47405 USA

iupress.org

Manufactured in the United States of America
First printing 2021

Library of Congress Cataloging-in-Publication Data

Names: Roberts, Jonathan (Historian), author.
Title: Sharing the burden of sickness : a history of healing and medicine
  in Accra / Jonathan Roberts.
Description: First printing. | Bloomington, Indiana : Indiana University
  Press, 2021. | Includes bibliographical references and index.
Identifiers: LCCN 2021014696 (print) | LCCN 2021014697 (ebook) | ISBN
  9780253057945 (hardback) | ISBN 9780253057938 (paperback) | ISBN
  9780253057914 (ebook)
Subjects: LCSH: Medicine—Ghana—Accra—History. | Traditional
  medicine—Ghana—Accra—History. | Medicine—Ghana—Religious aspects.
Classification: LCC R653.G4 R63 2021 (print) | LCC R653.G4 (ebook) | DDC
  610.9667—dc23
LC record available at https://lccn.loc.gov/2021014696
LC ebook record available at https://lccn.loc.gov/2021014697

CONTENTS

KEY TERMS[1]

adope: Invisible dwarves who offer magical and healing power to their followers, known in Akan languages as *mmotia*.

akon: Drumming cult derived from Akan cultures.

akutso, pl. *akutsei*: Quarter, division of a town.

Al-Tibb al-nabawi: Medicine of the Prophet.

Alufa: Islamic holy men, usually of Yoruba ethnicity, who infused the power of the Quran into charms.

amenye: Elder woman with many offspring.

awoyoo: Freelance pastors offering spiritual and herbal remedies.

ayε: Witch.

babanso: Gonorrhea.

bid'ah: Innovation to Islamic thought, breaking with tradition.

blofo tsofa: "White man's medicine."

---

[1] All *Ga* terminology takes its spelling from Mary E. Kropp Dakubu, ed., *Ga–English Dictionary with English–Ga Index* (Accra: Black Mask, 1999). The orthography of the terms is consistent with Dakubu's work, with the exception of the character of ɔ (representing the *o* sound in *hot*), which has been changed to *o* to prevent gaps in the formatting of paragraphs. All Ga terms are in italics, with the exception of the proper noun Ga, which can be used to refer to the Ga language, the Ga ethnic group, and the city of Accra (by Ga speakers).

cassarerte: An antiquated Portuguese term meaning "to take into one's house," referring to relationships between Europeans and African women in Accra.

deus otiosus: A so-called idle god who is no longer involved in the daily events of life.

feitiço: An antiquated Portuguese term referring to the material culture of sorcery and witchcraft, transliterated in English as "fetish."

gbaja: (lit. pouch.) Venereal disease, syphilis.

gbeshi: Individual fate, or personality.

gbomotso: Body.

Gov'ment: Margaret Field's transliteration of a local pronunciation of *government*.

Hauka: Hausa term for "crazy," and also used to describe deities of possession.

hela: Disease, illness, sickness.

hela folo: Ordinary illness.

helatsalo: Doctor, physician.

hewalɛ: The vigor and strength of a person in a physical and mental sense.

hiatso: A medicinal herb (*Fagara zanthoxyloides*).

hijama: A cupping technique used for bodily maladies.

Homowo: (lit. the time to "hoot at hunger.") The annual harvest festival in Accra.

jemawoŋ, pl. *jemawoji*: A lesser god attached to a geographical location, usually a shrine. The major *jemawoji* in Accra are Nae, Sakumo, and Korle.

kita: Oath.

kitakalo: Swearer of an oath.

kitatomo: Oath breaking.

kitatomono: An object presented as pacification, in atonement.

kla: Spirit residing within the living body.

Kolebu: General Ga name for a hospital or clinic.

Kolebu awula: General Ga name for a nurse.

kpele: Drumming cult of the Ga people.

mallam: General term for Muslim healer or priest.

maŋ: City, or urban area under the jurisdiction of chiefs and priests.

maŋtse, pl. *maŋtsemei*: Chief.

mumo hela: Spiritual illness.

mumo kroŋkroŋ: Holy Spirit.

nyanyara: A medicinal herb (*Momordica charantia*).

Nyoŋmo: Supreme God, Divine Creator.

otofo: Ghost of someone who dies unnaturally (violently, by accident, unexpectedly, or when young).

otutu, pl. *otutui*: A mound filled with consecrated objects that serves as a shrine or a point at which to worship spirits.

ruqyah: Islamic charms to protect against harm by spiritual forces, such as *jinn*.

sisa: Ghost or ancestral shade of someone who died a natural death (in sickness or old age).

susuma: Soul, shadow, or subconscious.

ti: Consecrated healing powder made from the charred remains of herbs and symbolic reagents.

tsofa: Drugs, herbs, roots.

tsofatse, pl. *tsofatsemei*: (lit. "father of the roots/drugs.") Herbalist.

wanzamai: Hausa surgeons who were adept at barbering, circumcision, ritual scarification, herbal remedies, and the creation of Islamic apotropaics.

woŋ, pl. *woji*: Lesser god, normally contained in medicinal ingredients.

woŋtse (m), *woyoo* (f), pl. *woŋtsemei/woyei*: Spirit medium and herbalist.

woŋtsulo: Herbalist who uses spiritual skill to harm, poisoner.

wulomo, pl. *wulomei*: Priest and caretaker of the shrine of a *jemawoŋ*.

Yesu Kristo: Jesus Christ.

zoŋo: A neighborhood established by Muslim immigrants, usually multiethnic.

ACKNOWLEDGMENTS

THIS HAS BEEN A TWENTY-YEAR project, so the number of institutions and persons involved is lengthy, to say the least. The research was supported financially by the University of Toronto Department of Graduate Studies, the Social Sciences and Humanities Research Council of Canada, the Ontario Graduate Scholarship Program, and the Hannah Institute for the Study of the History of Medicine, as well as by grants through Hartwick College in Oneonta, New York. The most important ongoing support has been offered through Mount Saint Vincent University in Halifax, Nova Scotia—my professional refuge and my academic home. Thank you to the family of scholars at this unique institution, with a special mention to Adriana Benzaquen, Elizabeth Church, Ken Dewar, Frances Early, Roni Gechtman, Janet Guildford, Arthur McCalla, Corey Slumkoski, Brook Taylor, Martha Walls, and the late Reginald Stuart.

The folks at the Ghana National Archives (PRAAD) were immensely important in bringing out enough sources to make this possible—namely, Judith Botchway, Killian Onai, William Ashaley, and particularly Bright Botwe, whose retreat from farming has allowed him to become a masterful archivist.

I would also like to offer a heartfelt thank you to all the people who offered comments on drafts of this book, including Amal Ghazal, Gary Kynoch, Nakanyike Musisi, and Ato Quayson. Also special thanks to Timothy Brook, Marty Klein, Chima Korieh, Colin Mitchell, Joey Power, Stephen Rockel, Andra Thakur, and the eternal Chris Youe.

To my academic coaches I offer the deepest gratitude: Myron Echenberg, who sparked my interest in bubonic plague and taught me how high a flea can jump (answer: it depends on the species); Sean Hawkins, who trained me up from a blue dot to a yellow dot in squash and opened my eyes to the creative methodologies that made this book plural rather than singular; and most importantly to Phil Zachernuk, who showed me how to slide out of the hack with enough draw weight to get it into the house, which is the precise curling metaphor for how he helped me finish this project.

To everyone in and around Bukom who assisted me with this research, *nyɛ yi wala doŋ*, in particular to Ebenezer Abiase, Abigail Quaye, and Ellis Nkrumah. But it is to Richard (Gorgeous George) Nii Oshiu Codjoe, a stalwart friend, that I owe the most gratitude. He taught me the dos and don'ts of Ga culture (do shake hands clockwise, don't cross your legs in front of a priest, do take your shoes off before entering a shrine, don't talk back to a goddess), and he always had my back—in Bukom and beyond.

Finally, to my beloved wife, Mary Nkrumah, whose legendary patience with this project has sustained me through its completion.

NOTE ON SOURCES

IF THERE WAS A MOMENT of genesis for this book, it was a visit to the Nae We Shrine in Ussher Town, in the heart of Accra, in 2003. On the wall of the inner courtyard of the shrine is a painting of the Nae We Coat of Arms, depicting a meeting between Jan Pranger of the Dutch West India Company and Nii Boi Tono, priest of the Ga goddess of the sea. The mural makes an argument for priestly sovereignty, acknowledging Nii Boi Tono as the "king of Akra," a spiritual and political leader of the Ga people.[2] The priests of Nae still declare their preeminence as contributors to the functioning of the Ga state, but during the twentieth century they are better known as coordinators of social healing in the city. Nae We has always been a rendezvous point for herbalists, spirit mediums, and ritualists in the city, making it a rallying ground for local healing practitioners, especially during the annual harvest celebration of *Homowo*. The paramount role of the priest of Nae is contested by other shrine priests and by Ga chiefs, but the history of the shrine demonstrates that there has always been a loosely coordinated, plural network of African healers in Accra. Subsequent inquiries revealed the continued existence of a diverse set of shrine priests (*wulomei*), dozens of spirit mediums

---

[2] Nae Wulomo, interview with the author, August 5, 2003.

XV

(*wontsemei*), and hundreds of herbalists and ritualists (*tsofats-emei*). Over the course of the next decade, I conducted interviews to trace the history of the construction of shrines, the aesthetics of fetish production, and the profession of herbalism, all under the rough heading of Ga healing. The interview process began through simple visits to the three major shrines of Nae, Korle, and Sakumo, where I was given names of people in Accra who were practiced in ancestral arts of religion and healing. Almost all of these encounters took place in Ussher Town and James Town, the old quarters of Accra, which have been a site of performance for African healing for centuries. However, as people have moved out and around the city, I found myself moving into the suburbs also, tracking down elders knowledgeable in the history of African healing traditions.

While I had started by seeking out the Ga-ness of healing, the many interviews I conducted revealed the use of Christian prayer, Islamic therapies, market medicines, and medical techniques, without any necessary referent to Ga practices. This led to further interviews with pastors, *mallams*, pharmacists, itinerant vendors, and, of course, doctors and nurses. The voices of these people reverberate through this book, including Naa Korle, a *wulomo* who walked me around the *otutui* of the lesser gods of the city; Obolo Ama, a *woyoo* who channels the husky speech of the river deity Nsaki; Thunder, a ritualist who heals with Islamic slate wash; Carlos Santos, a shop owner selling Christian and Islamic spiritual medicines; Comfort, a woman who sells both herbs and packaged sex medicines from a basket on her head; Otia Badu, a veteran who wore a sticky cape to catch mosquitos during the antimalarial campaign of World War II; and Dr. Quartey-Papafio, a surgeon descended from the first African physician to practice privately in Accra. These are the real people who make up the tableau vivant of Accra's healing past.

Oral memories provide the foundation for therapeutic pluralism, but interview and observational data contain historical gaps that can only be bridged by documentary sources. Anthropological texts are particularly useful when they reach back over a hundred years, and Accra is blessed with several extant works, including the foundational *History of the Gold Coast and Ashanti*, written by Carl Christian (C. C.) Reindorf in 1895, as well as the reflective autoethnographies of A. B. Quartey Papafio and the lyrical accounts of Ga songs and customs by Marion Kilson.[3] But it is Margaret Field's ethnographies that offer the richest descriptions of healing in Accra. Indeed, one of my most profound research insights came in 2005, with the priest of Nae at the rocks of Osekan, throwing bottles of schnapps into the Atlantic as the waves crashed around us. At that moment, I recalled that Margaret Field had participated in that exact ceremony almost seventy years earlier, demonstrating the strength of continuity within Ga healing culture.[4] But works of anthropology, even when written by insiders, are never free of their essentializing tendencies. All of these sources must be read at three levels: first, for what they can provide *prima facie* about healing customs; second, as artifacts of a colonial project to classify the inhabitants of the British Empire; and third, for the insight they offer into change and hybridity within the therapeutic cultures of Accra.

Early European texts are also essential to understanding the history of healing in West Africa because oral memories begin to peter out beyond a couple of hundred years. European travel accounts, slave trade records, and missionary journals portray Africans as exotic heathens, objects of exchange, or colonial subjects, but they nevertheless offer valuable knowledge about ideas, practices, and material cultures of healing. All of these European sources are soaked in discourses of racial difference, but in odd passages and throwaway sentences, the story can be found—in

---

[3] Carl Christian Reindorf, *History of the Gold Coast*; Quartey Papafio, "Ga Homowo Festival," April 1920; Quartey Papafio, "Ga Homowo Festival," January 1920; Kilson, *Kpele Lala*.

[4] Field, *Religion and Medicine*, 91.

the tribulations of Ga patients who sought out more than one healer when sick, in accounts of sailors who abandoned ship to seek help from African healers, or in the letters of Basel missionaries who thanked God for being saved by African herbalists. Some textual materials are less mediated than others, such as the records of the high and circuit courts of Accra, where one can find quests for therapy within the testimonies of litigants fighting over the costs, efficacies, and dangers of medicines. The medical ideas of the elites of Accra, many of them physicians, are also readily available in twentieth-century newspapers and autobiographies. And as a final supplement, statistical material collected by the colonial government offers a lens on the will of patients, en masse. It makes for heavy reading, but the subaltern voices of healers and patients can be found within this eclectic colonial archive.

SHARING THE
BURDEN OF
SICKNESS

INTRODUCTION

Historicizing Therapeutic Pluralism

Pluralitas non est ponenda sine necessitate—plurality is not to be posited without necessity.

Occam's razor

Hela tamo jarawoo—sickness must be put out for sale.

Ga aphorism

IN THE EARLY SEVENTEENTH CENTURY, the city of Accra was a small fishing outpost, one of many along the coast of West Africa. It was a Ga village of perhaps a few hundred people who made their living in the immediate surrounding area but were also connected to villages in the hinterland by footpaths and to towns along the coast by canoe. Those who got sick in Accra had the option to visit a handful of herbalists and spiritualists, who used plant medicines and spiritual remedies to counter illness. Patients might also, through great effort, venture out of Accra to visit healers in nearby villages, but their therapeutic horizon did not reach beyond a regional network of ideas about disease causality, local practices, and the local herbaria. More than three hundred years later, Accra is a metropolis of over three million people. The city now offers patients a choice among five major

1

therapeutic traditions: West African, Islamic, Christian, Western, and over-the-counter medicines. Each of these traditions had a historical point of arrival in Accra, each of them has endured over the generations, and each of them remains. If someone falls sick in Accra today, they can shop around among these traditions to find a cure.

The five healing traditions of Accra should not be understood as antique lifeways that stand in opposition to progress. On the contrary, they are vibrant collections of ideas, practices, and material cultures that are always adapting to new circumstances while at the same time maintaining their cultural integrity. Over the decades and centuries, they have changed so much that one might speak of them as continuously modernizing, in the sense that they have regularly adapted to the circumstances of a growing West African city. Their practitioners have been innovators, bringing new methods of healing to Accra, while at the same time policing ancestral boundaries of lexica, ritual, and aesthetics. All traditions change over time, but they find ways to become, as Kwame Gyekye has put it, "symphonic with forms of life in the new era."[1] No major tradition has disappeared, nor has any major tradition gained hegemony. Rather, patients have supported and sustained these five healing traditions, giving birth to a plurality of historical narratives about healing, each with its own characters and plotlines.

The oldest and most diverse subgroup of healing traditions in Accra today is uniquely West African. Until the twentieth century, the majority of the healers in Accra were Ga, members of the same ethnic group that founded the city. In the kitchens and markets of the city, Ga herbalists prepared draughts, salves, and powders, using recipes passed down through generations. Meanwhile, Ga priests and spirit mediums built shrines in homage to the local deities and harnessed occult powers to cast diseases out of their patients. Yet even the Ga-ness of healing contained a deeper plurality, based on Guang gods and traditions that

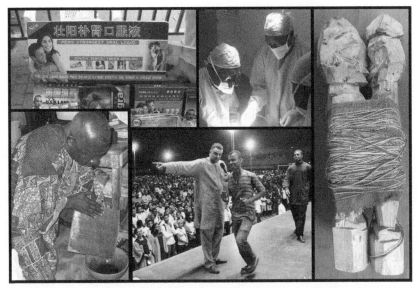

Introduction 1.1. Five traditions of healing in Accra today (*clockwise from top left*): (a) potency medicines from a street vendor in Accra (Source: author); (b) a patient undergoing reconstructive surgery at Korle Bu TeachHospital (Source: ReSurge Africa); (c) love medicine prepared by a Ga spirit medium (Source: author photo); (d) Bishop Dag Heward of the Lighthouse Group of Churches healing attendees (Source: Lighthouse Chapel International. Healing Jesus Crusade, https:// bit.ly /31LI6rK); and (e) a mallam preparing a Quranic slate wash (Source: author photo).

inhabited the land before the Gas arrived, along with Akan, Ewe, and other ethnic palimpsests. The Gas of Accra had always accommodated settlers from other parts of West Africa, a process that supplemented the healing classes of the city with practitioners from around the Gold Coast; from Nigeria, Togo, and Benin; and even from the distant savanna lands to the north. Over hundreds of years, novel concepts of illness have been added to the Ga healing lexicon, innovative practices have been brought to the city, and new plants, paraphernalia, and spirits have been incorporated into the local materia medica. The West African healing traditions of Accra have never fallen into the category of disappearing customs. Rather, they continue to proliferate as a mix of holistic therapies that heal the body, repair family relations, quell social disputes, and facilitate spiritual harmony.

A second major group of therapists in Accra comprises Muslim healers, spiritualists who conduct healing rituals and produce healing objects based on the word of God as written in the Quran.[2] For centuries, Accra has been home to clerics who fabricate amulets, charms, and geomantic squares to aid people suffering from bodily and spiritual ailments. The techniques for producing Islamic medicines can be traced back to traditions that crossed the Sahara Desert centuries ago, and for many centuries, promulgated by a small but devout cadre of *mallams* and soothsayers. But the Islamic healing culture in Accra rapidly increased in prominence toward the end of the nineteenth century, as migrants from the Hausa, Brazilian, Yoruba, and Zabarima communities gradually increased the size of the Muslim community and as the number of Ga and Akan Muslim converts began to grow.[3] The power of the Arabic language and of Quranic text magnified in the twentieth century, as patients from all walks of life in Accra began to seek out advice from Islamic healers. In response, *mallams* reconfigured their practices again and again to address local concerns. Today, people still buy Islamic charms to cure illnesses, but they also purchase them for contemporary concerns: to pass exams, to avoid car accidents, or to receive a visa to travel abroad.[4] In the twenty-first century, Islamic medical tradition continues to adapt itself to the needs of the residents of Accra, creating medicines embedded in local aesthetics of consecrated medicine production.

A third group of healers falls under the broad rubric of Western medicine, a tradition derived from Europe that now has firm roots in Africa. Ships' surgeons were the first European healers to arrive, followed by missionary lay healers. Both groups struggled to propagate their ideas in Accra. They had little curative help for African patients, and by the end of the nineteenth century,

Accra had only a tiny, poorly equipped colonial hospital. This changed dramatically in 1923, when the government of the Gold Coast Colony built a major institution dedicated to scientific healing on the outskirts of the town, to the west of the sacred Korle Lagoon. The Gold Coast Hospital, as it was officially known, was a medical complex designed to facilitate the growth of a working population and exhibit the benevolence of paternal colonialism. Not surprisingly, patients in Accra were skeptical at first, but they quickly found that the hospital provided efficacious cures for illnesses like yaws and malaria, and the hospital soon became so integrated into local culture that it took on the moniker of Korle Bu, a term that literally refers to the lowlands near the lagoon but figuratively echoes the respect that people developed for the hospital. Once its reputation was established, Korle Bu became an avenue of upward mobility for the aspirant classes of Accra, whose sons and daughters joined the institution as a new generation of physicians, nurses, and colonial dispensers. Today, as a full-fledged teaching hospital, Korle Bu remains a pivot point in the cycle of life for residents of Accra: hundreds of thousands of people were born there, millions have sought treatment there, and many will have their corpses stored there before burial. Many other clinics and private hospitals have sprung up in the city, filling in the gaps of a weak national health care system, but Korle Bu is still the largest medical institution in Ghana.

A fourth major tradition is Christian faith healing. Every week, hundreds of worshippers flock to the Protestant charismatic Christian churches of the city to conduct ceremonies for sufferers of physical and spiritual ailments. Many churches have built their reputations on their ability to heal, and megachurch founders like Nicolas Duncan-Williams of Action Chapel, former physician Dag Heward Mills of Lighthouse International, or the self-proclaimed Prophet Salifu of Jesus Is Alive Ministry have become faith-healing superstars.[5] The roots of church healing rituals go back to the mid-nineteenth century, when missionaries at the Basel Mission translated the Holy Bible into Ga, offering a new narrative of healing based on the miracles performed by Jesus Christ. After a slow start with modest congregations, African churches saw dramatic growth during the 1930s and 1940s, as part of a broader West African Christian revival spurred by the Aladura movement in Nigeria. Since then, the fortunes of the so-called mainline churches (Catholic, Anglican, Methodist, and Presbyterian) have waned as they have resisted engaging in public events of faith healing.[6] Meanwhile, charismatic and Pentecostal congregations splintered and multiplied to dominate the religious landscape of the city. At these churches, patients marshal the physical strength to fight everything from migraines to cancer and gather the spiritual fortitude to ward off attacks by demonic forces.

The fifth tradition is the common-sense practice of self-healing with herbal remedies and over-the-counter medicines. Because the medicinal flora of West Africa is so robust, sufferers of illness have always been able to acquire leaves, roots, and barks to prepare their own cures, without the help of professional healers. Patients have also been keen to try out new reagents, including herbs imported from around the world, which are now indistinguishable from the local medicinal flora. The consistent search for new and appropriate cures stimulated the growth of the patent medicine trade in the nineteenth century and the proliferation of the pharmaceutical market in the twentieth. These medicines were initially designated as cures for particular maladies conceived of by Europeans, and as such they have been presumed to be part of a larger oeuvre of Western medicine. However, the efficacy of imported nostrums was regularly challenged by the medical profession, and British physicians cast them out of the medical fold in the early twentieth century. When these nostrums landed in Accra, patients soon detached them from their Western meanings and redeployed them to suit local health needs. Today, chemist shops and medicine stalls dot the neighborhoods of the city, and patients can choose from thousands of different generic drugs from Nigeria, India, and China. More recently, neatly packaged Ghanaian brands of bottled herbal draughts have also taken their place on the shelves of chemist shops. Accra has always been an open market for medical products because government control over the distribution and sale of medicines has never been strictly enforced, but the site is now home to the rapid commodification of healing goods, some made locally and some imported. As a result, "self-care" with over-the-counter medicines is a widespread practice, operating beyond the scrutiny of healing professionals, just as herbalism has always been practiced in Accra.[7]

The coexistence of five major therapeutic traditions in a twenty-first-century city should not be surprising. Healing traditions have been crossing borders and spreading around the world for centuries. In India, the state-funded biomedical system competes with Vedic medicine, Unani Tibb, and herbal folk remedies, as well as imported practices such as homeopathy.[8] In China, traditional medical practices such as massage, acupuncture, moxibustion, and herbalism have been rationalized through programs of scientific certification and now operate side by side with the national medical system.[9] Even in the West, where biomedicine is the dominant tradition, practices formerly regarded as quackery are becoming mainstream. Over one-third of patients in the United States regularly use therapies deemed alternative or complementary to treat their ailments.[10] A short list compiled by the US Centers for Disease Control includes homeopathy, naturopathy, osteopathy, chiropractic, hypnosis, energy therapies, and faith healing. They also mention the grab bag of treatments offered by *curanderos* at a growing number of *botanicas* around the country.[11] These so-called alternative therapies face ongoing criticism from biomedical practitioners who insist on evidence-based therapeutics, but the trend is clear—patients in the West, as in other parts of the world, shop around by exploring a plurality of healing options rather than adhering to the conventions of a state-endorsed medical regime.[12]

Africa has always been home to a plurality of therapeutic traditions. In every region of the continent, multiple systems of healing abound. In Southern Africa, migration patterns have brought together a unique mix of African, Indian, and European practitioners, each with their own particular subsets of healing knowledge and practice.[13] In East Africa, herbalism practices and drumming cults share the market with Islamic and Chinese medicines, as well as state-funded Western medicine.[14] In North Africa, Islamic healers share patients with herbalists and government-funded clinics and hospitals.[15] And in West Africa, traditions of herbalism and spiritual healing proliferate alongside Christian faith healing, Islamic healing, and state medical systems.[16] No longer can we think of Africans as possessing indigenous ethnomedicines; the healing landscape of the continent has been changing for so long that it is now a place with clusters of therapeutic regimes competing in each region.

Therapeutic diversity may be a global phenomenon, but explaining how it became so is harder than one might think. For almost a century, historians of medicine in Africa ignored evidence of pluralism, preferring to circumscribe their topic within the singular idiom of scientific medicine. They hoped that the progressive nature of medical research could offer knowledge about the human body that was universal and verifiable rather than relative and cultural. Put another way, chroniclers of the story of healing in Africa have been reluctant to abandon the parsimony of Occam's razor, the logical principle that obliges us to assert a singular hypothesis rather than propose a complex set of explanations. Anything broader would require scholars to allow for a comparison of incommensurable etiologies, the parallel existence of diverse practices, and a bazaar of different material cultures. Moreover, the simplicity of the thesis of scientific progress has always been seductive because it offers a tidy three-part narrative sequence to the history of medicine: a beginning point of ignorance to the scientific etiologies of disease; a middle point when medical discoveries are unveiled; and a climax via the success of medical reforms. Throughout the twentieth century, the wedding of universal science with the progressive trope of medical triumph was hard to resist, and it came to dominate medical historiography.

Furthermore, Africa provided an ideal setting with useful characters for the story of medical triumph. It became a place where Europeans, empowered with the gift of medical science, could vanquish the diseases that impeded civilization. So certain was the narrative of medical advance in African historiography that it naturalized the expectation that Western medicine, if not already preeminent, would eventually surpass all other traditions to become the definitive, universal healing practice on the continent. Indeed, wherever a European medical narrative was established, deep traditions of African herbalism and spiritualism were abandoned to the ethnographic present, and imported traditions like Christian and Islamic healing were relegated to the status of alternative, complementary, holistic, or spiritual therapies.

Evidently, it is time for a new approach to the history of healing. This book positions itself as a narrative intervention, one that will challenge the Western medical metanarrative while at the same time creating enough discursive space to explore four other story lines, each with its own early beginnings, periods of growth, and adaptations to the particular locale of Accra. The goal is to provincialize Western medicine as a tradition that emerged in Europe but was compelled to adapt in order to fit into the healing landscape of Africa. Indeed, from the perspective of African patients living in Accra over the past three hundred years, Western medicine has been something of a healing outlier. The naval surgeons, colonial doctors, laboratory technicians, and public hygiene officers of the Western tradition were like a cast of minor characters walking on and off the stage of Accra, forming only a subplot within part of the larger narrative of therapeutic pluralism. Only when it reshaped itself as colonial medicine, and associated itself with a desire to name and control bodies and illnesses, did European healing gain ground as a significant tradition, but even then it remained one of many therapeutic choices. As the centuries wore on, other traditions transformed and adjusted to their circumstances. African healing changed with each immigrant deity, each influx of migrants, and each exchange of healing material, forming the longest subplot within the story of therapeutic pluralism. Other traditions surged in the late nineteenth century, as different ideas and peoples began to spread around the Atlantic world. By the twentieth century, the world of healing in Accra was so dynamic that one can speak of the ascendance of colonial medicine in the twentieth century while at the same time telling the story of the diversification of African herbalism, the revival of Christian faith healing, the spread of Quranic therapeutics, and the boom in patent medicine consumption. Indeed, this book will show how the twentieth century witnessed the conjunction of many flourishing healing traditions, rather than the singular triumph of Western medicine.

The city of Accra is an ideal setting to study how patients tied together different traditions of health and healing. Home to the Ga people, the city has pluralist beginnings that can be traced back hundreds of years. The city also has an open healing culture, one that has appropriated healing ideas, practices, and goods from both African and Atlantic circuits. The healing culture of Accra is best understood via the Ga saying *hela tamo jarawolo*, which, as Kodjo Senah has argued, "likens illness to a piece of merchandise which must be advertised as widely as possible until it is bought (that is, until a cure for it has been found)."[17] This means that a sufferer must shop their sickness around, seeking help from as many people as possible to find a cure. More broadly, it implies that problems are a burden that must be shared with others to find a solution. Not all patients in Accra have felt compelled to adhere to this maxim. Many arrived in the city with preconceived notions of health or later adopted antisyncretic dispositions toward healing. But by focusing on how people have shopped around for cures, sharing the struggle against illnesses with family, friends, and different healers, this book aims to capture the complex experiences of patients in ways that the linear metanarrative of medical progress has never been able to do.

CONFRONTING NARRATIVES OF
EUROPEAN MEDICAL HEGEMONY

The celebratory historiography of medicine in Africa began in the nineteenth century, with popular accounts of the exploits of White missionaries such as Robert Moffat, David Livingstone, and Emin Pasha. Though these men were medical amateurs who relied on rudimentary techniques such as tooth pulling, boil lancing, and smallpox inoculation, the reading public of the British Empire regarded them as "heroes of the dark continent."[18] The story line of the missionary-doctor was further perpetuated in hagiographies of Albert Schweitzer, which venerated him as a savior of bodies and souls.[19] The link between Christianity and the provision of medical care continued after the Second World War, typified by the writing of physician-turned-historian Michael Gelfand in publications like *Tropical Victory* and *The Sick African*.[20] These paternalistic accounts lauded the triumphs of medicine at the cost of nullifying other healing traditions, thereby reducing Africans to unwell masses in need of both spiritual and medical salvation.

The three major works that form the historiography of medicine in the Gold Coast have followed more or less the same pattern. Two foundational studies of medical history by Dr. David Scott and Dr. K. David Patterson, written in the 1960s and 1970s, were groundbreaking for their time and continue to offer the backbone to the medical historiography of the Gold Coast Colony, but they are products of an era when a belief in medical progress was unquestionable.[21] The work of Patterson and Scott was followed two decades later by a textbook written by Ghanaian professor Stephen Addae, a comprehensive account of the history of Western medicine in Ghana, with chapters on epidemic disease, colonial medicine, military hospitals, and auxiliary medical services. Addae sharply criticized the curative bias of the Gold Coast and Ghanaian biomedical tradition but again relegated nonmedical healing practices to the realm of anthropology. Most notably, he did not venture to search for the pluralistic leanings found in patient behavior.[22]

In the late twentieth century, historians began to discard the teleology behind the medical metanarrative in an effort to critique the work of missionaries and physicians in Africa. These secularized accounts, written mostly by former physicians, pointed out that some of the gains made by Western medicine in Africa had been overstated, but they still adhered to a positivist narrative that assumed that physicians would eventually bring "medicine to the African masses."[23] Even up to the late 1980s, historians remained wedded to the idiom of the "magic bullet" cure, which naturalized medicine as a universal healing force.[24] But by the 1990s, some historians had begun to challenge assumptions about the triumph of colonial medicine by highlighting the disastrous effects of epidemics in twentieth-century Africa.[25] By proving that colonial activity increased, rather than decreased, the death rate in some parts of Africa, historians such as Philip Curtin, Myron Echenberg, Meghan Vaughan, and Gwyn Prins finally put to rest the notion that colonial medicine had vanquished illness on the continent.[26] This new wave of revisionist histories identified "colonial medicine" as a unique part of healing culture—one that offered cures for the very diseases that colonialism helped to spread.[27] Unfortunately, the narrative structure of colonial medical intervention relied upon an imposition-response paradigm, reducing African healing practices to a backdrop for the larger story of European agency. These authors never intended to generate an African ethnomedical present, but after the focus on colonial medicine, there wasn't much room left to describe how indigenously generated healing ideas, practices, and material cultures had changed over time.

For the most part, the changing world of therapeutics in Africa has been consigned to the realm of anthropology, where scholars, unburdened by the heritage of medicine, have been able to assess ethnic and regional healing practices on their own terms. In the mid-1970s, Ghanaian medical sociologist Patrick Twumasi made pluralism a standard framework for understanding the mixing of scientific, herbal, and spiritual medical systems.[28] His research indicated that traditional healers were far from irrelevant in late twentieth-century Ghana, as they continued to innovate in their herbal and spiritual practices to deal with contemporary health concerns, and that Western medical professionals were far from dominant, as they found it difficult to win the trust of patients seeking the deeper causes of illness. In the United States, the idea of medical pluralism was popularized by two American anthropologists, Charles Leslie and Arthur Kleinman, who traced the interconnections between Unani, Ayurvedic, Chinese, and Western medicine in Asia.[29] The team of John Janzen and Steven Feierman brought the notion of medical pluralism back to the continent in the late 1970s, through the study of patient behavior in East and Central Africa. In a major study of Kongo healing practices, Janzen argued that sufferers and their "therapy management groups" (made up of family, trusted friends, and acquaintances with health expertise) sustained several therapeutic options in one region.[30] By seeking help from more than one healer, Janzen noted, patients and their retinues conducted "quests for therapy," without a prescribed beginning or end and without privileging medical care.[31] In an accompanying work,

Janzen historicized healing pluralism by showing the emergence of the Central African Lemba drumming and healing cult—a system whereby the sufferers who were cured of the Lemba sickness (a mixture of bodily, social, financial, and spiritual ills) became the healers of future patients.[32] Steven Feierman also historicized change within the culture of healing in preliterate Shambaa society, where he argued that "peasant intellectuals" generated a subaltern rainmaking discourse that challenged royal authority to heal the land.[33] Feierman opined that a long-standing focus on scientific medicine had obscured a plurality of "systems of explanation and treatment" that competed to define the meaning of health and healing in Africa.[34]

Since then, historians and anthropologists have continued to refine the notion of medical pluralism in order to better understand relations of power between healers and patients. New concepts such as "medicoscapes," "medical landscapes," and "medical diversity" have emerged, offering ways to better track how patients borrow and combine medical ideas and, conversely, how therapists police the boundaries of their practices.[35] Unfortunately, the awkward term of *medicine* still colonizes the subject matter, acting as a yardstick against which other therapeutic traditions are measured. This book will exchange the term *medical* for *therapeutic* as a way to avoid privileging the European-derived metrics that are used to assess healing outcomes. This terminological shift is a necessary step toward decentering the study of healing in Africa, but it cannot entirely detach itself from the larger biomedical metanarrative.

Historians in Africa have followed Janzen and Feierman's lead in the search for pluralism, using local chronologies of change to write about traveling witch-finding gods, the material culture of Islamic healing, the rise of Christian faith healing, and other therapeutic subcultures.[36] However, most of the recent work on healing in Africa has focused on single strands of healing practice. There are two recent exceptions, exclusively from South

Africa. Anne Digby has traced the historical "patterns of resort" taken by sufferers in South Africa, finding that patient eclecticism was the norm because "no one had overall authority to act as a gatekeeper in accessing a pluralistic provision of health care."[37] And in a remarkable composite work, Karen Flint's *Healing Traditions* demonstrates how Zulu, European, and Indian practices operated in parallel in the Natal Colony during the nineteenth and twentieth centuries.[38] This new generation of historians has dared to tell more than one story at the same time in order to recreate a deep history of patient behavior. That is the goal of this book: to reveal the shifting and changing world of Accra's major therapeutic traditions, including as much insight as possible into relations of power between healers and patients.

HISTORICIZING PLURALISM

Incorporating multiple traditions into the story of healing in Africa should be a straightforward task. Anthropologists have provided ample evidence that Africans commonly form kinship-bound therapy management groups and embark on quests for therapy among many healing traditions.[39] So the question remains: When will historians recognize the significance of therapeutic pluralism in the daily lives of Africans? The answer is more complicated than one might initially think because a historian of therapeutic pluralism is faced with three substantial challenges. The first is an obvious lack of indigenous documentary sources. While historians of early modern England can rely on accounts like the *Diary of Samuel Pepys*—as Roy Porter so famously did in his groundbreaking essay "The Patient's View"—robust documentary sources about patient decision-making in Africa are extraordinarily rare.[40] In order to accumulate information about healing in a place like the Gold Coast, a historian must sift through fragments of the oral, written, and material past just to piece together a basic outline of therapeutic pluralism. The work of gathering these disparate sources can be prohibitively time-consuming and sometimes overwhelming, especially since almost all of them are mediated through a Eurocentric, colonial lens. But with persistence, written accounts with diverse provenances can be compiled and compared to the oral memories of healers and patients. Together, these sources can reveal the outlines of therapeutic pluralism, and often much more.

A second, more significant challenge arises from expectations that curative efficacy can be proven with historical data. Medical history has been teleological in its construction, starting with calamity, leading toward discovery, and finishing with triumph, a plotline that hinges on the development of curative efficacy. The story of victory over smallpox, for instance, serves as a model of medical historiography because it has a data set of progressive curative success leading to disease eradication. However, ever since the work of Thomas McKeown called into question the fundamental assumptions of medical curative efficacy, historians have uncovered many instances of accidental medical outcomes in which medical success emerged through trial and error rather than through scientific medical rigor.[41] Even today it is difficult to explain scientifically why some medical therapies work, a challenge that has given birth to the new field of effectiveness studies.[42] Without robust laboratory data, without evidence from clinical trials, and without even a readily available discourse of medical efficacy, it is impossible to compare the curative outcomes of healing traditions in the past, Western or non-Western, on equal terms. To overcome this impediment, this book abandons the universal notion of curative efficacy and adopts a framework of *perceived* efficacy—a concept used in medicine today to refer to an assessment of health outcomes as judged by the patients or the caregivers.[43] For instance, if supplicants attend a shrine to cleanse themselves of an illness caused by spiritual forces, there may be no way calculate the medical outcome of their actions, but it may be possible to assess the perceived curative value of the therapy. After all, in the pluralistic healing environment of Accra, the question of curative value has always been relative rather than universal because patients moved between healing traditions, adopting more than one sense of efficacy during the course of a single illness. The historian's responsibility is to trace the quotidian acts of patients and healers to show how, in the aggregate, they reveal contingent, contextualized, perceived efficacies.

The third, and most troubling, challenge faced by a historian of therapeutic pluralism is the potential to negate the agency of African patients. While contemporary anthropological studies provide evidence that Africans *tend* to emphasize spiritual health, *tend* to form kinship-bound therapy management groups, and *tend* to "explore all avenues of a cure," it is not possible to build a historical narrative on such a contemporary behaviors.[44] To do so would simplify human decision-making in the extreme, potentially replicating the Enlightenment stereotype of the capricious African *bricoleur*—the patient who is willing to try any old thing to heal themselves, regardless of logic or efficacy.[45] This is not to say that contemporary analyses of patient behavior cannot help us understand African therapeutics in the past. Indeed, patients in Accra did tend to follow a quest for therapy framework, using their social capital to seek out therapies from multiple practitioners. However, a historian must demonstrate that there has been a balance of forces at work in determining patient choice. Most evidence points to patients playing the field by seeking treatments from multiple sources, but there is also proof that many others wholeheartedly committed themselves to single therapeutic avenues. African elites, for example, might have adhered strictly to colonial medical treatment on the basis of their perceived notion of social class, while Ga patients living in central Accra might have felt obliged to follow only the advice of their Ga ritual advisers. Christians might have wanted to demonstrate their piety by taking counsel only from their pastors, while Muslims might have adhered rigidly to the dogma of the medicine of the Prophet to outwardly demonstrate their faith. Additionally, a new migrant to Accra might have arrived with little social capital, which would leave them with incomplete knowledge of the wide variety of healing options available. A historian simply cannot ignore the fact that, even within a pluralistic healing culture, many people either doggedly conformed to a singular therapeutic tradition or simply did not know whom to ask for help.

One way to address tendencies toward pluralism, without projecting rigid models of behavior on patients, is to heed the advice of Steven Feierman, who argued that an understanding of therapeutic pluralism in Africa must include a deep inquiry into the "fundamental social institutions which control therapeutic choice."[46] This means that the power relations between practitioners and their patients must be carefully studied to understand when patients have the capacity to choose their own route to health, and when they feel constrained to follow a specific therapeutic pathway. This book takes on that challenge, by highlighting the passions, impediments, and aspirations that altered the way that patients planned out their quests for therapy. In particular, three major social forces played a key role in the story of healing in Accra because they generated rapid change within the healing networks of Accra.

The first is the fervor of religion, which filled many residents with a desire to isolate themselves entirely from other therapeutic traditions. Although the healing networks of Accra were traditionally hybrid and tolerant of new forms of spirituality, many devout members of the Ga, Christian, and Islamic communities chose to adhere only to practices that aligned closely with their faith. Some Ga healers insisted that their patients stay confined to their compounds and reject all other healing options. The Basel missionaries took this restriction further, geographically isolating themselves in a Christian village north of Osu known as the Christian Salem. Muslim communities also carved out territory for themselves on the periphery of the city, occupying grazing lands and villages near military installations, propagating their own philosophies about healing. Within these religious communities, the choices a person made when sick were regarded as an indication of their piety and loyalty, and some religious leaders forbade their followers from seeking care outside the group. It seemed that religious zeal, and the spatial segregation it entailed, might sever the intimate ties that bound together the therapy management group. But the power of antisyncretism was constantly challenged by the willingness of patients to seek out new ideas, practices, and material cultures of healing.

The second force that had a dramatic impact on the composition of therapeutic pluralism in Accra was colonialism, or more specifically, the emergence of a medicalized colonial state. By the late nineteenth century, British physicians and sanitary engineers had commenced a series of campaigns to usurp the right to name and manage states of bodily health in Accra, on the basis of the transformations that had taken place in the arena of medical science in Europe. So bold were these interventions that they beg for examination as instances of what Michel Foucault named "bio-power," the ability of the state to "take charge of life" through "continuous regulatory and corrective mechanisms."[47] Bio-power in Africa was both discourse and practice in the sense that colonial subjects were assessed as having a quantitative value for the larger imperial project, and colonial governments made efforts to enhance their utility by enhancing the vital and reproductive capacities of the labor force. During the colonial era, when labor was no longer being extracted into servitude in the Americas, the government of the Gold Coast found itself compelled to manage the aggregate health of its subject population, in part by dividing the population into groups that would be granted larger or smaller doses of colonial medical care.

One might protest that Foucault "never came to Africa"[48] in the sense that, as a scholar, he did not directly address the transposition of bio-power in the form of policies like racial segregation. Nevertheless, his ideas have been indispensable to Africanists trying to understanding the intersections between racial theory and colonial power.[49] In particular, Foucauldian analysis has been used to understand the generation of pseudo-scientific knowledge about racial difference that became part of the power/knowledge matrix of the colony, leading to concepts such as racial ecology and the sanitation syndrome, which vilified Africans as members of an unclean race.[50] Racialized medical discourse is most evident within the legacy of Southern African apartheid and the history of segregation in French African cities, but bio-power was also present in Accra. The history of the Gold Coast was characterized by a weak regulation of healing practices, making it an awkward fit for the application of social constructivism, but the specter of bio-power did emerge. During the first half of the twentieth century, a flurry of laboratory tests, clinical trials, and medical examinations turned many colonial subjects into medical subjects in Accra. Indeed, at some points, it appeared that the colonial state would become the preeminent social force in assigning states of health to the bodies of its subjects, thereby guiding therapeutic choice.

But the will to power of colonial medicine proved to be practically weak on the ground. The grand schemes of colonial medical officials faced many barriers to implementation. British governors were always wary of medical and sanitary interventions, mainly because of the expense involved but also because of the fear of local rebellion. It was easier to do things on the cheap by keeping the White population well housed, supplied with quinine, and tucked away in their own neighborhoods than it was to fritter away political capital on bonification schemes for the colonized. More significantly, in a city where patients and healers were comfortable with incommensurable disease etiologies, the expansion of the colonial medical infrastructure was regarded by many patients in the city merely as an enhancement of yet another therapeutic option rather than the imposition of a singular pathway to universal health. In Accra, the bio-power of colonial medicine was never capillary in the sense that it reached into all aspects of people's lives. Nor was it arterial (except for brief moments during epidemics and wars). Rather, it was an auxiliary expression of healing power, compelled to coexist with other healing traditions without assuming a hegemonic role.[51]

Moreover, as Foucault's critics have argued, the overweening power of the state seemed to evaporate when subjects dared challenge the connections between knowledge and power, taking charge of the meanings of their corporeal selves.[52] Indeed, it was the persistence of patients in defining their search for a cure that allowed for the emergence of a third major social force related to healing: the desire for social distinction. Throughout the history of Accra, patients have boldly exhibited their right to choose their therapies, consuming healing goods and services as a means of publicly displaying their sense of taste. Using the ideas of Pierre Bourdieu as a guide, we can think of sickness as a time in life when people attempt to position themselves vis-à-vis others by consuming types of health care that assert their rank within a social hierarchy.[53] For instance, identifying with a particular ethnic group in Accra might mean seeking aid from healers of that same ethnicity, whereas identifying with colonial modernity might mean feeling obliged to visit a new colonial hospital. Being a pious Christian or Muslim might also entail specific types of performances when sick, such as placing faith in a pastor or *mallam*'s healing advice or denying the need for a secular cure. The patients' goal is to get better by trying as many cures as possible, but that doesn't mean they can't differentiate themselves from other patients in the process. The will to distinguish oneself while playing a sick role is not recognizable as a direct challenge to medicalized governmentality, but it should be understood as an expression of agency. In the twentieth century in particular, medicines could be equated with class and status, and patients in a sick role sought to position themselves favorably within the social strata via the consumption of imported salves, patent medicines, and over-the-counter pills.

In sum, it is not enough to simply say that Africans have always sought out multiple healing options. Individual decisions, as well as religious, social, and political forces, filtered patient choice in unique ways that changed over time. Patients showed strong tendencies toward pluralistic behavior, yet no essential cause for pluralism is evident. And though powerful regimes of healing did appear briefly, no hegemonic episteme emerged. In other words, telling the story of how quests for therapy and healing traditions changed over time in Accra takes some subtle maneuvering. The goal of this book, then, is to historicize therapeutic pluralism, era by era, tradition by tradition, to uncover the lived experiences of patients and healers in the dynamic cultural setting of urban West Africa.

PARAMETERS OF HEALTH AND HEALING: CAUSES, PRACTICES, MATERIAL CULTURES, AND SPACES

According to the World Health Organization, "health is a state of complete physical, mental and social well-being and not merely the absence of disease or infirmity," a definition that demonstrates that the international medical community is aware that health must be understood holistically rather than just physically.[54] However, international regimes still abide by the belief that there are universal parameters with which to measure states of health. As an institution founded on the principles of Western medical thought, the WHO remains dedicated to evidence-based policies and spends much of its time identifying the presence of Western-defined diseases within individuals and societies. This top-down model of assessment breaks down quickly in the context of a city like Accra, where notions of illness evade any universal definition precisely because they are plural. Well-being in Accra has always been assessed situationally, contingently, and comparatively rather than being judged against a singular definition of health.

Rather than adhere to globally determined standards of health and healing, this book breaks down health and healing into four constituent parts, including *causes* (notions of disease etiology), *practices* (actions and intentions of generating health), *material cultures* (symbols and equipment associated with healing practice), and *spaces* (the geographic divisions of healthy and unhealthy spaces). Assessing information about healing according to these four parameters makes it easier to understand how healing traditions were constituted in the past and how demand for each tradition has waxed and waned. Unpacking the meanings of health and healing will help to avoid slipping into scientific judgments about outcomes or efficacy and show how patients had the option of accessing particular components of different traditions, mixing and matching therapies in different ways.

The first category, causes, is foundational because notions of disease etiology undergird therapeutic actions. The Ga language, for instance, contains two basic categories of illness. The first is natural illness (*hela folo*), sicknesses with accidental causes, like colds, coughs, constipation, worms, stomach troubles, rashes, and malaria. The second is social or supernatural illness (*mumo hela*), sicknesses caused by human-made curses or by malicious spirits.[55] Sufferers who think about illness within these categories understand that the causes of their maladies progress along a continuum: initially, an illness might be considered to be natural, something treatable with basic herbal remedies, but if it is chronic, recurring, or lingering, it might be regarded as unnatural, requiring a cure involving the powers of the gods.[56] In such cases, patients and their therapy management groups might seek aid from local deities, *mallams* who heal with the Quran, or pastors who channel the healing power of Jesus. Within a conceptual framework of natural and spiritual illness, it is irrational for patients to follow a single therapeutic route because the illness could leap suddenly from one state to the other. A sick person is better off using many different healers as "helpers," each with their own notions of causality that can help find the cause of the disease.[57]

A diversity of practices is also important to the story of therapeutic pluralism in Accra. In some other African polities, political leaders accumulated healing power to supplement their political influence, as in the use of *muthi* by Zulu chiefs, the accumulation of *nyama* by Mande rulers, or the creation of the *ajalela* national war medicine by the chiefs of Dahomey. In Accra, Ga chiefs never attempted to appropriate the power to heal.[58] On the contrary, the first chief of the Ga state, Ayi Kushie, is said to have purposely surrendered the sacred rites of the state to medico-religious experts in the fifteenth century, as a means of freeing himself from taboos associated with the local deities.[59] The division of the Ga political sphere from the modes of healing created room for a wide variety of practitioners to name, explain, and fight illness in Accra without interference from the state. And unlike in Europe, where state-endorsed medical systems gradually marginalized competitors like astrologers, Paracelsians, homeopaths, cunning men, wise women, and lay healers, the colonial medical system of the Gold Coast never did achieve hegemony.[60] Though British medical officials established medicine as a legitimate therapeutic option by the mid-twentieth century, a number of factors, including financial limitations, political disinterest, and dubious efficacy, weakened the gains made by Western medicine in Accra.

Third, the material cultures of medicine have always played an essential role in the history of healing in Accra. As a port city on the Atlantic coast, Accra became a hub for the import of goods such as cloth, guns, and alcohol.[61] To these commodities were added healing reagents, such as herbs, roots, tree barks, and animal parts, carried north and south along the inland trade routes. Over time, herbalists in Accra adopted medicinal flora from Asia and the New World, and by the twentieth century, the residents of the city started buying and selling patent medicines and pharmaceuticals from Europe. Additionally, sufferers of illnesses sought aid from migrant deities in the West African littoral, the Guinea rain forest, and the savanna beyond, making Accra a commercial hub for the trade in spirits with therapeutic powers. Rather than one product line of healing goods displacing another, in Accra a diversity of healing products could be bought and sold in a mostly unregulated market. Not only did goods accumulate, but their meanings did too, as different classes of society adapted and appropriated them for their own uses.

Fourth, spaces are a key parameter with which to measure the relative power of healing traditions over time. Since its founding as a Ga capital in 1677, Accra has slowly aggregated into a series of neighborhoods, or *akutsei*, each with ethnic lineages. Over the course of generations, these urban quarters have been subsumed under the umbrella of the Ga nation, but the residents of each quarter remain loyal to their own healing practices, expressed through the worship of the deities that they brought to Accra. For example, Fante sojourners brought their own gods and goddesses related to fishing, while Akwapim migrants brought spirits used to fight witchcraft. Each neighborhood, in turn, participated in the annual *Homowo* harvest festival as a means of healing and celebrating the Ga nation. In the nineteenth century, the city became further subdivided into spaces that dictated health status. In 1827, the Ga Christian population segregated itself into the Basel Mission Salem, isolating themselves from the world of "fetish" that they believed surrounded them in order to institute Christian ideas of physical and spiritual health.[62] In the 1850s, the Muslim *zoŋo*, a multiethnic neighborhood of Hausa, Yoruba, and Ga residents, started to grow just north of Ussher Town, establishing the healing culture of Islam in Accra.[63] And in the 1880s, the British built a sanitized "European reservation" for White officials, followed by the walled campus of the Gold Coast Hospital in 1923.[64] These new neighborhoods demarcated the city according to both religious and medical lines and created domains within which healers could distinguish themselves geographically and professionally. The segmentation of the city according to the contours of healing knowledge and power did little to restrict the mobility of patients. Those who were suffering with sicknesses found ways to move among therapeutic spaces, tying the five major healing traditions into a loosely articulated network. However, as this book will show, the variety of healing spaces that emerged in Accra became like a series of mises en scène, stages with props, where the assessment of health and the performance of healing could be acted out, as they still are today.

CHAPTER BY CHAPTER

This book starts with an initial incident: the fall of Great Accra, the inland Ga capital at Ayawaso in 1677. It then traces the major events of political consolidation, migration, colonialism, and war, all of which altered the healing practices of the city over the course of three centuries. It ends in 1957, the year Accra became the capital of a newly independent state and the Ghanaian government took full control of the national Department of Health. Each chapter covers a distinct era in the history of healing, but because of source limitations and the varied intensity of social change over the past three hundred years, some chapters are longer than others. Nevertheless, all of the chapters offer the social, economic, and political background needed to place the actions of patients and healers in context. Sometimes the chapters follow distinctly global or colonial temporal frameworks, as in the case of the Second World War. At other times it is epidemic disease, like the bubonic plague of 1908, that defines the end of one era and the start of another. At the heart of each chapter are one or two vignettes that feature characters who embody the spirit of therapeutic pluralism during each particular era. At the end of each chapter is an interlude, connecting each major period together by highlighting a specific historical incident.

Chapter 1, entitled "The Roots of Therapeutic Pluralism in Accra, 1677 to the Mid-1800s," begins with the demise of the inland market town of Ayawaso, which at the time had an estimated population of twenty thousand people. Known to Europeans as Great Accra, Ayawaso was sacked by the armies of the Akwamu in 1677, a traumatic event that triggered the flight of thousands of Ga refugees. Many relocated to the seaside village of Little Accra, which, by default, became the new capital of the Ga state. At this time, the vast majority of residents in the new Accra conceptualized illness and health within a Ga lexicon, but notions of disease causality from Akan, Ewe, and Hausa quickly became part of local healing terminology. During the seventeenth and eighteenth centuries, the European presence in the city was economically substantial but medically insignificant; high death rates for Europeans and the brutal nature of the slave trade restricted the exchange of ideas and practices between Africans and Europeans. What did occur, however, was a subaltern exchange of herbal and spiritual material cultures. Included in this chapter is a discussion of the medicinal flora from Asia and the Americas that the residents of the city incorporated into their local herbaria. Also included is a description of the use of consecrated medicines through the eyes of a merchant called Noyte, who had his own collection of medico-spiritual devices. This section ends with an interlude describing how the Battle of Katamanto crystalized Ga religious culture during the 1820s and how the arrival of European scientists laid the groundwork for a medical gaze that would soon infiltrate the city.

The second chapter, "The Convergence of the Five Healing Traditions in the 'Healthy' Capital of the Gold Coast: Mid-1800s to 1908," covers a period when Islamic, Christian, and European healing practices were in ascent. Muslim therapists arrived in the city in the late nineteenth century, when trade links with Yorubaland, Brazil, and the Sahel began to grow. At the same time, Europeans at the Basel Mission converted a small group of Gas to Christianity and translated the healing terminology of the

Bible into Ga. The choice of Accra as the new capital of the Gold
Coast Colony in 1877 should have enhanced the professional status of European surgeons, but colonial medical ideas and practices remained mostly on the margins. While East and Southern
Africa witnessed the rise of segregation based on racial hygiene,
and French West African cities were being forcefully remade as
showcases for the so-called *mission civilisatrice*, the colonial discourse on hygiene in Accra was a muddle of sanitation theory and
laboratory science. The chapter is followed by an interlude about
the bubonic plague epidemic of 1908, a crisis that resulted in riots
against British sanitation crews, the death of many African healers, and a strangely successful inoculation campaign that may
have stopped the disease in its tracks.

The third chapter, "Therapeutic Pluralism during the Cocoa
Boom, 1908–1930s," covers a period of rapid economic growth fu-
eled by a rise in exports from the port of Accra. This was a time
when British medical officials aspired to rebuild the colonial capital according to the dictates of sanitary science. In practice, however, the finances of the Gold Coast government did not permit a
radical rezoning of the city. In a desperate effort to fight malaria
and yellow fever, the cash-poor Town Council resorted to segregation, relocating the White population to a suburban European
reservation, a mosquito flight away from the city center. Meanwhile, African healing practices continued to thrive, as demonstrated by the work of British anthropologist Margaret Field, who
revealed how Ga healers adapted to their new status as subjects of
a British colony.[65] The movement of patients between European
and African systems of healing is exemplified in this chapter by
the curious story of Olivia, a young woman who received treatment from both a local healer and a European-trained physician.
The dramatic expansion of the market for patent medicines is also
covered here, in order to show how patients repurposed imported
medicines according to their own health needs. The chapter concludes with an interlude introducing the dashing new governor

of the interwar Gold Coast, Gordon Guggisberg, and his effort
to produce a culture of modern medicine in Accra.

Chapter 4, entitled "Colonial Medical Culture at Korle Bu, the
Gold Coast Hospital, 1923–1945," documents early activities at
the Gold Coast Hospital, the largest medical institution in British
West Africa. Physically removed from the city core, the hospital
represented an attempt by the Medical Department to offer a
distinct practical and spatial alternative to West African healing.
Most patients attended the Gold Coast Hospital for cures for
specific illnesses like yaws and syphilis, but the institution also
gave birth to a professional class of African doctors, nurses, and
dispensers. Despite the gender and racial divisions inherent in
the colonial medical system, the African men and women working at the hospital appropriated European-derived practices to
establish their own type of urban medical culture, affectionately
referring to the institution by its Ga name. Korle Bu also became
home to a new method of child rearing known as "mothercraft,"
a British imperial style of parenting that spread outward from the
maternity branch of Korle Bu and into the homes of mothers in
the city. This chapter follows something of a standard periodiza-
tion, chronicling the growth of Western medicine in the city, but
does so only because African patients and medical workers were
so invested in the story of Korle Bu and the clinics. In concludes
with an interlude that introduces the goddess Korle, the significance of the Korle Lagoon to the menology of the Ga people, and
interwar attempts to reengineer the Korle waterway.

The fifth chapter, "The Creation of an African 'Bloodstream':
Malaria Control during the Hitler War, 1942–1945," is about a singular, dramatic event in the history of Accra—the short-lived success of an Allied antimalaria campaign during the Second World
War. This instance of medical technocracy was unprecedented in
Accra and will be used as a case study to ask why colonial sanitation
and medicine failed to achieve hegemony in the city. In 1942, when
the Gold Coast became a transit hub for Allied aircraft destined

for North Africa, British and American malariologists tried to eradicate the mosquito population of Accra by reengineering the Korle Lagoon and spraying the city with DDT. Fear of epidemic malaria allowed a new type of medical discourse to emerge, one that reduced the inhabitants of Accra to a reservoir of disease with malaria in its so-called "bloodstream."[66] The immediate effect of the dredging and spraying campaign was a rapid decline in malaria among Allied soldiers, but despite its short-term success, the British Army abandoned the project when the Americans (and their seemingly endless capacity to spend) left in 1944. This chapter shows how the technocratic dream of rebuilding the city according to the rules of medical science almost became a reality but collapsed when the fiscally constrained colonial government refused to make it a priority. Central to this chapter are interviews with retired soldiers, whose accounts of unrestrained medical authority during a time of martial law spurred the inclusion of this chapter in the book. It ends with an interlude vignette of the release of Jean Rouch's *Les Maîtres Fous*, a film about the Hauka cult that offers insight into how migrants attempted to heal the sickness of colonialism in Accra.

The sixth chapter, "The Resilience of Therapeutic Pluralism on the Eve of Ghanaian Independence," is a review of the diversity of healing cultures present in Accra when it became the capital of Ghana. This chapter draws on a 1958 sociological report entitled *Accra Survey*,[67] which made the dramatic assertion that colonial medicine was the first choice of the residents of Accra in times of illness. A deeper investigation into the data of the survey reveals that, despite the construction of several hospitals and clinics, colonial medicine was still only one choice among many for patients in Accra. A strong network of African healers—which now included practices such as Afa divination, acupuncture, and Zabarima cults of affliction—was still active in the city. Islamic and Christian healing options also flourished, as did the availability of patent medicines and pharmaceuticals. This chapter is supplemented by the recollections of retired African-born physicians, who recalled how they struggled to assert their authority to heal within a crowded marketplace of healing traditions.

The book ends with an epilogue that demonstrates continuities of healing pluralism during the demographic boom of the late twentieth century. Domestic growth and in-migration increased the population of Accra from 350,000 in 1964 to over three million by 2000,[68] multiplying the number of African healing traditions in the city, reducing Ga healers to a minority, and creating a scandalously dangerous sanitary situation for the city's residents.[69] Key events during the postcolonial period—including President Kwame Nkrumah's efforts to Africanize the medical system; the rapid expansion of the market for pharmaceuticals from Europe, India, and China; a proliferation of charismatic healing churches; the rise of private medical care; and the rapid growth in demand for locally produced bottled herbal remedies—have led to several changes in the way that quests for therapy are now conducted.[70] This concluding chapter will discuss trends in health and healing and suggest that Accra remains an open medical culture where patients, rather than medicine, will define the culture of healing in the twenty-first century.

Interlude: Therapeutic Pluralism in Little Accra by the Sea

One might begin an inquiry into the nature of therapeutic pluralism in Africa in many places. At first blush, Accra is not an obvious place to start. As a fishing village on a stretch of surf-bound shoreline, Little Accra was not initially well suited to sustain a large population. Accra receives only minimal rainfall in comparison to the fertile forestlands to the north and west, and the lands around the city offer only modest agricultural output. Nevertheless, Accra was thrust into the spotlight through upheaval caused by wars in the Akan forestlands, making it a sudden capital for both the Ga people and the growing transatlantic trade.

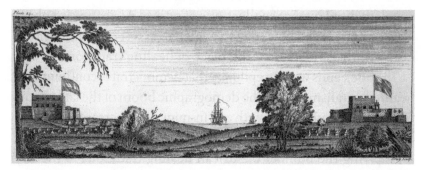

Introduction 1.2. "North Prospect of the English and Dutch at Akkra, by Smith, 1727." Though the villages of "Little Accra" on the Guinea Coast were probably not as neatly defined as they appear in this stylized print, each village in the shadow of each fort held to a distinct ancestral identity. At the base of Fort Crevecoeur is the village of *Kinka*, whose inhabitants claim first-comer status as the original Ga-speaking inhabitants of the city. Their oral traditions recall a strong trading connection with the Dutch. Across the small valley to the right is the village of *Ngleshi*, a local pronunciation of "English," which was established when James Fort was built. Both of these towns also had different sub-divisions, each with a distinct history connected to the ethnicity of its founders. Christiansborg Castle and the village of Osu are not shown here, but they were similarly arrayed on a headland approximately three kilometers to the east. (Sources: interview, Nae Wulomo, August 5, 2002; image from Thomas Astley, *New General Collection of Voyages and Travels*, Vol. 2 (London, 1745), 616–7.)

Oral tradition and archaeological evidence suggest that Ga speakers established their first capital city around 1400 at Ayawaso, at the base of the Akwapim Ridge.[71] From this inland entrepôt, Ga merchants were able to control the gold trade moving south from the Guinea rain forest and the salt trade moving north from the lagoons of the coast. The commercial exchange of these two major commodities supported a large marketplace, which made Ayawaso a crossroads for Guang, Ga, and Akan cultures.[72] Europeans were eager to establish trade links with the Ga capital, which they called Great Accra, and the Portuguese established a trading post near the Korle Lagoon sometime during the 1570s.[73]

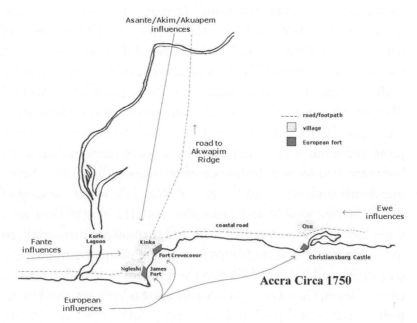

Map 1.1. Map of Accra in 1750.

The Portuguese monopoly on trade in West Africa held sway for over half a century, but other European merchant houses arrived in the city by the mid-seventeenth century. The Dutch built Fort Crevecoeur on a cliff near the old quarter of Accra in 1642, the Danish built Christiansborg Castle at the nearby village of Osu in 1661, and the English built James Fort to the west of the city in 1672.[74] The new fortresses transformed Little Accra into a competitive outpost for the traffic in slaves in West Africa, making it a key part of what archaeologist James Anquandah has called a "slave trade economic revolution."[75] The new commerce in slaves also encouraged merchants and laborers to settle in Accra, bringing in Ewe migrants from the East and Fante migrants from the west.[76]

The inland capital of Ayawaso prospered until the end of the seventeenth century, when, weakened by internal political disputes, the Gas were unable to defend themselves against an uprising by the vassal state of the Akwamu.[77] In 1677, the armies of the Ak-wamuhene marched south from the rain forest and, after a series of battles, sacked Ayawaso and took control of the trade routes from the coast to the interior.[78] Refugees from the ruined city fled south, with the majority seeking shelter in the villages of Little Accra.[79] Their respite was brief. In 1680, the Akwamu armies attacked again, sacking and burning the Ga coastal villages. The Dutch and British protected some of the inhabitants by housing them in their forts, but many fled to neighboring chiefdoms along the coast.[80] Some merchants took refuge to the east at Whydah, while the king of Accra traveled west to seek protection with the king of Fetu, near Cape Coast.[81] These years of exile and turmoil are memorialized in Ga songs and oral traditions as a period of mixing of peoples, languages, and cultures.[82] When the refugees returned to rebuild their villages, Ga merchants became increasingly involved in ex-porting slaves and gold and importing cloth, guns, and liquor. Quite suddenly, Little Accra replaced Ayawaso as the political and commercial capital of the Ga people.[83]

The new coastal version of Accra was subdivided according to associations with European slave traders: James Town at the base of James Fort; Kinka at the base of Fort Crevecoeur; and Osu at the base of Christiansborg Castle.[84] Each of these neighborhoods was, in turn, made up of a patchwork of quarters known as *akutsei*, each with a chiefly stool and a clan lineage that led back to the founding of Accra, the arrival of Ga refugees, or the settlement of immigrant groups.[85] Though the lineages of the people living in the *akutsei* differed, they all spoke Ga, they all nominated chiefs to represent them within a broader Ga polity, and they all participated in the annual harvest festival of *Homowo*.[86] Nonetheless, each neighborhood held true to its own religious and ethnic composition, a situation that allowed for a diversification of healing practices.

Ga was the majority language of Accra, but Akan languages were also prominent because of intermarriage, immigration, and commercial ties.[87] Accra-based traders maintained connections with Akan merchants in the interior, and some traveled regularly to Aburi, about forty kilometers north of Accra, where they exchanged cloth, guns, and brandy for gold, slaves, and ivory at a thrice-weekly market.[88] Trade links along the coastal littoral were also significant. For instance, Akoda, a Fante merchant resident in Accra, made his fortune dealing up and down the coast in cattle, gold, slaves, pottery, beads, and clay pipes.[89] Ewe speakers were also prominent in the city because the Dangme-speaking territory (with a language similar Ga) was coterminous with the Ewe lands across the Volta River.[90] Over two hundred years of linguistic mixing made Accra a polyglot "speech field," a multiethnic commercial center open to newcomers.[91] The welcoming spirit of Accra is aptly expressed in the hybrid Ga/Akan saying "*Ablekuma abakuma wo*" (may people come and join us).[92] It was in this setting that the pluralistic healing culture of Accra began to flourish.

NOTES

1. Gyekye, *Tradition and Modernity*, 287.

2. Healers from northern Nigeria and immigrants from Brazil brought new forms of herbalism and Quranic healing to Accra in the nineteenth century. See Stock, "Traditional Healers in Rural Hausaland"; Amos and Ayesu, "'I Am Brazilian,'" 46.

3. Silverman and Owusu-Ansah, "Presence of Islam," *History in Africa* 16 (1989); Maier, "Nineteenth-Century Asante Medical Practices," 79; Pellow, "Power of Space," 435.

4. Tsofatse Thunder, interview with the author, December 22, 2006.

5. Gifford, *Ghana's New Christianity*.

6. Baeta, *Prophetism in Ghana*; Cephas N. Omenyo, "New Wine in an Old Wine Bottle? Charismatic Healing in the Mainline Churches in Ghana," in *Global Pentecostal and Charismatic Healing*, ed. Candy G. Brown (Oxford: Oxford University Press, 2011), 231–49.

7. Bernhard Bierlich uses the term *self-care* to describe how patients in Northern Ghana diagnose and treat their own illnesses with bottled medicines. Bierlich, *Problem of Money*, 182. Kristine Krause has argued that healing in Ghana today is defined by competition among a plurality of healing traditions. Kristine Krause, "'The Double Face of Subjectivity': A Case Study in a Psychiatric Hospital (Ghana)," in *Multiple Medical*

Realities: Patients and Healers in Biomedical, Alternative, and Traditional Medicine, ed. Helle Johannessen and Imre Lazar (New York: Berghahn Books, 2006), 57. Kodjo Senah has noted that health care in Ghana is provided at diverse places, including "shrines, healing homes, spiritual churches, hospitals, clinics, health posts, materiality homes, and pharmacies or drugstores." Senah, *Money Be Man*, 48, 196.

8. Minocha, "Medical Pluralism and Health Services in India"; Attewell, *Refiguring Unani Tibb*; Hausman, "Making Medicine Indigenous"; Dinges, *Medical Pluralism and Homeopathy in India and Germany*.

9. Andrews, *Making of Modern Chinese Medicine*; Fang, *Barefoot Doctors and Western Medicine in China*.

10. Nahin et al., "Costs of Complementary and Alternative Medicine (CAM)," 1; Firkins et al., "Use of Complementary and Alternative Medicine."

11. Nahin et al., "Costs of Complementary and Alternative Medicine (CAM)," 11–14.

12. For more on the epistemological debate over the assessment of the efficacy of alternative medicines, see Tonelli and Callahan, "Why Alternative Medicine Cannot Be Evidence-Based"; also, *Evidence-Based Complementary and Alternative Medicine* (Oxford University Press, published since 2004) contains dozens of articles that evaluate the scientific merits of alternative therapies.

13. Hokkanen, "Quests for Health and Contests for Meaning"; Langwick, "Devils, Parasites, and Fierce Needles"; Schumaker, Jeater, and Luedke, "Introduction"; Livingston, "Productive Misunderstandings."

14. Beckerleg, "Medical Pluralism and Islam"; Rekdal, "Cross-cultural Healing"; Vinay R. Kamat, "The Anthropology of Childhood Malaria in Tanzania," in *Anthropology and Public Health: Bridging Differences in Culture and Society*, ed. Robert A. Hahn and Marcia Inhorn (Oxford: Oxford University Press, 2009), 35–64; Jennings, "Chinese Medicine and Medical Pluralism."

15. Gran, "Medical Pluralism in Arab and Egyptian History"; Obermeyer, "Pluralism and Pragmatism."

16. Keita, *Political Economy*, 27.

17. Senah, *Money Be Man*, 198. This saying has an analog in Twi, the language of Akan cultures to the north of the city: "*se wo anton wo yaree a wo enya ayaresa*" (you must sell your disease if you want to find a cure).

18. Quote taken from the title of Buel, *Heroes of the Dark Continent*. European missionaries in Africa quickly discovered that basic surgical

techniques attracted African patients to mission stations, aiding (sometimes) in the process of conversion; see Comaroff and Comarofff, *Of Revelation and Revolution*; Landau, "Explaining Surgical Evangelism"; Landau,
Realm of the Word; Seth Quartey, *Missionary Practices on the Gold Coast*.
The missionary doctor became a heroic figure in the European public
imagination in the late nineteenth and well into the twentieth centuries
in works such as *Scenes and Services in South Africa*; Elliott, *"Nyaka" the
Doctor*.

19. Marshall and Poling, *Schweitzer*, 238. Schweitzer has been since criticized for his "Moral Paternalism" (Davenport, "Moral Paternalism of Albert Schweitzer"), and his "benevolent racism" (Mazrui, "Dr. Schweitzer's
Racism").

20. Lyons, *Colonial Disease*, 1; Gelfand, *Tropical Victory*, 247; Gelfand,
Sick African; see also Ransford *"Bid the Sickness Cease."*

21. Patterson, *Health in Colonial Ghana*, 105.

22. Addae, *Evolution of Modern Medicine*, 8–14.

23. Quoted from Ransford, *"Bid the Sickness Cease."* See also Azevedo,
Hartwig, and Patterson, *Disease in African History*; Sabben-Clare, Brad-
ley, and Kirkwood, *Health in Tropical Africa*; Wilcocks, *Aspects of Medical
Investigation*.

24. Prins, "But What Was the Disease?"

25. As in the work of McKeown, *Role of Medicine*. See also Ehrenreich,
Cultural Crisis of Modern Medicine, 2–16.

26. Curtin, *Disease and Empire*; Echenberg, *Black Death*; Vaughan, *Curing Their Ills*; Lyons, *Colonial Disease*.

27. Steven Feierman, "Struggles for Control."

28. Twumasi, "Social History"; Twumasi, *Medical Systems in Ghana*.

29. Leslie, *Asian Medical Systems*; Leslie, "Medical Pluralism in World
Perspective"; Arthur Kleinman. *Culture and Healing in Asian Societies:
Anthropological, Psychiatric, and Public Health Studies* (Boston: G. K. Hall,
1978); Kleinman, *Patients and Healers*.

30. Janzen, *Quest for Therapy*.

31. Janzen, *Quest for Therapy*, 7–8.

32. Janzen, *Lemba*.

33. Feierman, *Peasant Intellectuals*.

34. Feierman, "Change in African Therapeutic Systems," 277.

35. Hörbst and Gerrits, "Transnational Connections of Health Professionals"; MacConnaughey, *Medical Landscapes*; Krause, Parkin, and Alex,
"Turning Therapies."

36. Waite, *History of Traditional Medicine*, 11–12, 120; Maier, "Asante Medical Practices," 63–81; Allman and Parker, *Tongnaab*; Sundkler, *Bantu Prophets in South Africa*; Schoffeleers, "Folk Christology in Africa"; Schoffeleers, "Ritual Healing and Political Acquiescence"; Luedke, "Spirit and Matter"; Gifford, "Ghana's Charismatic Churches"; Gifford, *African Christianity*; Gifford, *Ghana's New Christianity*; Meyer, "Christianity in Africa"; Robinson, *Muslim Societies in Africa*, 52–58; Akhtar, *Health and Disease in Tropical Africa*, 286–88; Lambek, *Knowledge and Practice*; John Janzen and Edward C. Green, "Continuity, Change and Challenge in African Medicine," in *Medicine across Cultures: History and Practice of Medicine in Non-Western Cultures*, ed. Helaine Selin (London: Kluwer Academic, 2003), 1–26.

37. Digby, *Diversity and Division in Medicine*, 373, 391.

38. Flint, *Healing Traditions*.

39. Feierman, "Change in African Therapeutic Systems"; Janzen, *Quest for Therapy*; Mullings, *Therapy, Ideology, and Social Change*, 192; Krause, "Double Face of Subjectivity," 57; Senah, *Money Be Man*, 48, 196; Good, *Ethnomedical Systems in Africa*; Whyte, *Questioning Misfortune*; Fink, *Religion, Disease, and Healing in Ghana*; Lambek, *Knowledge and Practice*; Baronov, *African Transformation of Western Medicine*, 31; Sama and Nguyen, *Governing Health Systems in Africa*, 25.

40. Porter, "The Patient's View," 184.

41. McKeown, *Role of Medicine*; Winters, *Accidental Medical Discoveries*.

42. Gatsonis and Morton, *Methods in Comparative Effectiveness Research*, xv.

43. Maly, et. al., "Perceived Efficacy"; Klooster et al., "Further Validation."

44. Ashforth, "Epidemic of Witchcraft?," 133.

45. Pietz, "Problem of the Fetish, I"; "Problem of the Fetish, II"; "Problem of the Fetish."

46. Feierman, "Struggles for Control," 83.

47. Foucault, *History of Sexuality*, 1:140.

48. Pesek, "Foucault Hardly Came to Africa."

49. Callewaert, "Bourdieu, Critic of Foucault," 91.

50. Vaughan, *Curing Their Ills*; Butchart, *Anatomy of Power*; Pesek, "Foucault Hardly Came to Africa."

51. Foucault, *Discipline and Punish*, 191; Cooper, "Conflict and Connection," 1533.

52. Punday, "Foucault's Body Tropes." See also Giddens and Sutton, *Modernity and Self-Identity*, 57. For the contrasts between Foucault and Bourdieu, see Callewaert, "Bourdieu, Critic of Foucault."

53. Bourdieu, *Distinction.* See also Echtler and Ukah, *Bourdieu in Africa;* Iqani and Kenny, *Consumption, Media and Culture.*

54. World Health Organization, *Constitution of the World Health Organization: Basic Documents,* 45th ed. (Geneva, 2006), accessed May 5, 2015, http://apps.who.int/gb/bd/PDF/bd47/EN/constitution-en.pdf.

55. Mullings, *Therapy, Ideology, and Social Change,* 66; Senah, *Money Be Man,* 141.

56. Janzen and Green, "Continuity, Change, and Challenge in African Medicine," 6. See also Krause, "Double Face of Subjectivity," 56–57.

57. Twumasi, "Social History," 351.

58. Flint, *Healing Traditions,* 67–89; John Johnson, *Epic of Son-Jara,* 43–45; Niane, *Sundiata,* 70–71; Kaba, "Pen, the Sword, and the Crown," 250; David Ross, "European Models and West African History," 296; Burton, *Mission to Gelele,* 21.

59. Samuel S. Quarcoopome, "Impact of Urbanization," 115.

60. Feierman, "Change in African Therapeutic Systems," 281; Keith Thomas, *Religion and the Decline of Magic;* Gentilcore, "Was There a 'Popular Medicine'?"; Lindemann, *Medicine and Society in Early Modern Europe;* Moore and McClean, *Folk Healing.*

61. Ruth A. Fisher, ed., "A Description of the Castle's Forts and Settlements Belonging to the Royal African Company of England on the Gold Coast," in *Extracts from the Records of the African Companies* (New York: Association for the Study of Negro Life and History, 1930), 107; Kea, *Settlements, Trade, and Polities,* 216–23; Anquandah, "Accra Plains," 4–5; Bosman, *New and Accurate Description of the Coast of Guinea,* 70.

62. Miller, *Missionary Zeal and Institutional Control.*

63. Odoom, "Document on Pioneers," 3. Spelling from Dakubu, *Ga–English Dictionary,* 76.

64. Dumett, "Campaign against Malaria," 170; Carl Christian Reindorf, *History of the Gold Coast and Asante,* 218; Parker, *Making the Town,* 157; Odoom, "Document on Pioneers," 3; the spelling of *zoŋo* is from Dakubu, *Ga-English Dictionary,* 76; *Korle Bu Hospital,* 141.

65. Field, *Religion and Medicine of the Gā People.*

66. NARA, R. 705, Vickery, "History of the Medical Section Africa-Middle East," 213.

67. Acquah, *Accra Survey.*

68. Acquah, *Accra Survey,* 31; Accra Metropolitan Assembly, "MCE's Message," accessed March 1, 2011, http://www.ama.ghanadistricts.gov.gh /?arrow=dce&_=3.

69. Acquah, *Accra Survey*, 123. By 1958, Ga healers made up only 45% of all "traditional" healers in Accra. In 1948, the Ga made up 52% of the population of Accra. Considering the growth in immigration and the birth rate of the non-Ga population, by 1957, the Gas would have certainly been in the minority.

70. Patrick A. Twumasi and Dennis Michael Warren, "The Professionalisation of Indigenous Medicine: A Comparative Study of Ghana and Zambia," in *The Professionalisation of African Medicine*, ed. Murray Last and G. L. Chavunduka (Manchester: Manchester University Press, 1986), 122; Senah, *Money Be Man*, 4; van Dijk, "Contesting Silence"; Govindaraj et al., "Hospital Autonomy in Ghana," 15–16, 21–22.

71. Odotei, "Pre-colonial Economic Activities of the Ga," 67.

72. Carl Christian Reindorf, *History of the Gold Coast*, 97. See also Wilks, "Rise of the Akwamu Empire," 104; Kea, *Settlements, Trade, and Polities*, 36; Dakubu, *Korle Meets the Sea*, 105; Anquandah, "Accra Plains," 3.

73. Barbot, *Barbot on Guinea*, 430; Justesen and Manley, *Danish Sources for the History of Ghana*, 12; Anquandah, *Rediscovering Ghana's Past*, 117. Slightly different dates (according to when construction commenced or was completed) are given in van Dantzig, *Forts and Castles of Ghana*, 8; Carl Christian Reindorf, *History of the Gold Coast*, 24.

74. Parker, *Making the Town*, 10; de Marees, *Gold Kingdom of Guinea*, 85.

75. Anquandah, "Accra Plains," 3.

76. Carl Christian Reindorf, *History of the Gold Coast*, 40; Kilson, *Kpele Lala*, 269.

77. Carl Christian Reindorf, *History of the Gold Coast*, 33–34.

78. Carl Christian Reindorf, *History of the Gold Coast*, 20, 25. The precise date of the fall of the inland capital of the Ga is disputed: see Carl Christian Reindorf, *History of the Gold Coast*, 34; Odotei, "Pre-colonial Economic Activities of the Ga," 69.

79. Carl Christian Reindorf, *History of the Gold Coast*, 38–39.

80. Astley, *New General Collection*, 618; Carl Christian Reindorf, *History of the Gold Coast*, 36–43; Dakubu, *Korle Meets the Sea*, 147.

81. Daaku, *Trade and Politics on the Gold Coast*, 154; Bosman, *New and Accurate Description of the Coast of Guinea*, 61.

82. Kilson, *Kpele Lala*, 259–60; Rømer, *Reliable Account of the Coast of Guinea*, 116–21; Bosman, *New and Accurate Description of the Coast of Guinea*, 70.

83. Bosman, *New and Accurate Description of the Coast of Guinea*, 70; Fisher, ed., "Description of the Castle's Forts and Settlements," 107; Kea, *Settlements, Trade, and Polities*, 216–23; Anquandah, "Accra Plains," 4–5;

Ruth A. Fisher, ed., "Winnebah 21 Dec. 1773. Thomas Westgate to 'Dear Dick' (Richard Brew at Annamaboe)," in *Extracts from the Records of the African Companies,* ed. Ruth A. Fisher (New York: Association for the Study of Negro Life and History, 1930), 92.

84. Astley, *New General Collection of Voyages,* 619.

85. For further detail on the quarters of each town, see Carl Christian Reindorf, *History of the Gold Coast,* 24–28, 38–48; Samuel S. Quarcoopome, "Impact of Urbanization," 119–122; Wilks, "Akwamu and Otublohum," 391–404.

86. Field, *Religion and Medicine of the Gā People,* 64–65, 87–88.

87. Dakubu, *Korle Meets the Sea,* 105; Meredith, *Account of the Gold Coast of Africa,* 217–18.

88. Astley, *New General Collection of Voyages,* 619–20.

89. Kea, *Settlements, Trade, and Polities,* 221; Ruth A. Fisher, ed., "David Mill to Richard Miles. Cape Coast Castle. July 19, 1774," in *Extracts from the Records of The African Companies,* ed. Ruth A. Fisher (New York: Association for the Study of Negro Life and History, 1930), 95; Wisnes, *Letters on West Africa and the Slave Trade,* 133; Adam Jones, ed., "Wilhelm Johann Müller's description of the Fetu Country, 1662–9," in *German Sources for West African History, 1599–1669,* ed. Adam Jones (Wiesbaden: Steiner, 1983), 209.

90. Carl Christian Reindorf, *History of the Gold Coast,* 9; Dakubu. *Korle Meets the Sea,* 114–15.

91. Dakubu, *Korle Meets the Sea,* 162. Dakubu uses Hymes's definition of *speech field* as "a total range of communities within which a person's knowledge of varieties and speaking rules potentially enables him to move communicatively," from Gumperz and Hymes, *Directions in Sociolinguistics,* 18–19.

92. The word *ablekuma* is a name for a neighborhood, but etymologically it is a conjunction of the Ga word for corn and an Akan diminutive form.

ONE

THE ROOTS OF THERAPEUTIC PLURALISM IN ACCRA, 1677 TO THE MID-1800s

IN 1680, JEAN BARBOT, THE agent-general of the French Royal African Company, noted that "it . . . often happens that one doctor is discharged with a good regard, and another called in his place, knowing well how to manage the superstitious simplicity of his patient. His first act is to condemn all the former physician has done, whereupon new offerings are made, cost what they will, to get what may be had, for fear of being also turned away very shortly, as his predecessor was, and another again brought in, in his stead. For this change of doctors, or physicians, will happen twenty times or more successively."[1] At first glance, this passage may seem like just another racist account of Africans by a chauvinistic European merchant. It is lazy reportage in the sense that it uses a derisive and exaggerated tone, portraying the West African healer as a cynical charlatan and the African patient as a credulous fool without any details for proof. However, as objectionable as this quip from Barbot may be, it offers two key insights into the history of healing in Accra. The first is the basic fact that a plurality of African healers worked in the towns and villages of the West Coast of Africa, each offering different types of therapies. Barbot's mistake was to assume that the succession of doctors was a band of fraudulent quacks, lining up to deceive credulous patients. Within the context of therapeutic pluralism, such an assertion is clearly a mistake. If Barbot had bothered to distinguish between the different types of healers he described, he would have more carefully enumerated the diversity of herbal remedies, consecrated medicines, and spiritual therapies circulating around West Africa.

Barbot's second insight is that patients had the power to choose between practitioners and healing systems. In an era of therapeutic pluralism, patients had the luxury to patronize healers who promised to cure and dismiss healers who failed to do so. They did not "change doctors" because they were capricious, as Barbot wants us to believe, but because they had the power to choose. West Africa, it seems, was an open arena for therapeutic services. It was a patient's market, and if Barbot had bothered to ask patients why they kept dismissing their healers, they might have told him they were "selling" their sickness.

Jean Barbot failed to recognize this diversity of therapies because, like other Europeans during the transatlantic slave trade, he believed that Africans lived in a world beholden to so-called "fetish." Derived from the Portuguese *feitiço*, the word *fetish* became a pejorative term that associated idol worship with diabolism and malificium.[2] The use of the term was a mistake, of course, because West Africans did not worship idols per se, but rather sought guidance from innumerable lesser deities, spiritual forces and consecrated objects. Ideas about fetish worship pose a discursive barrier that still impedes an understanding of the history of therapeutic pluralism in West Africa today, but European travelers' obsession with African religious practices and material cultures has, fortunately, also left behind rich archival material about healing traditions.[3] In fact, when European travel accounts are correlated with data derived from linguistics, archaeology, and botany, their discussion of so-called fetish practices shows that the healing culture of West Africa was both dynamic and pluralistic.

This chapter sketches out an early era of therapeutic pluralism, evident within the language, practices, and material cultures
of the Ga people. As the city grew, it became a polyglot capital,
and the Ga healing lexicon became an aggregation of core Ga-
Dangme terms and Akan, Ewe, and Hausa loanwords. Accra
also became home to multiple healing practices, including deity
worship, spirit possession, dancing, drumming, animal sacrifice,
libation, and ritual surgery, which took hold in the city as different ethnic groups carved out distinct neighborhoods within the
Ga capital. Material culture also played a crucial role in making
Accra a hub of therapeutic pluralism, as the city became a clear-
inghouse for herbal ingredients and consecrated medicines from
around West Africa and a marketplace for medicinal flora from
Asia and the Americas. Diversity reigned within the African healing culture of Accra. When European surgeons first appeared in
Accra, they did little to alter the context of pluralism. Far from
being agents of change, European healing traditions survived
only as a marginal component of the larger pluralistic network
of Accra, one choice among many for patients in the city, and not
a very good choice at that. Even European sailors were quick to
abandon their shipboard surgeons to conduct their own quests
for therapy among the African healers of the city.

THE LINGUISTIC INFLUENCES ON HEALING IN ACCRA

The roots of therapeutic pluralism are embedded within the Ga
language. At the core is a set of terms drawn from early iterations
of Ga, known to linguists as Proto-Ga-Dangme (PGD). Within
this core word list is a group of foundational sounds and shapes
identified as uniquely Ga and labeled with a system of starred
forms. At the heart of this healing lexicon is *hewalε*, a word that
contains the PGD starred form of *wā, a basic component of
many terms relating to a normative state of health, strength, and
hardness.[4] As Ga speakers understand it, *hewalε* flows through

the body as a type of essential vigor, but it can be diminished by blockages, which may result in illness.[5] The goal of the healer is to remove these blockages by treating the body and, if necessary, by purifying the spirit of the patient.[6]

Within the Ga language, common illnesses fall into the category of *hela folo*, or ordinary illness. A case of indigestion, for example, might be read as a common illness caused by putrid food or intestinal worms, and so a patient suffering from stomach trouble would not need to theorize about the deeper causes of the illness.[7] But the Ga understanding of the corporeal self has always gone beyond bodily illness. The definition of the word for body, *gbomotso*, exemplifies the intertwining of the physical and the spiritual. As a concatenation of *mo* (PGD: *mɛ-), the term for person, and *tso* (PGD: *tse-), the word for tree, the *gbomotso* operates as a mask covering the spiritual essences of the individual.[8] The implication here is that the outward body is a surface that can be read and interpreted. If a patient suffered from a chronic illness, for instance, a Ga healer would be obliged to inquire about the deeper causes of the malady. After investigating, they might suggest that the disease is a spiritual illness caused by rogue spirits known as *woji* or by named deities known as *jemawoji*, words derived from core Ga terminology (PGD: *wode).[9] If a healer has divined that a person is being attacked by spirits, they might resort to the use of ritual and consecrated medicines to combat the assault.

Whether a disease has been deemed natural or spiritual, the primary weapon used to fight it has always been herbal medicine, known in Ga as *tsofa* (PGD: *tse-). Speakers of Bantu languages will note that the core sound within this word matches the Bantu starred form of *ti, which suggests a deep continuity within the medical lexicon of sub-Saharan Africa.[10] The most common form of *tsofa* was derived from the leaves, twigs, roots, and bark of local plants. Patients consumed plant medicines as herbal drafts and poultices, usually without any deep contemplation of the source of their healing power. Lingering illnesses required additional therapies, containing both material and ritual elements. A common example of this sort of aggregate medicine is *ti*, a collection of charred herbs mixed into poultices, suspended in potions, or rubbed into cuts in the skin. The production of *ti* differed from the preparation of individual herbs because it was made by specialists who conducted rituals as part of the fabrication process. Ga speakers have traditionally regarded *ti* as an elevated form of *tsofa* because it includes both herbal ingredients common to the scrublands of the Accra Plains (such as *hiiatso* and *nyanyara*, two medicinal plants that have been used by herbalists for centuries) and ground-up minerals and animal parts.[11]

Consecrated ritual objects make up another category of medicine used in Accra. Europeans referred to these items as fetishes and were confounded by their spectacular diversity. As European records show, Ga healers have been producing amulets, charms, and figurines as devices of healing for several hundred years at least. Pieter de Marees, a Dutch traveler who visited Accra several times during the late seventeenth century, recorded seeing consecrated devices used to prevent ailments such as insomnia and indigestion, and Danish botanist Paul Isert noted in the late eighteenth century that all members of society wore amulets made of leather, gourds, beads, and shells as protection against illness and misfortune.[12] The owners of these amulets often rubbed them down with charred *ti* to incorporate the spirits of the forest into the object of healing. They bound multiple spiritual forces into a single *tsofa*, creating a mobile, personalized packet of healing power. One of the better-known consecrated medicines in Accra is knife medicine, or *kakla tsofa*, which has been known to prevent injury. Others have come and gone, like the mysterious "Arkah truth fetish" mentioned in past court records.[13] But whatever form they took, Ga medicines were designed to protect the body, clear harmful blockages, purify the spirit, thwart illness, and restore the flow of *hewalɛ*.[14]

The core concepts of healing can be expressed within the Ga lexicon, but imported Akan terminology has added further depth to the healing language of Accra. In particular, the imported notions of *susuma* and *kla* offer unique ways to explain spiritual causes of imbalance in the body and the soul. *Susuma* is defined broadly as an individual spirit, shade, or shadow.[15] An assistant to *susuma* is *kla*, sometimes defined as the part of the human being that endures into the afterlife.[16] As borrowed terms, *susuma* and *kla* have operated independently from PGD terminology. For example, if a person had feverish convulsions, a healer might have explained that their *kla* and *susuma* were fighting each other.[17] The *susuma/kla* framework has been especially useful for understanding the ravages of witchcraft, known in Ga as *ayɛ*.[18] According to ethnographic accounts of witchcraft, witches have used their *susuma* to leave their bodies and fly off at night to join their coven, with the intent of devouring the *kla* of their victims. As Margaret Field noted, the "*kla*, though invisible, has arms and legs and bodily organs corresponding to the visible body, and the witches cut it up, share it round, and eat it. When it is completely eaten the victim dies."[19] Attacks by witches, within this linguistic framework, can be countered through healing rituals that focus on cleansing the malicious *susuma* or defending the ravaged *kla*. Additionally, a Ga speaker might conjoin Ga and Akan terminology to generate hybrid forms of witch-fighting discourse. A powerful Ga *jemawoŋ*, for instance, could be mobilized as a healing force to cleanse a witch's *susuma* or defend the *kla* from attack by witchcraft.[20]

Other significant Akan contributions to the Ga healing lexicon are concepts related to ghosts, specters, and invisible dwarves, terrifying supernatural forces that could foment sickness. The activities of lingering spirits have been thought to influence health because they can take on benevolent or malicious personalities. Generally speaking, a *sisa* is the spirit of someone who died peacefully or of old age, while the vengeful *otofo* is the ghost of someone who died a violent or unnatural death.[21] These forces have expanded the Ga notion of ancestral spirits, which were previously understood simply as aggregate powers that could either heal or harm.[22] Another linguistic import is the concept of the *adope* (a borrowed Akan term for "ape"), known in Akan languages as *mmotia*.[23] The power of the *adope*, who have been thought of as migrant spirits from the rain forests to the north of the city, could only be harnessed by those with a special connection to the supernatural forces in the Twi-speaking territories.[24] Developing a relationship with invisible dwarves could be advantageous, providing a healing knowledge that could make a person wealthy. Conversely, ignoring the designs of the dwarves could make one ill.

Terms from the Ewe and Hausa languages have also been adopted by Ga speakers, though to a lesser degree than Akan terminology. Two Ewe loanwords within the healing lexicon of Ga, *gbaja* (syphilis) and *babanso* (gonorrhea), form a pairing related to venereal and skin diseases.[25] Despite the established presence of Ga words for venereal disease, these Ewe loanwords were adopted as typologies of disease, suggesting a history of intimate contact, both verbal and physical, between Ga and Ewe speakers. Another borrowed word commonly used to understand illness and misfortune is *kita*, a Hausa term for oath.[26] In contemporary spoken Ga, *kita* forms the root of a larger set of borrowed terms for the process of making oaths, which includes the swearing of oaths (*kitakalo*), the breaking of oaths (*kitatomo*), and the material object presented in atonement for a broken oath (*kitatomono*). How these words were adopted by Ga speakers is unknown, but they have played a role in the generative health of oath making and, as a consequence, the negative outcomes of oath breaking.

The Ga language, as linguist Mary Esther Kropp Dakubu demonstrated, "arose in a multilingual context and has existed in one ever since."[27] The Ga healing lexicon naturally followed suit, bringing together ideas about medicines, consecrated objects, witchcraft, vengeful spirits, invisible dwarves, new diseases, curses, and oaths. So diverse are the ideas contained within Ga terminologies of healing that anthropologist Kodjo Senah has argued that "there is no such thing as a fixed and systematic Ga canon of ideas on body and illness."[28] Indeed, Ga healing never did coalesce into an ethnomedical dogma but instead found its expression within a plural set of ideas that came to the city via historical processes of conflict, exile, migration, and commerce.

A PANTHEON OF DEITIES AND A
REPERTOIRE OF PRACTICES

When Portuguese mariners began to explore the Guinea coast in the fifteenth and sixteenth centuries, they showered derision on African religious and medical practices by labeling them as *feitiço*, a late-medieval Portuguese word for sorcery.[29] The denigration of African practices continued through the seventeenth century, as the Dutch, Danish, and English used the concept of fetish as a shorthand for irrational superstition. Slave trader Willem Bosman, for instance, characterized "fetish" practices as displays of "whim" and "caprice" by depicting them as the random worship of "a stone, a piece of wood, or anything else of that nature."[30] Barbot concurred, noting that fetishes were made from almost any element or compound.[31] These travel accounts, written by Europeans who only briefly passed through West Africa, are problematic in the sense that they generated racial and cultural hierarchies that were later codified in Carolus Linnaeus's *Systema Naturae*.[32] However, the irony of the European obsession with so-called fetish is that it offers historians tremendous insight into the workings of medical and religious practices on the Gold Coast. European travelogues contain a wealth of information about the practices conducted in towns along the Atlantic coast, including worship of deities, spirit possession, drumming rhythms, animal sacrifice, libation pouring, and ritual scarification. These European commentaries reveal that, like the Ga lexicon, the repertoire of healing practices in Accra expanded over the course of several centuries according to patterns of economic, social, and cultural change.

Because they have responsibility for the general well-being of the Ga people, the deities of Accra have always played a role as arbitrators of physical and mental health. According to oral traditions compiled by C. C. Reindorf, Accra was once a "fetishcracy" where political, social, economic, and cultural power was wielded by the priests of the major shrines, known as the *wulomei*.[33] After the conquest of Accra by the Akwamu, chiefly authority began to grow and secular power accumulated in the hands of merchant families.[34] Nonetheless, the divinities of Accra continued to play a major role in urban affairs, and a triumvirate of paramount deities soon emerged: Nae, the goddess of the sea; Korle, the goddess of the lagoon; and Sakumo, the god of war.[35] The priests of the paramount shrines claim that their deities were the first to animate the bodies of spirit mediums in Accra, the first to reside in permanent sanctuaries, and the first to be consulted by the Ga state before any major national endeavor.[36]

But though Nae, Sakumo, and Korle are understood as a founding triumvirate today, it may not have always been so. Some oral traditions indicate that the original three gods are attached to local bodies of water, making them indigenous to the city, but other oral traditions describe them as immigrant deities who were brought to Accra by Ga settlers. Their conflicted identity is complicated by the fact that while all three speak Ga, they also speak smatterings of broken Obutu, the language of the Guang people who lived on the Accra Plains before the arrival of the Ga. This dual persona, as both indigene and immigrant, suggests that the founding triumvirate had to struggle to assert themselves vis-à-vis other deities as the leaders of the Ga spirit world.[37] Moreover, none of the three major deities is mentioned in the European journals of the seventeenth and eighteenth centuries—a hint that they may have been minor players on the spiritual landscape of Accra prior to the nineteenth century.

Like the founding gods and goddesses, the lesser deities of the Ga pantheon have been subject to fortunes that have risen or fallen over time. For hundreds of years, the people of Accra have worshipped a "multitude of sub-godheads," with new gods springing forth from the landscape, usually in the physical form of a freshwater spring or a termite mound.[38] Conversely, old gods can decline or disappear because of neglect. Olila, a deity worshipped by the first chief of the Ga, Ayi Kushi, is only a minor figure in Accra today.[39] Another deity, the once-powerful figure of Klan the hyena god, has been reduced to the status of a house medicine.[40] Oyeni, a water spirit and child of Nae, ascended to power during the transatlantic slave trade but fell into rapid decline when the British locked up its shrine in James Fort after abolition in 1808.[41] As if to fill the gaps left by the retreat of local spirits, migrant gods have established themselves in the city over the centuries, including Fante-speaking deities like Bentum and water spirits like Mami Wata.[42] These deities prospered along with the new inhabitants of the city by aiding in the development of fishing culture in Accra and by offering a way to understand the social and spiritual risks of engaging in the slave trade.[43]

Like gods and goddess, spirit mediums, known as the wontsemei and the woyei, have also been ubiquitous. In Accra, a person can become possessed when they experience an illness, usually a lingering, debilitating physical or mental affliction, which may climax with a sudden attack by the spirit. Once a person realizes that they are possessed, they must be trained by an elder spirit medium to recover from their malady and learn how to manage the occult forces controlling their body.[44] When effectively trained, spirit mediums can gain insight into the causes of disease, learn about the healing properties of herbal remedies, and master the material culture of consecrated medicines.

European accounts of West Africa abound with descriptions of spirit possession, including graphic depictions of mediums wearing ceremonial cloth, decorated with white paint and ritual scars, and dancing in ecstatic states.[45] A description of possession written by Danish merchant Ludvig Ferdinand Rømer in 1760 emphasizes how the spirits could readily dictate the behavior of the possessed: "With staring eyes they foam at the mouth, gasping for breath. They usually enter this [state] suddenly and unconsciously... [they can] at times be walking with a water pot or something else on her head, talking to someone walking beside her, and in an instant she is possessed. I have seen some who have made all these contortions, and yet kept the water pot on their heads."[46] This account of sudden clairvoyance might have been shocking to a European onlooker, but possessed mediums were a common sight at major religious events in the city (just as they are today), and the residents of Accra understood themselves as living, interacting, and moving through time with a changing cadre of local gods and goddesses. Today, the spirit mediums of Accra channel dozens of different gods and goddesses, and different deities can be identified by the languages they speak. Many communicate in glossolalia, usually in language fragments derived from the original Guang dialects of the Accra Plains. But the spirits of Accra speak other languages too, including Ga, Dangme, Fante, Twi, and Ewe, and their biographies tie them to immigrant groups who have settled in Accra.[47] Like the Ga healing lexicon, the speech acts of the gods express the accumulation of regional ideas about religion and healing.

Deities can also be identified by the rhythms they dance to. Historical accounts indicate that Ga spirit mediums congregated during public ceremonies such as the harvest festival of *Homowo*, dancing and singing to rhythms to ensure that the gods and goddesses of Accra would provide a good harvest and peace within the Ga state.[48] The Ga claim that the pentatonic *Kpele* rhythms used in Accra today are traditional tempos, dating as far back as when Ayawaso was the capital, and there is reason to believe that these rhythms dominated the religious music scene in Accra during the seventeenth and eighteenth centuries.[49] The major Ga gods and goddesses, for instance, dance to *Kpele* beats. However, the heptatonic *Akon* rhythms from Akan and Fante influences are also an integral part of Ga drumming today, and many foreign gods dance to these rhythms.[50] New patterns of percussion have been added in the twentieth century, offering a wide variety of rhythms for individual and group healing practices in the city.

The sacrifice of animals is another historical practice that has been intimately connected to health and healing in Accra. European travelers on the Gold Coast reported that religious ceremonies often required the ritual slaughter of chickens and goats and that the blood of an animal was believed to give sustenance to ancestral shades and spiritual entities.[51] Such practices could be both religious and medicinal. Ferdinand Rømer mentions that the inhabitants of Accra paid ritualists to sacrifice animals for them as a means of placating the spirits. A wealthy merchant, Rømer claimed, might ask a shrine priest or a spirit medium for a diagnosis every month and, upon receiving a clean bill of health, sacrifice a goat to the local deities. The meat from the animal would be shared among friends and family, and the entrails would be left at an urban crossroads to supplicate vengeful ghosts known as the *otofo*.[52] To European observers like Rømer, this type of sacrifice was a throwback to a pre-Christian era, but within Ga cosmology it was congruent with beliefs that animal spirits could maintain harmony between the physical and metaphysical worlds. For people who could afford it, animal sacrifice was preventive medicine that healed social relations and kept evil spirits at bay.[53]

Like possession and animal sacrifice, libation pouring has long been a fundamental component of religious and healing ceremonies in West Africa.[54] In many cultures of the Gold Coast, communication with the world of the supernatural required the pouring of drink on the ground, an offering that was believed to attract the interest of ancestors and spirits.[55] So widespread was the practice of pouring libation that it is not necessarily connected to priestly power or spirit possession. Anyone could pour libation to seek aid from ancestors or spirits, and alcohol was not always required. Before the growth in transatlantic commerce in West Africa, water was preferred, even above corn wine or palm wine. However, as the trade in brandy, rum, and gin increased, the residents of Accra began to use imported liquors in libation rituals.[56] The intoxicating spirit within *da ni na waa* (PGD: *dã-, meaning "strong drink") was believed to act as a sort of "fast water," lubricating communication between human beings and their deities, and it became a necessity when requesting the assistance of gods and ancestors.[57] Over time, healers started to mix imported liquor with herbs and roots to make restorative medicinal tinctures.[58] Today, the walls of herbalists' shops in Accra are lined with bottles of schnapps for libation, as well as liquor infused with herbs and roots. In particular, malaria tonics that follow traditional herbal remedies mixed with alcohol are evidence of the way that the changing practices of libation have altered the fabrication of traditional herbal remedies.

Another set of healing techniques prevalent in Accra involved cutting and incision. Surgeries practiced by therapists in Accra were minor in comparison with the amputations and internal operations common to Europe (which, incidentally, would have been quite deadly in a tropical climate without knowledge of sepsis or recourse to antibiotics), but they were nevertheless medically, socially, and spiritually significant. For instance, specialist lay healers learned how to remove Guinea worm by making vertical incisions on the leg. Most people in Accra, whether European or African, probably endured this painful procedure at some point in their lives.[59] There is also some evidence that healers in the region performed smallpox variolation, perhaps as

Muslim practitioners began to settle along the coast of West Africa, but there is no proof that Ga healers systematically adopted the practice.[60] Female circumcision was not practiced in Accra, but elder male members of the community did circumcise young boys as a means of distinguishing them as members of the Ga ethnic group.[61] Ritual scarification was another common practice, conducted by priests, spirit mediums, and herbalists who made incisions on the skin and rubbed them down with the ashes of charred herbs. Woodcut prints in the documentary record display patients bearing the scars of ritual incisions, darkened with dry herbal *ti* as a means of inoculating them against attacks by malicious spirits.[62] Some incisions also marked a person as ethnically Ga, and some people argue today that a single horizontal stroke or a cross on the cheek has always been a mark of Ga tribal identity.[63] Paul Isert mentioned that the practice of making Ga "tribal marks" had been discontinued by the 1800s and that he encountered only one old man, who was over ninety years old, with a small cross on each cheek.[64] Moreover, there are so few references to so-called tribal markings during this period that it is difficult to argue that scarification has been a long-standing tradition.

As this collection of practices shows, patients in Accra found themselves bound up in a world of spirits that inhabited bodies of water, buried mounds, crossroads, and dark sanctuaries. Dealing with long-standing illnesses and chronic problems meant abandoning oneself, as a patient, to the care of experts who used divination and possession to harness the occult powers that surrounded them. Most practitioners operated independently, but many were also loosely connected by their allegiances to local gods, as witnessed in their performances in spirit and their oblations to the deities, particular in the old quarters of the city during the *Homowo* harvest festival. Yet despite its religious underpinnings, this sophisticated set of traditions was neither fetish caprice nor random worship. Rather, it was a repertoire of healing actions, often (but not always) with deeply held spiritual meanings.

Herbal remedies have always been the medicine of first resort in Accra. Medicinal curatives, harvested and traded in Accra, could be used in a variety of ingestible forms. Common to Accra were many concoctions, potions, decoctions, and suspensions, which were put to work as laxatives, emetics, diuretics, analgesics, and antimalarials.[65] Some were combined with palm oil to make ointments, while others were mashed together to make herbal paps. There was even a market, as there is today, for chewing sticks and tooth scrubs.[66] Many of the more complicated herbal remedies prepared in Accra were composed by experts who held an encyclopedic knowledge of the medicinal flora of West Africa, but the occupation was not restricted to professionals—anyone could practice herbalism. Most mothers and grandmothers in Accra today have some knowledge of healing herbs, and knowledge of what Europeans have called "kitchen physick" was probably passed down from mother to daughter.[67] However, there are no hard and fast gender delineations. Knowledge about medicinal herbs has always been diffuse, and family members of every variety would try to heal their kin at home before seeking help from professionals.

After the fall of Ayawaso, Little Accra on the coast was well positioned to become a market for medicinal flora because it occupied the seaport at the end of the Akyem trade route, the commercial pathway leading from the Guinea coast to the Guinea rain forest and the Western Sudan.[68] The extent of the exchange in medicinal flora is evident in the diversity of plants that appear in a compendium of herbal reagents compiled by Danish surgeon and botanist Paul Isert, who lived in Accra for several years in the late eighteenth century.[69] Isert came to the Gold Coast to tend to the medical needs of slaves and Danish officials at Christiansborg Castle, but he was particularly interested in the flora of the region. During his free time, he traveled through nearby villages, collecting hundreds of samples of plants to send back to Denmark.[70] Isert's collection is still held at the Natural History Museum in Copenhagen, and it represents the earliest assemblage of medicinal simples from the Gold Coast.

Isert's collection contains many common weeds found in fields around Accra, like the all-purpose *Momordica charantia* (*nyanyara*) and the versatile *Fagara zanthoxyloides* (*hiatso*), the two most commonly used herbs in Accra today. Other plants collected by Isert were used less frequently, and he mentioned some plants specific only to the microclimates of the Gold Coast, such as an unnamed parasitic flowering red plant that grew exclusively in the roots of one species of tree and was used locally for the treatment of venereal disease.[71] We may never know what plant that was, but recent chemical analyses of Isert's listed curatives show that many of them, not surprisingly, contain potent medicinal compounds. The ubiquitous *nyanyara*, for instance, contains alkaloids that make it a useful purgative and anthelmintic, while the common weed *hiatso* has antimalarial properties.[72] The most famous of the herbs that Isert gathered, *Aframomum melegueta*, latterly known as grains of paradise, became celebrated in Europe for its properties as an aphrodisiac.[73]

Part of Isert's motivation to catalog the medicines of the Gold Coast came from the hope that he would find a cure for malaria. At a time when Peruvian cinchona bark was expensive and surgeons had not yet perfected its dosages, Isert hoped to find a local remedy for the disease that had impeded European settlement in West Africa for so long. As soon as he arrived, he heard rumors of a "wonder cure" for malaria that was reputedly known by herbalists in Accra and by some of the Europeans who had managed to survive on the Gold Coast.[74] In fact, so steadfast was the belief in local antimalarials that the "older Coastmen" had little regard for Isert's talents as a surgeon.[75] Unfortunately, Isert never did find his singular cure for malaria and in his frustration he later lashed out at the temerity of laypersons who suggested that such a panacea existed. His reaction was strange because there were indeed many herbs in the area that could be used to cure malaria. His informants might have been referring to any number of plants, including *Cryptolepis sanguinolenta*, a yellow root that contains antimalarial alkaloids; *Rauvolfia caffra*, a type of milkweed; or the barks of the *Khaya senegalensis*, *Sarcocephalus esculentus*, or *Crossopteryx febrifuga* trees.[76] Oddly, none of these plants made it to his list of medicinal herbs, perhaps because he did not have enough time to find them or maybe because local herbalists refused to divulge their secrets.

When Isert compiled his list of healing plants, he probably assumed that all of his specimens were native to the region. However, what is most surprising about his compendium is that it contains plants that were not native to West Africa, including the West Indian Bahama tea (*Lantana camara*, used for snakebites), a South Asian anthelmintic (*Cissus quadrangularis*, used to fight Guinea worm), and a South American tropical plant (*Physalis angulata*, used as a skin salve). How exactly these plants arrived in Accra is uncertain. There is no record of them being traded formally as commodities, so they must have been part of a subaltern exchange in medicinal reagents. They may have arrived via shipborne trade as seeds or saplings, to be propagated in gardens or encouraged to grow in the wild. They may also have wandered their way across the African tropics, ending up in Accra from distant parts of Africa. Unfortunately, the human agents behind these exchanges are unknown, but whatever the means of exchange, the existence of foreign medicinal flora growing in and around Accra in the late eighteenth century speaks to the scope of trade and exchange in the early modern era, as well as the willingness of healers to incorporate novel herbal simples into their remedies.

Though we cannot trace the precise arrival of foreign plants growing in Accra, there is a record of one particular plant medicine arriving as a commodity in the city. During the slave trade, Europeans brought Central American sarsaparilla root to trade along the Guinea coast.[77] Jean Barbot noted in 1680 that Africans immersed the root in alcohol to make a cure for venereal disease,[78] and Pieter de Marees noted in his journal that "they often use Salsaparille, which is brought to them by the Dutch ships, against the Pox and the Clap. They boil this Ointment in fresh water and drink it as a draught against the Pox and similar diseases, and also against the Worms which they get in their legs"[79] The "Pox" that de Marees described was probably yaws, an ulceration of the skin caused by bacterial infection.[80] Isert also noticed the endemic nature of yaws and was adept enough to ascertain that it was different from a venereal disease because most of the people he spoke to on the Gold Coast had contracted the disease at least once.[81] The worms that de Marees mentions were almost certainly Guinea worms, whereas the mention of "the Clap" was likely a reference to gonorrhea.[82] The effectiveness of sarsaparilla against these diseases is unquantifiable, but the mention of the clap is significant here—as sailors spread venereal disease around the ports of the Atlantic Ocean, they also spread knowledge of the one medicinal root that offered hope for a cure.[83]

Apart from sarsaparilla, there is no historical record of a trade in herbal reagents between Europeans and Africans. This is surprising considering how widely cinchona, the progenitor to the drug quinine, was traded around the Atlantic.[84] Cinchona became an indispensable febrifuge in the tool kit of surgeons traveling through West Africa, yet the documentary records do not mention local demand for cinchona bark on the Gold Coast or cultivation of the tree among West Africans.[85] There are many possible reasons for this. It may have been that cinchona did not grow well on the Gold Coast, or that the aforementioned antimalarials were deemed sufficient by African patients, or that the Spanish restricted the supply of seeds and saplings across the Atlantic, or that the British and the Dutch found it easier to build cinchona plantations in India and Java.[86] Nevertheless, the absence of cinchona either as a commodity of exchange or as an indigenized plant remains an oddity in a region where foreign medicinal plants were so quickly adopted.

Apart from herbal simples, a number of composite spiritual objects also appear in European records as so-called fetish medicines. These consecrated objects were compilations of things, including plants, animal parts, minerals, and symbolic components found in and around Accra. They could also include imported goods, like brass bowls, cloth, knives, guns, buttons, and coins, because the material culture of healing was profoundly influenced by the movement of goods and people in and out of the city. During his tenure on the Gold Coast, Jean Barbot noted that even European men wore consecrated objects and encouraged the worship of local spirits and deities among their colleagues and clients.[87] In particular, Europeans adopted the custom of making pledges before a mobile consecrated object to guarantee business deals in Accra. According to Rømer, who lived at Christiansborg Castle in the late eighteenth century, Europeans often employed local ritualists to mediate their oath-taking ceremonies. His account of "eating fetish," though racist and patronizing in its tone, demonstrates how Europeans were beholden to consecrated medicines as a means of guaranteeing honesty in business dealings:

> According to the laws of the land, we can force a Negro who has swindled us or stolen from us to eat fetish [to prove that] he had not done it. We pay two rixdaler to the fetish of our broker Adoui. Together with the fetish there usually come into the Fort a whole swarm of old Negroes, so that it costs us an additional two rixdaler to serve them brandy. This fetish is carried on a mat covered with an old cloth. The fetish consists of a stuffed snake skin, without head or tail, but in their stead, the hair from an

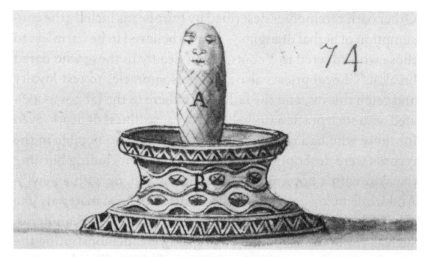

Figure 1.1. A consecrated oath object sketched by Jean Barbot in 1680. The figurine brought together spiritual and material power through a composition of local and imported items, including cloth, "glassware, beads, herbs, clay, burnt feathers, tallow and threads of bark from the fetish tree, all pounded and kneaded together." This particular oath object resided in Christiansborg Castle and was maintained by an employee there. It would have been one of many different consecrated medicines and shrines in Accra that could be used to seal business contracts or personal relationships. (Source: Barbot, *Barbot on Guinea*, fig. 49 between 580 and 587. See also Silverman and Owusu-Ansah, "Presence of Islam," 333.)

elephant's tail, or a cow's or wolf's tail, mingled with the feathers from a cock, so that it looks horrible. By custom it is made like a necklace, with threads at both ends, so that the individual who wishes to wear it can tie it at the back of his neck. This is placed at the feet of the Europeans who are present, the old cloth is taken from the sausage-like fetish and a crumb of dough as large as a pea placed on it. The accused then comes forward, goes down on his knees, holding his hands behind his back, and utters this oath: "If I have done that" or "If I have stolen this or that, then let the fetish kill me." With his mouth he takes the dough from the snake skin, holds it on his tongue, and by opening his mouth, proves that he really has it there. Then he swallows it. He has thereby been freed of the accusation.[88]

Other oath ceremonies described by Europeans include the consumption of herbal draughts—drinks believed to be harmless to those who adhered to a contract but deadly to those who dared break it.[89] Local priests also used poison oracles to test loyalty and catch thieves, and the failure to adhere to the taboos associated with such oracles was believed to cause illness or death, even for those who had not committed crimes.[90] Also notable in the records were descriptions of trials by ordeal, including burning the skin with a hot knife or piercing the tongue with an awl.[91] And while many oath fetishes were made of local materials like clay, hair, and feathers, many others included European items, such as cloth, beads, pottery, and glassware, demonstrating the significance of transatlantic commerce.[92] Not all oath fetishes properly fit the category of healing in the European context, but the rituals performed around oath fetishes were socially medicinal because they tied the health of a business relationship directly to the health of the body. Breaking a business bond when under oath could result in financial ruin, sickness, or even death.

Accra was also home to a network of hundreds of minor shrines, spirit mounds, and mobile consecrated objects. An example of the diversity of objects imbued with supernatural power can be found in an account of a cabinet of knickknacks owned by Noyte, a slave trader who worked with the Danes at Christiansborg Castle in the eighteenth century.[93] By chance, Ludwig Ferdinand Rømer passed by Noyte's home and found him

> sitting among many thousands of knick-knacks, among which I saw the heads of elephants, oxen, sheep, and other animals. He did not see me before I had stuck my head and half my body in through the narrow door, thus casting a shadow inside. He stood up and asked me to leave. I did not wish to do this, but promised him that I would come no closer, if he would tell me what it all meant. He swore by his father—a great oath among Negroes— that he did not know one hundredth part of the amount of good that had come [from the collection of sacred objects], but that all

of it (perhaps with the exception of some one hundred items) had been collected by his forefathers, and each piece which I saw had helped his forefathers in some way, because of the help of God and the fetish. . . . This was also Noyte's way of celebrating morning prayers, by sitting for an hour among these knick-knacks and rummaging among them.[94]

Their dialogue further revealed that Noyte had protected his collection of objects as part of his ancestral heritage, moving them several times to save them from invading armies and even burying them to save them from destruction. Rømer, wanting to make a point to his readers about the capricious nature of African worship, challenged Noyte on the value of one particularly innocuous object, a small stone the size of an egg, arguing that it could not possibly be of any use. Noyte objected, stating that the stone was clairvoyant and could warn him of trouble in the future. The stone, he said, had saved his collection because he had tripped over it just days before his village was attacked by the armies of the Asante; the accident had somehow reminded him to bury his curios to protect them. Since then he had kept the stone in his pocket and squeezed it when he needed spiritual protection. The stone had been particularly useful for Noyte when he was accused of an unscrupulous business arrangement before a magistrate at Christiansborg Castle. Rømer even had to admit that he had seen Noyte squeeze the stone right before he was declared innocent by the magistrate.[95]

A historian could never recount the millions of individual biographies of consecrated objects in Accra. Even if such artifacts could be passed down through time, without an account of their meaning at the particular moment that they were produced, they become mute relics of a distant past.[96] Indeed, even Noyte had lost track of some of the stories embedded in his inherited fetishes. Nevertheless, his curio cabinet offers a glimpse of the diversity and dynamism of the material culture of religion and medicine in Accra in the eighteenth century. Noyte's bones and stones were everyday objects, but when he joined them together, he could multiply their power in unique ways. By working with local understandings of spirituality, and by improvising accord- ing to his own intuition, Noyte was able to perpetuate Accra's open, changing, and pluralistic material culture of religion and healing.

PARTIAL ADAPTATION: EUROPEAN SURGEONS AND EUROPEAN PATIENTS

Western healing practices eventually became a major component of the healing culture of Accra, but they were adopted in histori- cal slow motion. Three major factors limited the early integration of European medicine into the city's networks of healing. The first was the tropical disease environment, which posed a major barrier to intercultural contact because it killed off Europeans at such a high rate.[97] The second was the commerce in slaves, which created hierarchies of power that acted as a barrier to cultural exchange. The third factor was the chauvinism of European sur- geons, who were so deeply invested in notions of race and fetish that they were unable to see how African therapies might help them survive. Such limitations make it difficult to demonstrate any impact that Europeans had on the culture of healing in Accra, or vice versa. However, a new era of cultural mixing did begin when European patients, the sailors and merchants of the trans- atlantic trade, began to leave their ships and fortresses to seek help from African healers.

During the era of the slave trade, there were never more than a few dozen Europeans living in the port cities of West Africa at any given time, and they were mostly afraid to leave their ships. If they did go ashore, they stayed cloistered within Danish, Dutch, and English forts. Most Europeans who visited the coast were struck with fever within a few weeks. Of these, half were dead within the first year.[98] Those who survived their first bout of malarial fever might gain a temporary immunity to the disease, but they were still vulnerable to yellow fever, typhoid fever, Guinea worm, and gastrointestinal illnesses. Waves of illnesses swept through garrisons on the Gold Coast, often leaving forts in the hands of African merchants.[99] As Danish chaplain H. C. Monrad noted in 1822, "Europeans never grow very old in Africa, and I know of none who have reached an age of much over 50 years. The climate and the way of life work against them."[100] It is no wonder that by the nineteenth century the Gold Coast became known as the "White Man's Grave."[101]

The notorious climate of tropical Africa made it difficult for Europeans to staff their forts with medical professionals.[102] The training for a ship's surgeon was cursory, composed of a short apprenticeship and a perfunctory examination.[103] Moreover, the duties of surgeons in West Africa were reduced mostly to evaluation of the physical health of slaves.[104] Their employers judged their success by how many slaves survived the journey, and rewarded them with a salary and a share of the ship's revenue (often in the form of slaves to sell for their own personal profit).[105] Since so few surgeons could survive long enough to disseminate their understanding of health and disease, and because they were co-opted into the business as slave traders, the influence of European surgical practices in West Africa was inevitably limited. The largest trading concern on the Gold Coast, the Royal West Africa Company, tried to keep a surgeon on staff at Cape Coast Castle, the fort with the largest slave dungeons, but in many years there was simply no surgeon available. Europeans who fell sick at James Fort in Accra were expected to sail west to Cape Coast for medical attention, and if they could not find help there, they would wait for the service of a shipborne surgeon.[106] Most slave ships had one surgeon on board when they left European ports, but there was no guarantee that the surgeon would survive his visit to Africa.[107] A recent study of the Dutch slave trade between 1751 and 1797 revealed that, of the twenty-nine surgeons found in shipping records, only one made more than two voyages to West Africa. This meant that they either died during their voyages or were afraid to risk their lives in Africa more than once.[108]

Moreover, the few surgeons who did stay on the Gold Coast were ill equipped to deal with tropical illnesses. In order to tackle the efficient cause of humoral imbalance, they relied heavily on phlebotomy (draining excess blood from the body) and blistering (burning the skin to draw malevolent humors to the surface). Bleeding was used as a preventive therapy in hot climates, while blistering was a curative intervention of last resort, applied to the skin only if a person was close to death.[109] Paul Isert, the same Danish surgeon who combed the Gold Coast for a cure for malaria, held firmly to the belief that bleeding and blistering could save a patient. His program for fighting tropical fevers had three stages. If a surgeon noticed the fever immediately, he bled the patient and offered an emetic. If the illness continued, he prescribed a decoction of cinchona bark, sulfur, camphor, and musk, steeped in Madeira wine. If this did not work, he proceeded with blistering, using vesicant plasters. He stuck rigidly to this program throughout his tenure on the Gold Coast, despite admitting in his private journal that only rapid treatment within the first hours could check malarial fevers.[110]

The inability of surgeons like Isert to come to terms with the disease environment around them can be explained by their belief in the ill effects of miasma, a noxious gas believed to emanate from decomposing matter. Contact with miasma was understood to cause inflammation of the constitution, and in the heat of the tropics, miasma appeared to be everywhere. To check the debilitating effects of miasma, surgeons kept their patients on strict diets, advised them to live healthy lives, and, of course, bled them regularly. It was generally believed that patients who ignored this advice would bring illness upon themselves.[111] Surgeons also traveled with chests of medicines containing minerals (like calcium carbonate, arsenic, and mercury) and plant medicines (like rhubarb, pennyroyal, and opiates). These reagents were used variously as carminatives, purgatives, diuretics, and emetics—again for the purpose of balancing the humors.[112] Yet despite carrying all of this gear with them, ships' surgeons were still mostly powerless to stop severe malarial fevers. Though cinchona bark was available, it was not yet understood to have prophylactic qualities, and effective curative doses of cinchona were not standardized until the late nineteenth century.[113] Nor did surgeons have appropriate treatments for maladies like amoebic dysentery, typhoid fever, sleeping sickness, yaws, or Guinea worm.[114] One wonders what Africans must have thought of the White doctors who stepped off their ships with so much equipment and bravado yet were helpless to treat even the most common of illnesses.[115]

The inability of the ship's surgeon to stave off tropical diseases compelled European sailors and soldiers to rely on West African healers.[116] Willem Bosman, a Dutch merchant who spent fourteen years trading along the coast in the seventeenth century, claimed to have seen several Europeans cured by African healers when the therapies provided by surgeons failed.[117] Christian Tychsen, the governor of Christiansborg Castle during the 1760s, had a policy of sending his sick to the village of Osu, next to the fort. The journals of Chaplain H. C. Monrad also mention how the Danes abandoned their surgeons for African healers near the castle.[118] Even ships' captains sent their sick sailors ashore if they felt it would aid in their recovery. William Woodville, the captain of a slave ship who traveled the coast in the 1790s, sent his sick slaves to African healers because he believed that his ship's surgeon could not treat them effectively.[119] These examples are striking, considering they are found within the same sources that denigrate the healing practices of West Africa as superstitious fetish. They reveal a parallel world of patient choice on the Gold Coast that included Europeans.

That European sailors and merchants would seek help from African healers should not be surprising. In the average early modern village or town in Europe, patients also lived in a world of therapeutic pluralism, able to choose among physicians, surgeons, herbalists, homeopaths, and an assortment of lay healers.[120] They were also motivated to seek out help from Africans because the majority of them were unmarried men, under thirty, who were in dire need of emotional support.[121] Following a social pattern established by Portuguese merchants, many of them arranged temporary relationships with local women, adopting domestic arrangements known as *cassarerte*, meaning "to take into one's house."[122] These marital unions could be made informally with slaves, but the families of free women demanded bride prices that linked the man to the kinship group of his wife.[123] Some of these formal marriages may have been economic arrangements to facilitate trade with powerful kinship groups, while others may have been genuine bonds of love. Joseph Wulff, for instance, survived as a merchant at Christiansborg for years with the help of his African wife, Sarah Malm, whom he wrote about with endearment in his final will and testament.[124] Having a matrimonial residence on the Gold Coast was an advantage—it meant access to nutritious food, herbal medicines, and a type of intimacy that was unavailable in the slave forts.

Though there is ample evidence that European patients abandoned surgeons to patronize West African healers, there are very few instances in which European surgeons appropriated the practices of West African healers. This is surprising because, as early as 1705, Willem Bosman had noted with astonishment the discovery of more than thirty roots, branches, and tree barks "impregnated with an extraordinary Sanative Virtue."[125] Bosman himself was surprised that European physicians had not made use of these plants, but with only a few minor exceptions, the broader community of naturalists ignored his call for further investigation into their medicinal qualities.[126] Ludvig Rømer mentioned the use of grains of paradise, hot pepper, and palm oil in his journals, but only in passing.[127] Two chaplains at Christiansborg Castle, Johannes Rask and H. C. Monrad, reportedly cured many illnesses with "a mixture of Grains of Paradise, Spanish pepper, palm oil, and lemons" and adopted a locally derived antidiarrheal made of mashed yam mixed with an unidentified yellowish tuber.[128] The surgeon of the slave ship *Fredensborg*, Joch Sixtus, desperate to stop the high rate of death among slaves on his ship, incorporated some of these medicines into his repertoire by giving slaves with dysentery a mixture of "millet and Spanish pepper,"[129] but he was an exception. In the main, ships' surgeons remained largely indifferent to the tools of healing used by the healers of West Africa.

The reluctance of European surgeons to exploit the healing potential found in West African plants is astonishing, considering naturalists in the New World were rapidly incorporating medicinal flora into the European pharmacopoeia. The Jesuit order was bioprospecting throughout the Americas during the early modern period, and by 1565 Nicolas Monardes, a Spanish physician who studied the arrival of American medicinal flora in Europe, was advocating that twenty-four New World medicinal plants be added to the European materia medica.[130] More than two hundred years later, many American plants had indeed been added to European medicine chests, but only Guinea pepper, gum arabic, plantain leaf, and palm oil had been taken from Africa, and even then they were only used as stand-ins for more common European ingredients.[131] Despite the obvious presence of dozens of African cures for the tropical illnesses, European naturalists barely noticed the medicinal qualities of African flora. Paul Isert did make his list of medicinal plants at the end of the eighteenth century, but by this time it was too late—the days of the transatlantic slave trade were numbered, and European interest in West Africa declined rapidly in the nineteenth century. Cities like Accra, alive with therapeutic pluralism and the exchange of materia medica, did offer refuge for European patients but African healing practices did not trigger any substantial change to the practices of European surgeons.

Interlude: Abolition, War, Sanitation, and the Colonial Gaze in Nineteenth-Century Accra

Over the course of the nineteenth century, Europeans gradually ended their participation in the transatlantic slave trade, and commerce on the Gold Coast began to stagnate. Slavery and the slave trade in Africa continued, but the movement of human cargo between the coast and the hinterland dwindled. A "legitimate" trade in products like ivory, palm oil and cocoa eventually replaced the sale of human beings, but it was slow to take hold. Many slave forts were abandoned or left in disrepair because the mercantile activity could not sustain their upkeep. From the European perspective, the first several decades of the nineteenth century were a period of marking time, and whole decades passed without any significant European medical activity in the city.

By contrast, the nineteenth century was also a time of feverish activity for the priests and soothsayers of the city. In the 1820s, conflict between urban dwellers of the Guinea Coast and the Asante Kingdom to the north boiled over into war. In 1826, the king of Asante marched southward toward Accra, taking control of the Akwapim Ridge, where he made an oath to destroy Accra. [132] On August 7, he ordered his army out of the rain forest and down the hills onto the Accra Plains, where they engaged a coalition of Ga, Adangme, Fante, Denkyira, Akwapim, and British forces at a Ga village called Dodowa, ten miles inland from Accra. Official histories claim that the British governor John Hope Smith won the battle by using Congreve rockets to shock and disperse the center of the Asante line. Ga histories see it differently, giving their gods credit for healing divisions within the city and offering prophecies of victory. As the Ga remember it, the battle was won when the priest of Sakumo marched into the fray, rallying the troops while two white cranes known as the "hornblowers of Sakumo" flew across the allied lines. Then the goddesses Nae and Korle emerged from the sea to overwhelm the Asante and ensure victory. Fallen soldiers were taken to the shrines to be healed, and the Ga capital survived. [133] To the Ga, the outcome of the battle was as much a medico-religious triumph as it was a military victory, and they believed that when the Asante lost, the king of the Asante made a second oath: never to invade Accra again. In Accra, the fight at Dodowa became known as the Battle of "Katamanso"—a corruption of the Twi phrase for publicly swearing an oath.

West African traditions of healing remained robust in Accra, but the nineteenth century also witnessed the arrival of new types of therapeutic traditions. Islam had long played a role in the healing cultures to the West, in places like Senegal and Sierra Leone, and to the east in Lagos, but there are scant records of its presence in Accra until the late nineteenth century, when herders and soldiers founded the small enclaves that would eventually make up an Islamic community. With the daily calls to prayer came a culture of Quranic medicines, offering a new option for healing. Christian missionaries also found their way to Accra, taking on the responsibility to save a continent that they believed had been corrupted by the evils of the slave trade. The pietist missionaries of Accra believed that health was granted by divine providence, and they encouraged Africans to seek bodily redemption through the Lord.

Over two hundred years, the city had grown from a string of loosely connected villages into a cluster of mini cities, each at the base of a major European trading post and each with several subdivisions housing newcomers. According to custom, the residents of the city kept their compounds and streets clean by sweeping every morning and by burning rubbish in open locations outside the town, as designated by local chiefs. They also managed their personal waste compound by compound, as was the norm in every city in West Africa, with a system of night soil pans and nearby latrines. Cattle were kept outside the city by herders, but sheep, goats, and pigs were allowed to scavenge around the towns. Trading stalls were kept orderly by the women who worked there, and all merchants were governed by queen mothers responsible for the sanitation of each part of the marketplace. But despite these efforts, it was clear that Accra had never been well suited to house a large population. Ramping up village sanitation methods to the scale of a city of approximately fifteen thousand people was proving difficult without help from the colonial government. Distant from a large lake or a running river, residents still had to gather fresh water by collecting rainwater, drawing from hand-dug wells, or fetching it from the nearby Odaw River. In the dry season, water collection had always been a trial, and people were compelled to draw from stagnant sources, leading to high rates of Guinea worm. As the population grew, keeping the city clean became an ongoing trial for Ga leaders, who lacked support for such endeavors from their European counterparts. Additionally, Africans in Accra began to witness the rise of European racial theory, which othered the people of Accra as primitive and unsanitary.

The arrival of a new type of racialized sanitary gaze is evident in the reports of a group of naturalists who passed through the city briefly during the Niger River Expedition of 1841. As they rolled around the streets in handcarts pulled by young African men, these naturalists from several different European nations made notes on the streetscape, initiating a new type of urban discourse that envisioned Accra as divided into a landscape of stone warehouses filled with imported goods, and "dirty" swish huts filled with personal fetishes. After only a few days, they left, but their vision of Accra foreshadowed colonial aspirations for a new type of racialized and sanitized urbanity. Their depiction of the city would soon be replicated, decade after decade, by other European visitors, including missionaries who sought to abandon what they saw as the avarice and degeneracy of the colonial port city.

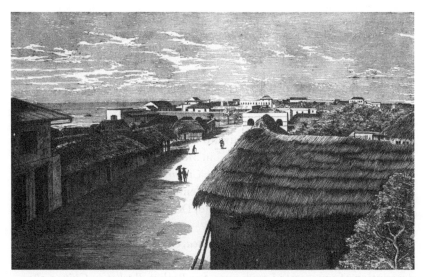

Figure 1.2. A street scene in Accra, around 1860. This sketch from a Basel Mission training booklet shows Accra during the mid-nineteenth century. The sun is setting, casting shadows on the sleepy thoroughfare between the African buildings in James Town and the merchant houses of Ussher Town. A forebearer of future landscapes of the urban health of Accra, the sketch divides the city into an African town of swish huts and a distant future of European stone buildings. (Source: Peter A. Schweizer and Otumfuo Osei Tutu, *Survivors on the Gold Coast: The Basel Missionaries in Colonial Ghana* [Accra: Smartline, 2001], 116, reproduced from a sketch in Wanner, Basel Handlers-Gesellschaft, 1859–1959, 104.)

NOTES

1. Barbot, *Description of the Coasts of North and South Guinea*, 280.

2. Pietz, "The Problem of the Fetish, I"; "The Problem of the Fetish, II"; "The Problem of the Fetish, IIIa."

3. Pietz, "Problem of the Fetish, I," "Problem of the Fetish, II," "Problem of the Fetish, IIIa."

4. Dakubu, *Ga-English Dictionary*, 66; Engmann, "Immortality," 156.

5. Field, *Religion and Medicine of the Gã People*, 111; Nii Oshiu Codjoe, interview with the author, February 23, 2005.

6. Senah, *Money Be Man*, 140.

7. Leith Mullings and Kodjo Senah both choose to distinguish ordinary illnesses and spiritual illnesses as a means of understanding how

people in Accra choose between Ga healers or biomedical practitioners, but both concede that seeking a cure is processual. See Senah, *Money Be Man*, 140–53, 174; Mullings, *Therapy, Ideology, and Social Change*, 46, 150–66.

8. Engmann, "Immortality," 156.

9. Field, *Religion and Medicine of the Gā People*, 4; Nii Cedi, interview with the author, February 4, 2004.

10. John Marvin Janzen and Edward C. Green, "Continuity, Change and Challenge in African Medicine," in *Medicine across Cultures: History and Practice of Medicine in Non-Western Cultures*, ed. Helaine Selin and Hugh Shapiro (Dordrecht: Kluwer Academic Publishers, 2003), 3.

11. Hepper, *West African Herbaria*, 30; Dokosi, *Herbs of Ghana*, 118–19.

12. De Marees, *Gold Kingdom of Guinea*, 69; Wisnes, *Letters on West Africa and the Slave Trade*, 118–19, 132. Jean Barbot also provides a lengthy description of consecrated medicines. See Barbot, *Barbot on Guinea*, 580.

13. PRAAD SCT 2/4/2, May 15, 1861–February 10, 1864, 5–7.

14. Woyoo Ankroh Ansa, interview with the author, June 21, 2007; Bentum, interview with the author, March 5, 2004.

15. Christaller, *Dictionary of the Asante*, 464; Salm and Falola, *Culture and Customs of Ghana*, 35–36.

16. Kwame Gyekye, "Person and Community in African Thought," in *Person and Community: Ghanaian Philosophical Studies I*, ed. Kwasi Wiredu and Kwame Gyekye (Washington, DC: Council for Research in Values and Philosophy, 1992), 114; Christaller, *Dictionary of the Asante*, 255; Salm and Falola, *Culture and Customs of Ghana*, 35.

17. Field, *Religion and Medicine of the Gā People*, 92; Nii Cedi, interview with the author, January 26, 2005.

18. Kotey, *Twi-English*, 45, 328; Rattray, *Religion & Art in Ashanti*, 28–31.

19. Field, *Religion and Medicine of the Gā People*, 93.

20. Nii Cedi, interview with the author, January 26, 2005.

21. Field, *Religion and Medicine of the Gā People*, 93–94.

22. Not all Akan concepts of body, soul, and illness have been appropriated by Ga speakers. Key terms such as *honam* (body), *hoham* (breath), *mogya* (blood), and *nkrabea* (destiny) have never been incorporated into Ga. For more information about the importance of these terms within Akan notions of body and soul, see Gyekye, *Essay on African Philosophical Thought*.

23. Bannerman-Richter, *Mmoetia*; O. B. Dokosi, "Some Herbs," 120; Amarh Amarteifio, interview with the author, July 18, 2003; McCaskie, "Innovational Eclecticism," 37.

24. Amarh Amarteifio, interview with the author, July 18, 2003.

25. The roots of these terms, found in Ga, are taken from Dakubu's *Ga-English Dictionary* and correlated with Kotey's *Twi-English Dictionary* and Westermann's *Ewe-English Dictionary*. See Dakubu, *Ga-English Dictionary*; Kotey, *Twi-English*; Diedrich Westermann, *Evefiala or Ewe-English Dictionary*.

26. Dakubu, *Ga-English Dictionary*, 80. *Kita* is derived from the Arabic term *kitab*.

27. Dakubu, *Korle Meets the Sea*, 5.

28. Senah, *Money Be Man*, 129.

29. Pietz, "Problem of the Fetish, I," 5–17.

30. Bosman, *New and Accurate Description of the Coast of Guinea*, 347.

31. Barbot, *Description of the Coasts of North and South Guinea*, 578.

32. Linnaeus, *Systema Naturae*, 22.

33. Carl Christian Reindorf, *History of the Gold Coast*, 105, 106; Korle Wulomo, interview with the author, February 16, 2005.

34. Parker, *Making the Town*, 12; Samuel Quarcoopome, "Impact of Urbanization," 115–17.

35. Carl Christian Reindorf, *History of the Gold Coast*, 39.

36. Sakumo Wulomo, interview with the author, November 17, 2002; Nai Wulomo, interview with the author, November 28, 2002; Korle Wulomo, interview with the author, February 16, 2005.

37. Nii Cedi, Nii Akramah, Lantey Rozer, and Nii Lantey, interview with the author, November 17, 2002; Korle Wulomo, interview with the author, September 2, 2003, February 16, 2005; Nai Wulomo, interview with the author, November 28, 2002.

38. Wisnes, *Letters on West Africa and the Slave Trade*, 138; Korle Wulomo, interview with the author, February 16, 2005; Robert Ayitey Quaye, interview with the author, December 30, 2005; de Marees, *Gold Kingdom of Guinea*, 85.

39. Kilson, *Kpele Lala*, 126.

40. Field, *Religion and Medicine of the Gā People*, 21–22, 77–78.

41. Carl Christian Reindorf, *History of the Gold Coast*, 100–101; Welman. "James Fort, Accra, and the Oyeni Fetish," 73–88.

42. Woyoo Ankroh Ansa, interview with the author, June 14, 2003; Rahel Roye, interview with the author, June 17, 2003; Kilson, *Kpele Lala*, 168; Drewal, "Performing the Other," 160–85.

43. Isichei, *Voices of the Poor in Africa*, 188–209.

44. Graeber, "Fetishism as Social Creativity," 418; Field, *Religion and Medicine of the Gã People*, 101–3; Woyoo Ogbame Rebecca Otoo, interview with the author, July 10, 2003.

45. De Marees, *Gold Kingdom of Guinea*, 71, 85; Monrad, *Description of the Guinea Coast*, 57; Rømer, *Reliable Account of the Coast of Guinea*, 92.

46. Rømer, *Reliable Account of the Coast of Guinea*, xiiv–xv, 92.

47. Dakubu, *Korle Meets the Sea*, 10; Rahel Roye, interview with the author, June 17, 2003; Bentum, interview with the author, June 17, 2003; Ankroh Ansa, interview with the author, June 14, 2003.

48. Rømer, *Reliable Account of the Coast of Guinea*, 90, 92; Field, *Religion and Medicine of the Gã People*, 104–8.

49. Collins, *Highlife Time*; Kilson, *Kpele Lala*, 13.

50. Nketia, "Changing Traditions of Folk Music in Ghana," 33.

51. Rømer, *Reliable Account of the Coast of Guinea*, 91.

52. Rømer, *Reliable Account of the Coast of Guinea*, 91.

53. Kilson, *Kpele Lala*, 145; Bentum, interview with the author, June 25, 2006; Ankroh Ansa, interview with the author, June 21, 2007.

54. Rømer, *Reliable Account of the Coast of Guinea*, 90.

55. Akyeampong, *Drink, Power, and Cultural Change*, 14.

56. Van den Bersselaar, *King of Drinks*, 44.

57. Van den Bersselaar, *King of Drinks*, 36–37, 44.

58. Adam Jones, *West Africa in the Mid-Seventeenth Century*, 97, 150, 322.

59. Wisnes, *Letters on West Africa and the Slave Trade*, 145; Herbert S. Klein and Stanley L. Engerman, "A Note on Mortality in the French Slave Trade in the Eighteenth Century," in *The Uncommon Market: Essays in the Economic History of the Atlantic Slave Trade*, ed. Henry A. Gemery and Jan S. Hogendorn (New York: Academic, 1979), 271. For an example of yaws inoculation, see James Maxwell, *Observations on Yaws on Acute Traumatic Tetanus on Tetanus infantum* (Edinburgh: Maclachlan, Stewart, 1839), 22–23, 37, cited in Sheridan, *Doctors and Slaves*, 87–88.

60. Wisnes, *Letters on West Africa and the Slave Trade*, 132.

61. Bosman, *New and Accurate Description of the Coast of Guinea*, 210, 353, 444.

62. Barbot, *Barbot on Guinea*, 237; de Marees, *Gold Kingdom of Guinea*, 175, plate 16; Monrad, *Description of the Guinea Coast*, 204.

63. Tsofatse Lamptey, interview with the author, June 9, 2003; Bentum, interview with the author, July 8, 2003.

64. Wisnes, *Letters on West Africa and the Slave Trade*, 140.

65. De Marees, *Gold Kingdom of Guinea*, 164; Hutton, *Voyage to Africa*, 386.

66. De Marees, *Gold Kingdom of Guinea*, 31; Wisnes, *Letters on West Africa and the Slave Trade*, 139, 174–75. Thonning and Isert did not name the species of the trees used as dental hygiene, but the Ga name for a chewing sponge is *taa kotsa*, and chewing sticks are known as *taatso*.

67. Curth, *From Physick to Pharmacology*, 3.

68. Anquandah, "Accra Plains," 5; Dickson, *Historical Geography of Ghana*, 42–44, 50–53.

69. Adam Jones, ed., "Michael Hemmersam's Description of the Gold Coast," in *German Sources for West African History, 1599–1669*, ed. Adam Jones (Wiesbaden: Steiner, 1983), 112; Hepper, *West African Herbaria*.

70. Brummitt & Powell, *Authors of Plant Names*.

71. Wisnes, *Letters on West Africa and the Slave Trade*, 165.

72. Grover and Yadav, "Pharmacological Actions"; Kassim et al., "Effects of Root Extracts."

73. Osseo-Asare, *Bitter Roots*, 87.

74. Wisnes, *Letters on West Africa and the Slave Trade*, 156.

75. Wisnes, *Letters on West Africa and the Slave Trade*, 156.

76. All of these plants have been used in the past as febrifuges. Oliver-Bever, *Medicinal Plants in Tropical West Africa*, 131; Iwu, *Handbook of African Medicinal Plants*, 37, 163–64; Hutchinson and Dalziel, *Flora of West Tropical Africa*, 325, 377–78, 396, 412; Maier, "Nineteenth-Century Asante Medical Practices," 67; Ankrah et al., "Evaluation of Efficacy and Safety"; Mshana et al., *Traditional Medicine and Pharmacopoeia*, 716–19.

77. Adam Jones, *West Africa in the Mid-Seventeenth Century*, 97, 150, 322; Barbot, *Barbot on Guinea*, 560.

78. Barbot, *Barbot on Guinea*, 576.

79. De Marees, *Gold Kingdom of Guinea*, 173–74.

80. De Marees, *Gold Kingdom of Guinea*, 11. The Ga language distinguishes between yaws and syphilis. *Ajito*, the observable skin disease of yaws, has two other terms associated with it. The first is *ajitofoi*, people who suffer from yaws, indicating that Ga speakers saw it as a common affliction, and *ajito gbowie*, a seed used for treating skin disorders such as yaws, indicating that it was the focus of healing practice. Syphilis is known by a specific term, the Ewe word for pouch, *gbaja*. The source and reasoning for this loan word are not known, but they likely relate to the fact that it was an American illness that arrived relatively recently in the city's history. The Latin word for yaws is *frambesia tropica*. This error of diagnosis was

repeated ad absurdum in Uganda during the colonial period. See Vaughan, *Curing Their Ills*, 138.

81. Wisnes, *Letters on West Africa and the Slave Trade*, 144.

82. The Ga word for gonorrhea is *babaanso*, from the Ewe-derived term *baba*, meaning skin disease with redness, and *babaaba*, a flowing and gushing out. *Babaanso* describes the visible symptoms of gonorrhea rather than the specific illness.

83. Sarsaparilla contains phytosterols that create testosterone and progesterone, chemicals that are believed to fight impotency and increase fertility, but it is not used today as an antibiotic. Dweck, "Internal and External Use of Medicinal Plants," 157. Trade in sarsaparilla is mentioned in Makepeace, *Trade on the Guinea Coast*, 9; Roller, "Colonial Collecting Expeditions."

84. Rocco, *Quinine*, 110–11, 246–48, 262.

85. Rocco, *Quinine*, 52. Cinchona appeared in the *London Pharmacopoeia* of 1677. Porter, *Cambridge History of Medicine*, 254. A detailed example of its use as a fever remedy can be found in Lind, *Essay on Diseases*, 54–72.

86. Rocco, *Quinine*, 110–11, 246–48, 262.

87. Barbot, *Barbot on Guinea*, 281.

88. Rømer, *Reliable Account of the Coast of Guinea*, 101.

89. Rømer, *Reliable Account of the Coast of Guinea*, 103; Wisnes, *Letters on West Africa and the Slave Trade*, 130; Monrad, *Description of the Guinea Coast*, 53–54.

90. De Marees, *Gold Kingdom of Guinea*, 69.

91. Rømer, *Reliable Account of the Coast of Guinea*, 101.

92. Barbot, *Barbot on Guinea*, 578–80.

93. Rømer, *Reliable Account of the Coast of Guinea*, 94–95. Though his biography is not offered by Rømer, it is likely that Noyte was a company slave who acted as the caboceer at Teshie. Justesen and Manley, *Danish Sources*, 613, 698, 717.

94. Rømer, *Reliable Account of the Coast of Guinea*, 94–95.

95. Rømer, *Reliable Account of the Coast of Guinea*, 94–95.

96. Pietz, "Problem of the Fetish, I," 12–13.

97. Curtin, *Disease and Empire*, 1.

98. Curtin, *Disease and Empire*, 1. See also K. G. Davies, *Royal African Company*, 256.

99. Justesen and Manley, *Danish Sources*, 103, 701, 789, 793.

100. Monrad, *Description of the Guinea Coast*, 266; Norregard, *Danish Settlements in West Africa*, 169.

101. Curtin, "White Man's Grave," 103. The phrase "White Man's Grave" does not have a distinct provenance but was probably coined during the establishment of Sierra Leone as a British colony during the nineteenth century; see Rankin, *White Man's Grave.*

102. Curtin, *Disease and Empire,* 16–17, 52–54; Crooks, *Records Relating to the Gold Coast Settlements,* 79, 132–33; Norregard, *Danish Settlements in West Africa,* 166.

103. Sheridan, "Guinea Surgeons," 611–12. Geoffrey Hudson suggests that surgeons sought positions in the navy or merchant marine to escape poverty at home and that the examination was largely a formality; see "Introduction: British Military and Naval Medicine, 1600–1830," in Hudson, *British Military and Naval Medicine,* 10. Paul Kopperman suggests that many surgeons were not examined at all or were allowed to pass even when they did poorly on the exam; see "The British Army in North America and the West Indies, 1755–83: A Medical Perspective," in Hudson, *British Military and Naval Medicine,*57–58.

104. Law, *Ouidah,* 141.

105. Hugh Thomas, *Slave Trade,* 307; Great Britain, "An Act to Regulate the Carrying of Slaves, 28 Geo. III, c. 54," in *Documents Illustrative of the History of the Slave Trade to America,* ed. Elizabeth Donnan (New York: Octagon Books, 1965), 2:582–89.

106. Metcalfe, *Great Britain and Ghana,* 210.

107. Christopher, *Slave Ship Sailors,* 33.

108. Hogerzeil and Richardson, "Slave Purchasing Strategies"; see also Donnan, *Documents Illustrative of the History of the Slave Trade,* 446.

109. Tanner, *Manual of the Practice of Medicine,* 56.

110. Wisnes, *Letters on West Africa and the Slave Trade,* 153–54.

111. Pickstone, "Fever Epidemics," 129, 138; Justesen and Manley, *Danish Sources,* 649; Cohen, "Malaria and French Imperialism," 26.

112. For a complete list of a surgeon's equipment, see Svalesen, *Slave Ship Fredensborg,* 70. For information on a surgeon's medicines, see Sheridan, "Guinea Surgeons," 615. For an example of a surgical kit used in West Africa in the early nineteenth century, see H. Tedlie, "Materia Medica and Diseases," in *Mission from Cape Coast to Ashantee,* ed. T. Bowdich (London, 1819), 376–79.

113. Curtin, *Disease and Empire,* 21–23, 26.

114. Svalesen, *Slave Ship Fredensborg,* 67; Sheridan, "Guinea Surgeons," 602.

115. Svalesen, *Slave Ship Fredensborg,* 88–89.

116. Ruth A. Fisher Fisher, ed., "R. Miles to Horatio Smith. Cape Coast Castle. Dec. 9, 1778," in *Extracts from the Records of the African Companies*, ed. Ruth A. Fisher (New York: Association for the Study of Negro Life and History, 1930), 99.

117. Bosman, *New and Accurate Description of the Coast of Guinea*, 225.

118. Svalesen, *Slave Ship* Fredensborg, 69; Monrad, *Description of the Guinea Coast*, 53, 204–7. Osu was known to the Danish as the "Negeriet."

119. "From Captain William Woodville of the Ship Rodney, to Messrs. James Rogers and Company in Bristol dated Bannee [Bonny Island], 16 May 1791, Rogers Papers, Chancery C. 107/14, Box No. 2, No. 21," in Sheridan, "Guinea Surgeons," 616.

120. Gentilcore, "Was There a 'Popular Medicine'?"

121. Ipsen, "Intercultural Intimacy."

122. Huber, *Ghanaian Pidgin English*, 25; Svalesen, *Slave Ship* Fredensborg, 96–97; Ipsen, "Intercultural Intimacy."

123. Justesen and Manley, *Danish Sources*, 302.

124. Wulff and Wisnes, *Danish Jew in West Africa*, 257.

125. Bosman, *New and Accurate Description of the Coast of Guinea*, 225.

126. Bosman, *New and Accurate Description of the Coast of Guinea*, 216.

127. Rømer, *Reliable Account of the Coast of Guinea*, 199.

128. Svalesen, *Slave Ship* Fredensborg, 70–71.

129. Svalesen, *Slave Ship* Fredensborg, 112. Svalesen records the date of their meeting as 1767, but this is not possible, as Rask and Monrad were at Christiansborg Castle in the first two decades of the nineteenth century; See Rask and Monrad, *Two Views from Christiansborg Castle*.

130. Norton, *Sacred Gifts, Profane Pleasures*, 10–11; Benjamin Schmidt, "'Imperfect Chaos': Tropical Medicine and Exotic Natural History c. 1700," in *Medicine and Religion in Enlightenment Europe*, ed. Ole Peter Grell and Andrew Cunningham (Burlington, VT: Ashgate, 2007), 145–71; Junia Ferreira Furtado, "Tropical Empiricism: Making Medical Knowledge in Colonial Brazil," in *Science and Empire in the Atlantic World*, ed. James Delbourgo and Nicholas Dew (New York: Routledge, 2008), 127–51; Daniela Bleichmar, "Atlantic Competitions: Botany in the Eighteenth Century Spanish Empire," in Delbourgo and Dew, *Science and Empire in the Atlantic World*, 225–52.

131. Adam Jones, *West Africa in the Mid-Seventeenth Century*, 186–89. The first listings of these items in European pharmacopoeia follow: guinea pepper: *British Dispensatory*, 128; gum arabic: *British Dispensatory*, 128; plantain leaf: *British Dispensatory*, 132 (plantain leaf was sometimes used

to bind wounds; see Mouser and Gamble, *Slaving Voyage to Africa and Jamaica*, 66); palm oil: *British Dispensatory*, 131; Murray, *System of Materia Medica and Pharmacy*. Murray's *System of Materia Medica* likewise mentions gums and aloes, and notes that the tropical gum of *Euphorbia officinalis* as a useful vesicant. Only Lindley's *Flora Medica*, published in 1838, contains any speculation about the potential value of West African herbal medicines, and that is still limited to discussions of peppers and gums. Lindley, *Flora Medica*, 28–29, 139–40, 485.

132. Kea, "GSGC Notes and Queries."

133. Carl Christian Reindorf, *History of the Gold Coast*, 205, 211.

TWO

THE CONVERGENCE OF FIVE HEALING TRADITIONS IN THE "HEALTHY" CAPITAL OF THE GOLD COAST: MID-1800s TO 1908

THE LATE NINETEENTH CENTURY WAS a time when all five of major healing traditions of Accra began to operate simultaneously. African healers continued to serve the vast majority of residents, but healing cultures based on monotheistic religion were emerging too. Muslim soldiers serving in the British Army and ex-slaves from Brazil settled in the new colonial capital, establishing neighborhoods where a new avenue of therapy based on the healing powers of the Quran began to develop. The late nineteenth century also witnessed a flourishing of medical missionary activity in the city, and the African catechists of the Basel and Wesleyan missions propagated new Christian concepts of spiritual health. Though their medical work was limited, Christian missionaries did lay the groundwork for a future when the Ga translation of the Bible would be used for faith healing. Also significant was the arrival of imported pills and bottled medicines. These portable curatives were initially brought to Africa by Europeans for Europeans, but Africans soon found ways to buy, sell, and consume these new medical commodities. As the century wore on, patients began to regularly move between all five therapeutic traditions in their quests for healing.

It would be easy to state that the Colonial Office's decision to move the capital of the Gold Coast to Accra was a historical watershed for Western medicine in the city.[1] Indeed, the arrival of the Medical Department in Accra did mark the end of an antiquated era when the city's surgeons conducted their business on ships or within former slave forts. One might also argue that the establishment of the new capital marked the dawn of bio-power, an era when medical discourse legitimized colonial control of subject populations.[2] And to take it even further, one might state that, as in Southern Africa, during the nineteenth century a uniquely clinical gaze was imposed on subject populations, resulting in hygienic anxieties similar to what Maynard Swanson has called the "sanitation syndrome."[3]

However, focusing on the creation of the new medicalized capital grossly overstates the impact of colonial rule in Accra. In the nineteenth century, Western therapies were still poorly suited for dealing with tropical illnesses because scientific notions of disease etiology were still intertwined with humoral theory, causing much confusion about whether illness could be blamed on constitutional imbalance or a biological pathogen. As a result, the actions of Gold Coast Medical Department officials were a muddled combination of medical and sanitary initiatives, intended primarily to make the colony a safe place for Europeans to live. Medical officials had little standing within a colonial regime obsessed with railways, mines, and other enterprises that would increase the profitability of the colony.[4] As a result, the colonial medical services in Accra operated "on the cheap" (to borrow a phrase from Ronald Robinson's assessment of indirect rule), with a set of half-hearted attempts to reduce death rates by governors who were more interested in commerce than public health.[5] Coercive bio-power did loom at times, but local residents violently resisted any plans to rebuild the city according to sanitary regulations, severely limiting the influence of Western medicine in Accra. What prevailed was the long-standing culture of therapeutic pluralism, one that sustained West African healing traditions and allowed novel approaches to healing to find a home in the growing capital.

There is little ethnographic or travel literature available from the nineteenth century, and oral memories rarely reach back that far. This means there is something of a gap in the source materials dedicated specifically to African healing traditions. Fortunately, details about healing pluralism can be found within the testimonies of African plaintiffs and defendants in court cases brought before British magistrates at Christiansborg Castle. Though fragmented, the small acts of healers and patients found within these trials demonstrate how African medico-religious traditions continued to dominate the healing culture of Accra and how African patients worked together with caregiving therapy management groups. As in the past, patients continued to understand that healers had the power to alter both bodily states of health and broader issues related to social and family health. Healers were still mixing herbs and patching up bodies, but they were also deeply involved in managing sexual reproduction, kinship relations, business agreements, rights to property, and many other aspects of the lives of their patients.

The most significant finding from the court records of the second half of the nineteenth century is that therapeutic pluralism continued to hold sway. Despite the arrival of Europeans, patients continued to embed themselves within the care of therapy management groups, seeking help from a wide variety of healers.[6] A key case that demonstrates this pattern of pluralism is the trial of a man named Odonkor, who was wounded in a knife fight in 1877. Odonkor's family shuttled him around to several different healers in Accra and even took him north to the Akwapim Ridge to seek help from a shrine priest in the village of Larteh. After several weeks of searching for physical and spiritual cures, Odonkor died from his injury. His sad story was related to a British magistrate while his family argued over who would pay for the expenses incurred while trying to save their loved one.[7] In another case about outstanding debts for healing services, a man fell sick and was taken by his wife to a nearby healer. She paid for the therapy, but the man did not feel any better, so a friend of the sick man paid another healer to cure him.[8] This treatment also failed, and the man died, but not until after his friends and family pursued several more therapeutic options. Once again, his sad tale came out when the family disputed, in front of a colonial magistrate, who ought to pay the expenses. These are just two examples from the court records but what they show that the old pattern of forming caregiving groups and the process of "healer hopping" strongly resembled the patient behavior described by Jean Barbot two hundred years earlier.[9]

Also evident in the nineteenth century was the continuity of the rich material culture of African healing, which included potions, salves, powders, and other aggregations of local medicinal ingredients. In many instances, these mixtures came in the form of *ti*, the carbonized dust made from herbal ingredients. In one case, a healer manufactured and consecrated *ti* and then blew it into the face of his patient to counter the malicious spirits causing the illness.[10] In another instance, a healer treated a woman with convulsions using *ti* mixed in rum, advising the woman to take the remedy orally over the course of three months.[11] In 1877, to cure a patient who was suffering from a snakebite, a priestess prepared *ti* comprising "candlewood, guinea pepper, the feather of a fowl, and other objects," which she administered as a purgative, and in a case from 1897, a healer shaved the head of a sick patient and rubbed a liquid suspension of *ti* on his scalp.[12] Unfortunately, few of the ingredients of these herbal reductions are known. Many of them would likely have been made of basic reagents like *nyanyara* and *hiatso*, but the practice of utilizing multiple ingredients to harness multiple healing spirits is also evident. Some recipes of *ti* were simple cures, while others were improvisations designed to challenge the spirits causing the illness. Clearly, the local material culture that undergirded African healing tradition was just as robust in the nineteenth century as it had been centuries before.

Trials by ordeal using herbal and consecrated medicines were also employed in Accra during the early colonial period. In 1867, a woman from Labadi accused a woman from Accra of stealing wood and cursing her so that she would die if she ate kenkey (a staple food made from fermented corn dough). In an attempt to save her life and clear her name, the accused went through a trial by ordeal in which she had to "eat fetish." She failed the trial, and the fetish priest found her guilty, ordering her to pay a hefty fine of rum and livestock.[13] So common were trials by ordeal during this time that some of them picked up nicknames, like the "Arkah truth fetish," which appeared to be circulating around the city as an oracle in 1861.[14] These types of trials were still expensive, costing a small fortune in gold dust, cowries, cloth, livestock, eggs, and knives. As the nineteenth century wore on, court cases showed that Liberian dollars and British pounds began to find their way into the means of exchange for healing, but the change in currencies did not diminish the cost of expensive rituals.[15]

Another continuity found in the court records is the abiding concern with spiritual reproductive health. In a city where infant mortality rates were high because of disease, one of the healer's most important roles was to link the generations by conducting puberty rituals, aiding conception with fertility medicines, caring for pregnant mothers, and ensuring healthy deliveries.[16] In some cases, people in Accra placed the blame for infertility on curses invoked by their enemies. As a means of defending themselves against such curses, some patients sought protective medicines from beyond the Accra Plains, as demonstrated by an 1874 case of a man who purchased a healing object, worth ten times the normal price of a local remedy, from an itinerant trader who had brought it from "very far in the interior." The expense was worthwhile in this instance because, as he attested in a colonial court, the object evidently cured him and one of his wives gave birth to twins shortly afterward.[17]

Witchcraft makes its first appearance in the colonial archive in reference to conflicts resulting from infertility. Desperate to protect their fertility and their offspring, women regularly sought out healing devices as protection from the ravages of invisible witch spirits, and one court case briefly mentioned an herbal potion used to wash children after birth as an inoculant against witchcraft.[18] In one trial, a man described how he had purchased an herbal prophylactic to ward off witchcraft and to prevent his wife from delivering another stillborn child.[19] Though witchcraft may have been present in the city centuries before, these cases represent the first documents that associate the affliction with infertility, which may represent a change in the way that reproductive health was understood in Accra. There is no way to trace the rise and fall of witchcraft panics in Accra at that time, but the rise of anti-witchcraft shrines in the Akan regions during the late nineteenth century suggests that an increasing amount of attention was focused on combating the forces of witchcraft on the Gold Coast during this period.[20]

Yet despite pervasive concerns about infertility, women in Accra did not always hold to a wealth-in-children stereotype. William Daniell, a traveler and ethnographer who visited Accra in the 1850s, reported to the ethnological society of London in 1856 that abortions in Accra could be "secretly induced by the assistance of powerful emmenagogues indigenous to the country."[21] Daniell noted that the demand for abortifacients was driven by the fear that pregnancy out of wedlock would "degrade the girl in estimation of the public" by creating "an indelible stain" on her reputation.[22] This theory was borne out during a scandal in 1899, when Basel Mission catechist Carl Christian (C. C.) Reindorf was accused of procuring an abortion for his daughter Christiana.[23] The details included in this case were sparse, but they suggest that while the inhabitants of Accra traditionally prized fertility, family patriarchs asserted control over reproduction to maintain the norms of the bourgeois classes.

Herbal remedies may have been ubiquitous in Accra, but not all concoctions were regarded as healthful. Some court cases reveal deep fears of being killed by the very medicines that were supposed to heal. This should not be surprising considering the established Ga maxim that deities and medicines could either be used to harm or heal. The official slogan for the deity Sakumo, for instance, is *Ofitee Osaa*, which translates roughly as "You spoil, You repair."[24] The black powdered *ti* also had this Januslike quality. Though it was a staple of the healing trade, it could also be used as a poison (or, in British colonial legal parlance, as an obnoxious medicine). In a case from 1900, a Mr. Larson claimed that he had been poisoned by a Mr. Bruce, a man who had previously prepared a healing draught for Larson's digestion and a fertility concoction for Larson's wife. Mr. Larson claimed that he had fallen ill after sharing beer with Bruce and that he was certain that some "black stuff" had been placed in the beer to change the "weight of the drink."[25] Mr. Bruce took the stand to defend himself, telling the magistrate that he was a practiced herbalist who never made poisons, and he was able to prove that no chemically active substances had been added to Larson's beer. Mr. Bruce went free, but it is clear from his case, and from others that followed, that it was easy for plaintiffs to bring charges against African healers by using the stereotype of the duplicitous fetish priest.[26]

But even when scapegoated as dealers in poisons, the voices of African healers ring out in court documents, as professionals with a sense of pride in their trade. An 1872 accusation of poisoning between employees at the Basel Mission serves as a vivid example. Theodor Wulff, the plaintiff, claimed that two of his colleagues, Lartey and Addor, had paid a medicine man a large sum of money to put a deadly poison in his drink. The medicine man, Tettey Amoye, stood in front of the magistrate to defend his reputation as a traditional healer and to tell the judge that he followed a strict code of ethics and felt compelled to warn Wulff of the peril he was facing: "I was promised thirty-two dollars to poison plaintiff. I did not agree so I came and reported to you. I did not agree because I had no bad feeling against you. I reported the matter to you about three times . . . I am a native doctor. I never practice Fetish. I never practice Fetish in this town. I do not know any medicine to injure people's life. I have no medicine to poison people I do not know any poison."[27] Amoye proudly differentiated himself from so-called fetish practitioners and explained that it was the perpetrators who had gathered toxic reagents and demanded he transform them into a poison. He refused their offer of thirty-two Liberian dollars, a tidy sum worth approximately one month's wages, as a slight to his honor.[28] In the context of the colonial courtroom, the derogatory meaning of *fetish* cropped up again and again, but healers like Bruce and Amoye were able to defend the virtue of their healing practices by distinguishing them from harmful criminal activities.

The commonality of African-derived therapies within the court records suggests that most patients in Accra still managed their health using herbal and consecrated medicines. Indeed, the records are jammed with references to African healing but are almost entirely silent on Islamic, Christian, or Western forms of healing. The only non-African therapeutics to appear of any significance are some mentions of European surgery, which suggests its growing influence in the city. In particular, an inquest into the death of a prisoner at James Fort is worth discussing because it shows the sharp contrast between the treatment of African and European healing methods in the courtroom and how the power was understood only on European terms within official circles.

In December 1877, two inmates at James Fort Prison were involved in a fistfight. One of the combatants was a fisherman named Commey, who walked away from the conflict with what initially appeared to be only minor injuries. However, in the days that followed, Commey's ribs became swollen and sore, and he was permitted to leave the fort to see a native doctor, who washed his wounds and rubbed them down with herbs. The local herbalist remained at his patient's bedside for seven days, but Commey's torso swelled so dramatically that he died from his injury. Because the incident occurred at a colonial prison, the government was obliged to conduct an investigation, and the transcript of the hearing offers an example of the asymmetry of African and European etiologies and practices during the late nineteenth century.

At the inquest, the presiding officer brought forward Dr. Anderson, assistant surgeon of the Gold Coast Colony, as an expert witness to determine the cause of death. The British surgeon offered the presiding officer an opinion on the injuries sustained by Commey.

> It is possible that the . . . injuries which he is said to have suffered from the [beating] might have disguised the pain—I knew an instance where a man had a rib broken by gunshot [and] his shoulder was also shattered and the injury to the shoulder might have disguised the pain of the rib. I have not known another instance where there was not pain felt very soon. There might have been internal injuries, but there are no symptoms described, whereas all the symptoms, the difficulty of breathing, the inability to sit up in bed, and the bloody spit all point to Pleurisy probably complicated with Pneumonia.[29]

Dr. Anderson made this assessment as a military surgeon, on the basis of his experience treating soldiers with bullet wounds. When he was asked if the herbal remedies of the local healer might have complicated Commey's injuries, he admitted that it would be difficult for him to comment because he did not know what sorts of herbs had been used, though he did mention that it was unlikely that any herbal remedy could hasten the death, considering it was applied on the outside of the body. In a city where surgeons rarely ventured outside the slave forts, Dr. Anderson might not have ever spoken to an African healer because of the language barrier involved, and even if he had, nothing in his testimony shows knowledge or interest in the African healing arts.[30]

After questioning Dr. Anderson, the presiding officer brought the (unnamed) herbalist to the stand to ask him whether his therapies had hastened the death of the patient:

Q. What medicine was used?
A. The medicine was root of the tree Oblijo.
Q. What was the purpose of applying the medicine?
A. Because he was [injured] and that was the proper medicine in such cases that is why I applied it.
Q. Was it to make him cool or hot?
A. It was to get down the swelling.
Q. Does it make the body hot or cold?
A. It makes him hot.
Q. Did you apply hot water or cold water?
A. Cold water. Hot water first, then cold water, then the medicine.
Q. Was there any peculiarity about the breathing?
A. He breathed like a sick man who is not expected to live.[31]

The responses of the herbalist are noticeably curt for several reasons. First, they were likely truncated by the court recorder. Second, the herbalist might not have fully understood the motives behind the questions, such as the implicit references to the humoral significance of hot and cold. Third, and most important, the herbalist probably decided to exclude as much information as possible to avoid any blame for the death. Also absent here is any mention of the recipe for the herbal remedy, the spiritual significance of the *oblijo* medicine, or his opinion about the spiritual cause of the illness.[32] Knowing well that the British magistrate might find him culpable in the death of Commey, he probably finished his statement by indicating that the patient was on his death bed anyway, suggesting he had merely made a last-ditch attempt to save him. Whereas Dr. Anderson felt quite comfortable speculating about the causes of death in front of the colonial legal authorities as a government-authorized medical expert, the unnamed herbalist did not. Indeed, the herbalist's careful release of information might have saved him from incriminating himself—when the inquest was concluded, the magistrate decided that the cause of death had nothing to do with the treatments he received.

What is most interesting about Commey's case is that it reveals two parallel evaluations of the health of the same patient, one European and one African. Dr. Anderson assessed Commey's illness along official medical lines as a humoral imbalance of bodily fluids caused by the trauma of the rib injury. The herbalist, on the other hand, saw a patient suffering from a bodily wound that needed the cooling virtues of local herbs, and perhaps a later spiritual inquiry into the illness. Neither of these healers could have kept the patient alive, but it is significant that the patient was sent to a local herbalist, even when he was imprisoned in a colonial institution and even when he had the option of European medical care. The tide of patient preference had not turned toward Western medicine, even at the end of the nineteenth century in the most colonial of institutions in the city.

THE EMERGENCE OF NEW THERAPIES: ISLAMIC AND CHRISTIAN COMMUNITIES IN ACCRA

Prior to the nineteenth century, there is no mention in any European accounts of a resident Muslim population in Accra. There were, however, Muslim slaves passing through Accra as early as the mid-eighteenth century, some of them literate. There were also Arabic texts, supposedly brought to Accra by Asante warriors who had taken the books as booty in wars with the Gonja.[33] However, the presence of Islam did not seem to have any influence on healing in Accra. Surgical techniques, like cupping, bleeding, variolation, and male circumcision, might have been present if a large Muslim population had resided on the coast. However, they are absent from European travel accounts, as are any instances of Quranic geomancy, slate wash, or amulets. In fact, Peiter De Marees, who visited Accra several times in the seventeenth century, stated explicitly that no barbers existed on the Gold Coast, and he did not once mention the presence of Islam.[34] Ferdinand Rømer argued that the barber-surgeons of the slave ships should never bleed slaves unless in an emergency because there was no knowledge of the benefit of phlebotomy at Accra.[35] Moreover, there do not appear to be any Islamic influences embedded in the Ga language of healing.[36]

Things changed in the late eighteenth century, when Paul Isert reported the widespread use of leather amulets, as well as the use of variolation (a technique that, he believed, dramatically reduced incidences of smallpox along the coast).[37] By the start of the nineteenth century, it is highly probable that Muslim apotropaics were available in Accra, considering their strong presence in the urban centers of the Kingdom of Asante. European envoys to Kumasi, the capital of the Kingdom of Asante, reported the presence of Islamic healing practices, noting that Kumasi contained a large Muslim population made up of Gonja, Dagomba, Mamprussi, Hausa, and Wangara immigrants and that their priests used Arabic script in the fabrication of charms and amulets, sometimes in combination with local herbal remedies.[38] Extant folios of documents in Arabic script used in Kumasi contain instructions for making amulets that protected the wearer from specific illnesses such as smallpox or leprosy, or conditions such as sexual impotency, infertility, migraine headaches, and bedwetting.[39] Amulets were in demand everywhere in Kumasi, "from the Asante palace to the slave's hut," but soldiers in particular were willing to pay for protective war charms. In 1807, the British governor of the Gold Coast, George Torrane, noted that every Asante soldier had a form of body armor fashioned out of a "little square cloth enclosing some little sentences" of the Quran.[40]

Although there is no direct evidence that the residents of Accra used such charms, they had been engaged in so many battles with the peoples of the rainforest that they would have been aware of their use and manufacture. In 1826, when the Asante fled the field after the Battle of Katamanso, they left behind a charm made from the skull of Sir Charles McCarthy "enveloped in two folds of paper, covered with Arabic characters," which was handed over to British officers.[41] After the battle, a collection of Arabic manuscripts taken from the Asante, many of them concealed within amulets, were archived at the Danish fort of Christiansborg, and they were eventually deposited in the Royal Library at Copenhagen.[42] In the aftermath of such a physically and spiritually challenging battle, the inhabitants of Accra must have become aware of the richness of the Islamic medico-religious world.

However, it was only in the mid-nineteenth century that a permanent Muslim community took hold in Accra. The first and most prominent group of migrants were Hausa-speaking soldiers from the Slave Coast (Nigeria), who were brought by the British Army to fight against the Asante.[43] By the 1850s, the Hausa population of Accra had increased to the point that they were able to form their own neighborhood, or *zoŋo* (from the Hausa term *zaŋgo*, meaning "camp"),[44] and by 1881 they had appointed their first leader, Idris Naino, a priest from Katsina in Hausaland.[45] The Hausa population was supplemented by the arrival of Yoruba migrants from Abeokuta, including Brimah the Butcher, who would later become a leader in the community.[46] By 1891, the Gold Coast Census stated that Muslims made up 8 percent of the population of Accra. They lived mostly along the eastern periphery of Ussher Town, and by 1900, some members of the Ga community began to convert to Islam.[47] Most Muslims worked as merchants in the livestock or kola nut trades, but a smaller number took up the role of priests within the Tijaniya Sufi brotherhood, offering Islamic education for the poor and marginalized of the city to attract converts.[48]

The coming together of Hausa and Yoruba Muslims might have allowed for the presence of the so-called *wanzamai*, surgeons/ healers who offered services like barbering, circumcision, and ritual scarification and products like herbal remedies, slate wash, and apotropaics.[49] The *alufa*, Yoruba holy men who used the spiritual power of Quranic charms to influence events, may also have been present during the late nineteenth century.[50] Unfortunately, the sources on this subject are few, offering no textual evidence of any particular school of thought about healing or any specific evidence of the use of *Tibb-ul-Nabbi* (medicine of the Prophet). However, considering the strength of the Muslim community in Accra, and considering the prevalence of Islamic medicines in Asante, some Islamic healing practices were almost certainly present in Accra by the mid-1850s.

The so-called Tabon, migrants who brought the Islamic faith back to Africa from Brazil, also influenced Islamic healing practices in Accra.[51] The first Afro-Brazilians arrived in 1829 and were received by the chief of Ussher Town, who gave them land in the Otoblohum quarter of the city.[52] In 1836, they were followed by about two hundred freed slaves from Bahia, and thereafter by Afro-Brazilian slave traders in the mid-nineteenth century. Many of the Brazilian immigrants cultivated herb gardens, and one particular settler, Abotchei Nassu, is known to have used herbs from his own garden to make a cure for Guinea worm, which would have been a medical innovation in a city with no prior record of an herbal remedy for this painful disease.[53]

In the nineteenth century, the Muslims of Accra began to form what Deborah Pellow has characterized as a "diverse collectivity," comprising various ethnic groups and backgrounds united though Islamic forms of worship.[54] They spoke many different languages, but used the West African lingua franca of Hausa to communicate with one another. They also shared the notion that healing authority could be vested in the holy language of Arabic. Practices such as divination via geomantic squares, slate washing of

Quranic script with consecrated black ink, and verbal incantations and recitations were present in nearby regions of West
Africa and may all have been present in the city. Non-Muslims
may have patronized these sorts of therapies to acquire spiritual
armor for battle, protection from malicious spirits, or help with
conceiving a child.

Another emerging religious force on the Gold Coast in the
nineteenth century was Christianity. The first outpost in Accra
was built by the Basel Mission Society in 1827, just a little north
of Christiansborg Castle. The German and Swiss lay preachers
who sailed to the city were filled with piety and ambition, but
they were also aware that they were entering a difficult disease
environment. As a newly formed mission, the leaders of the society were conflicted about whether to bring European medical
practices to Accra or whether to trust that the sick could heal
themselves through faith.[55] Some missionaries believed exclusively in healing via the laying on of hands, a practice that they
brought with them from Europe. However, the directors in Basel
decided it would be prudent to offer some rudimentary medical
training—such as basic humoral medical techniques like the use
of cold baths, bloodletting, and purging—to missionaries before
they left Switzerland. Not surprisingly, neither their faith nor
their basic training helped them much. Between 1828 and 1838,
eight of nine missionaries died, probably of malaria.

The lone survivor of the early years, Andreas Riis, fell sick like
the rest of his colleagues but was able to survive after a Ga healer
prescribed herbal remedies for his fevers. Riis subsequently became an advocate for African healing practices and claimed that
European remedies were useless in the tropical climate. African
converts followed the lead of Riis, shunning European medicine
and seeking help from African healers. It was not until the very
end of the nineteenth century, when Dr. Rudolph Fisch established a dispensary in Aburi, that Western medicines started to
compete with local Africa curatives. Even then, it was Western

medicines like quinine, rather than Western medical practices, that caught on, and both missionaries and converts continued to seek help within the African community when they fell sick.[56]

Missionary medicine had little to offer patients in Accra, but one Basel Mission convert did take up European surgical practice in the mid-nineteenth century. C. C. Reindorf, a catechist who would later become famous for writing a history of the Gold Coast, received a crash course in battlefield medicine, and during the Awuna and Akwamu wars of 1866 and 1870, he extracted three hundred slugs from the wounds of soldiers.[57] Reindorf later combined his surgical skills with an aptitude for producing local herbal medicines and tested a variety of local remedies until he devised an herbal concoction that cured several Europeans of dysentery. Later in his career, he used his experience to train several other catechists in basic surgery and herbal therapies. He hoped they would make use of their hybrid medical and herbal knowledge at the different stations of the Basel Mission around the Gold Coast.[58]

Oddly, Reindorf's medical endeavors petered out by the end of the century. His written work did not include information about missionary medicine, and there is no written record of his herbal remedies for dysentery. Though he trained other Christians in surgery, there is no evidence that European medical knowledge among converts was actively sustained, and no indigenous school of European surgical techniques emerged. The disconnect between mission activity and European medicine in Accra stands in contrast to other missions in Africa, where basic medical services, such as lancing boils or pulling teeth, became an essential part of attracting converts.[59] When Accra became the capital of the Gold Coast, it was institutions like the colonial army and the Gold Coast Medical Department, rather than the church, that propagated European-derived medical techniques.

The practice of medicine may not have been an important tool of conversion during the early years at the Basel Mission, but the missionaries did establish some key concepts about the healing power of God. In partnership with Ga catechists like Reindorf, Johannes Zimmerman translated the Bible in 1866, offering Ga speakers three new terms with which to conceptualize healing.[60] The first was a translation of the Supreme Deity as *Nyoŋmo*, a Ga word for both rainfall and a deity associated with the sky. Paul Isert had previously noted that *Nyoŋmo* was considered to be a type of *deus otiosus*—a deity "too eminent to be concerned with the activities of people"—which makes it a matter of speculation as to why Zimmerman assigned *Nyoŋmo* the status of creator.[61] In a dry area like the Accra Plains, he may have wanted to choose a term that would associate the Supreme Deity with rainfall and the health of the land, but it is more likely that he felt divine inspiration to redeem an obscure deity that he believed was once regarded by Africans as the almighty God.

When Zimmerman translated the term for Holy Spirit, he faced a different challenge. In Ga, the word for spirit is *woji*, an invisible force that can be harnessed to both harm and heal. In order to imbue the Holy Spirit with the purifying capacities of a divine force, while at the same time eliminating any possibility of malicious action, Zimmerman chose the term *mumo kroŋkroŋ*, joining the word for breath with a doubling of the word for purity.[62] To Zimmerman, this neologism was supposed to refer to an invisible force that cleansed the soul, but in Ga it could be more practically understood as a powerful healing energy, and in the churches of the twentieth century, it would be appropriated as a force that could clear spiritual blockages in the body and increase the flow of *hewalɛ*.[63] Translating the name of the son of God posed further problems, as Zimmerman wanted to avoid any confusion with ancestral spirits.[64] In the end, Zimmerman simply imposed the Greek name for Jesus Christ, *Yesu Kristo*, creating a new singular ancestral character with which all Christians could identify, irrespective of their ethnic or kinship ties.[65] By the end of the nineteenth century, a small subsection of the inhabitants of Accra, numbering in the hundreds, had been exposed to these terminologies of the Holy Trinity. The impact was modest at the time, but with these new conceptions of God, the Son, and the Holy Spirit, the tiny Christian congregation of Osu distinguished itself theologically from what they regarded as fetish worship. Moreover, Zimmerman's translations provided the tools Christians would later use to create a culture of faith healing in the twentieth century. The initiative to use Ga was unique to the Basel mission. Even when the Anglican, Methodist, and Catholic denominations preached against so-called fetish worship, they did so in English, limiting their outreach toward potential Christian converts. This left the Basel Mission as the preeminent Christian institution in the city.

For the Basel missionaries, defining the Christian world theologically was not enough. They also believed that African converts had to distinguish themselves spatially from the world of African spiritualism. The Basel Mission Salem (as it was known by the missionaries) was understood as a Christian refuge, purposely divided from the beliefs and practices of the Ga.[66] Converts were expected to divorce themselves from African therapies that drew on the healing spirits or risk expulsion from the church. This stance generated a conundrum for the new converts. At the Salem, there were no physicians, nurses, or pharmacists, and no prospect of any form of new therapy except prayer and the laying on of hands. How were they to distance themselves from African healing traditions if they had nothing to replace them with? Reindorf's hybrid practices of surgery and herbalism might have filled the gap, but there is no documentation to show conclusively that they did.

Intriguingly, under similar circumstances in Nigeria, Christians filled the therapeutic vacuum with imported medicines. For instance, Yoruba converts used Holloway's Ointment, a general-purpose patent medicine for skin ailments, in combination with an appeal to God to sanctify the medicine: "The medicine I use is

God's and to render it efficacious I must ask God's blessing upon it."[67] But in Accra, sources about the use of medicines at the Basel Mission are frustratingly thin, consisting of only one reference to the use of imported salicylic acid (aspirin) to fight fevers.[68] Nonetheless, it is hard to believe that the residents of the new Salem at Osu survived without any healers to care for them. It is more likely that they illicitly sought help from African healers or filled the therapeutic gap with the sorts of patent medicines that were becoming ubiquitous in the marketplaces of Accra.

NEW TOOLS FOR HEALING: PATENT MEDICINES

In the late nineteenth century, innovations in industrial production in the United Kingdom resulted in a flourishing of mass-produced commodities like alcohol, wine, foodstuffs, toiletries, and patent medicines. Branded consumer goods were markers of distinction, especially in the British colonies, where the rarity and value of imported products was much higher than in England. The medicine trade does not figure prominently in accounts of the legitimate trade of the nineteenth century, which is dominated by the discussion of cloth and alcohol, but for Europeans living West Africa, access to medicinal goods was vital to their survival. As they prepared for their travels around the empire, British officials and merchants packed their bags with all manner of drugs and medicines, thereby exposing people around the world to the medical matériel of the Industrial Revolution.[69] For patients in Accra, self-medication with patent medicines offered a way to heal oneself privately or, in a public sense, to define oneself as a member of a modern, urban, colonial society.

Of all the ingredients found in this new era of patent medicines, quinine sulfate was by far the most significant. In 1823, American chemists learned how to synthesize Jesuit's bark into quinine powder, and it quickly became available in tiny granules for sale around the world.[70] During the first Niger expedition in 1841, the British Army used quinine sulfate hoping it would ward off malaria among its soldiers, but the dosage was so low that it was ineffective. As a result, the crew suffered a 30 percent mortality rate, and the expedition was called off.[71] Undeterred, army doctors kept working on the dosage, and in 1845 the Medical Department of the British Army sent a circular to all British governors in West Africa recommending quinine as a prophylaxis to check malaria.[72] During the second expedition of 1854, no one died from malaria, and the use of the medicine gradually caught on. During the campaign against the Asante in 1873–74, army surgeons ordered the British soldiers to take large quantities of quinine per day, dramatically lowering the malaria rate during the expedition.[73] Though it took almost fifty years, the successful use of quinine allowed for the colonization of tropical Africa and dramatically changed the course of political and economic events in Accra.

Like their military compatriots, Europeans living in or traveling through West Africa took quinine pills to prevent malaria, though without any standard dosage. During his tenure as a minister for the Methodist Church in the Gold Coast, Dennis Kemp recalled that the amount of quinine one took varied according to individual preference: "[There are] those who are able to boast that they can dispense with the drug for five or six months at a time. Others take small quantities frequently—in the wet season, daily. A medical friend, of considerable experience and success, tells me that fifty grains, taken during three consecutive days once a month, gives a sudden and salutary check to all malarial tendencies."[74]

The use of quinine as a curative or a prophylaxis, it seems, was an imperfect process. The variation in dosage was attributable to the fact that patients did not understand that they were ingesting grains of quinine as a weapon against *Plasmodium falciparum*, a concept that would have been inconceivable until the parasite was discovered in 1898.[75] Rather, they took quinine as a check against miasmatic gases, a pathogen that was difficult to quantify. As a result, they had to be careful in its application—too much quinine produced side effects known as quininism, which included vertigo, tinnitus, nightmares, and nosebleeds.[76] As Kemp recalled, breaking a malarial fever often required "heroic doses of quinine" because the cure was almost as bad as the disease.[77]

By the mid-nineteenth century, European missionaries and colonial officials still traveled with the usual mix of chemicals and herbal treatments, but they soon began to add proprietary medicines to their kits.[78] During his travels through the Gold Coast in the 1860s, the famous Richard Burton passed through Accra with a kit containing quinine, sarsaparilla, and two patent medicines: Chlorodyne and Warburg's Tincture. Chlorodyne, devised by a British doctor in India as a treatment for cholera, was an addictive tonic made from opium, cannabis, and chloroform.[79] Burton likely used it as a painkiller, but it was advertised as a cure-all for a wide variety of ailments, from headaches to diarrhea. According to Burton, his use of Chlorodyne attracted so much interest during a visit to the Gold Coast that someone stole four large bottles from his medicine kit.[80] For fevers, Burton used Warburg's Tincture—a bitter concoction of quinine and various "aeromatic substances"—which he purchased directly from Dr. Warburg, an Austrian chemist living in London in the 1870s.[81] Burton advocated the use of Warburg's concoction among his friends and associates because he claimed it had saved his life many times. He even claimed that it had been bought by the crate for the navy and army during the Anglo-Asante war of 1873–74.[82] Methodist missionary Kemp also believed in the efficacy of Warburg's Tincture, despite its reputedly vile taste.[83] In the case of stubborn fevers, Kemp also used Anti-Febrin, an analgesic containing acetanilide, a strong chemical that, even by the late nineteenth century, was considered too toxic for regular use.[84]

Vegetable pills, bought by mail order and taken for gastrointestinal illnesses, were also a common type of patent medicine
on the Gold Coast. Archaeological evidence shows that Perry
Davis Vegetable Pills (a painkiller that likely included opiates)
were consumed in the nineteenth century in the African section
of Elmina, a major coastal trading center 250 kilometers down
the coast from Accra, and Dr. De Roos Vegetable Pills, an antacid
produced in England, were advertised in Gold Coast newspapers
in the 1880s.[85] These brands were the progenitors of a burgeoning mail-order medicine market, reflected in an 1881 advertisement in the *Gold Coast News* that listed throat lozenges, quinine
powder, laudanum, liver pills, iodine, and a variety of painkillers
for sale.[86] Branded medical kits, like the Burroughs Wellcome
Tabloid Medicine Chest, were also mass produced by the 1890s,
and they became de rigueur for colonial officials and missionaries traveling to Africa. These chests contained bottled remedies
like the aforementioned Warburg's Tincture, as well as less well-
known products like Dover's Powder, Easton's Syrup, and Livingston's Rouser.[87] The ubiquity of medicines is not surprising,
considering European newcomers to the tropics had to live with
the fear that a slight chill in the afternoon could lead to a raging
fever at night and death by morning.[88]

The rapid growth of patent medicine imports indicates that,
by sheer volume, they must have penetrated the African marketplace by the late nineteenth century. In 1890, an estimated
£3,000 worth of drugs and medicines were imported into the
Gold Coast, a modest quantity that was likely consumed exclusively by Europeans and African elites. But demand grew,
and by 1900, this number had doubled, and by the 1910s it had
reached £20,000.[89] The timing of the increased sales may indicate an increase in patent medicines' efficacy in fighting tropical illness. Certainly the varieties of brands containing quinine
must been useful in places like Accra. It may also have been
that many people became addicted to these medicines, which

contained healthy amounts of opium, cannabis, and alcohol. However, the best way to explain the sudden rise in demand for imported medicines is to suggest that Africans started to consume them en masse. After all, population growth in the city had been stagnant for several decades, for both the European and African populations. In 1911, there were fewer than 1,000 Whites living in Accra, in comparison to a African population of over 15,000.[90] The numbers dictate that it is almost certain that Africans on the Gold Coast had become the primary consumers of imported European medicines. This assertion is also supported by one definitive fact: in 1912, the chief medical officer of the Gold Coast noted that educated Africans were using patent medicines to cure gonorrhea.[91] We do not know whether the medicine they chose worked, but the hopeful use of new medical goods indicates that the quest for a cure was just as relevant as it had been in the past.

Africans would have adopted the use of patent medicines for many reasons. First, the markets of Accra were already clearing-houses for transcontinental herbal reagents and remedies, so it is not surprising that these items found their way into local commercial channels. Second, patent medicines and medicine chests could be ordered by mail, a method of purchase that the affluent African merchant classes might have taken advantage of.[92] Third, there is parallel evidence that African consumers were already buying imported gin as a medicinal product.[93] J. H. Henkes promoted their Star Brand gin by claiming on the label that it was recommended by physicians as a remedy for "Rheumatism, Gout, Gravel, Flatulency, Dyspepsia, Dropsy, Diseases of the Kidneys, Bladder, etc."[94] Another distiller, Blankenheym & Nolet, attached a medical certificate to every bottle that they exported to West Africa, hoping that their gin could carve out a niche as a medicinal tonic.[95] Since these spirits were produced specifically to serve African consumers, and since they were both available in Accra, it appears that Africans were looking for imported goods that were considered healthful.[96] Fourth, Gold Coast newspapers contained print ads for patent medicines. Though literacy rates were low within the general populations, a burgeoning class of African merchants and professionals were reading newspapers like the *Accra Herald,* the *Gold Coast Echo,* and the *Gold Coast Times.*[97] These periodicals offered news, commentary, and advertising for what Stephanie Newell has called the West African "reading public," a literate community that included many professionals who had traveled around the continent and to Britain.[98] Moreover, these newspapers may have been read aloud to those who could not read, expanding the market for patent medicine advertising exponentially.

The limits of historical source materials constrain what can be said definitively about how consumers in Accra appropriated patent medicines. But while Africans may not have been the target market, imported health products were clearly available, and there are plenty of hints to suggest that they were sought after. Because no regulations governed their distribution or consumption, patent medicines fit nicely into a stream of therapeutic self-medication that had been established for centuries, and they also could be acquired as a way of distinguishing oneself as a participant in the modernity of market therapeutics.

HOSPITALS, DOCTORS, AND NASCENT BIO-POWER IN COLONIAL ACCRA

The decision to move the capital of the Gold Coast Colony to Accra was part of a century-long period of sanitary reform in Britain. After spending several decades fighting cholera epidemics, Parliament finally passed the Public Health Act in 1875, making sanitation a national—and by extension imperial—concern.[99] The imperial quest to reduce the ravages of disease in Africa is evident in a speech to the House of Lords by the Earl of Carnar-von, the permanent undersecretary of state for the colonies, who lamented the miserable conditions at Cape Coast:

> The soil is saturated through and through with sewage. There is decaying vegetable matter everywhere about, and the houses are crowded on one another. . . . It deserves more than perhaps any other place the appellation of the white man's grave. (Hear!) This being the case, there must be a change; the seat of govern-ment must be moved, but for obvious reasons it must be on the sea coast. Now there is a choice of one or other of two places—Accrah on the east and Elmina on the west. Accrah appears to be a desirable place as regards health.[100]

The colonial officers on the Gold Coast agreed with the earl, and the move to the dry open plains of Accra was completed by 1877.[101] Unlike French policy, which forced sanitation on urban Africans at great expense and to the point of revolt, the British pre-ferred to make a fresh start in a different location.[102] Accra seemed just the place to establish a new capital, given the latest develop-ments in sanitary science.

But just as sanitation began to dominate the discourse of health and illness, a different perception of disease was emerging in Eu-rope. Starting in the 1880s, teams of laboratory scientists began to isolate the microbes responsible for epidemic diseases like an-thrax, tuberculosis, cholera, and bubonic plague. The search for microscopic pathogens broke from a long tradition of patient care that took into account the humoral balance of each individual pa-tient, and increasingly, sick bodies were being brought to clinics and hospitals where they could be observed en masse by medi-cal officers.[103] The unification of sanitary theory and laboratory science has been celebrated as an era when medicine finally be-came a progressive social force, but this viewpoint has been chal-lenged more recently by historians arguing that European states also used medicine to monitor and control their populations via institutions like clinics, hospitals, and asylums.[104] Considering the fact that Accra was a colonial capital founded on the promise of health, it is tempting to highlight discourses of bio-power within the colonial medical regime. However, any approach that relies on colonial records will almost certainly overestimate the significance of the work of the Gold Coast Medical Department. Unlike French West Africa, where sanitary discourse generated a "heavy-handed European paternalist rule" over the colonized, the new British colonial capital of the Gold Coast had a makeshift medical infrastructure, built mainly to protect the health of government officials.[105]

The story of the first hospitals of Accra shows both the gains and failures of colonial medical authority in Accra. In 1877, the only hospital in Accra was a cluster of huts beside the James Fort, and few records remain about the types of treatments offered there.[106] By 1882, the Medical Department had shifted this rudimentary hospital into the former home of George Lutterodt, a merchant who lived in the lee of Ussher Fort.[107] Little information exists about the early days of this first permanent institution, but it was evidently sparsely equipped and staffed by only one doctor. In 1883, Governor Rowe initiated the construction of a larger hospital building inside an old bungalow in Victoriaborg and placed the institution under the direction of Dr. J. Desmond McCarthy, a physician who would later become the chief medical officer of the Gold Coast. The hospital opened with some promise, with two segregated wards consisting of a large twelve-bed room for Africans and a smaller four-bed enclosure for Europeans, along with a small dispensary and living quarters for the nursing staff.[108] But it was never meant to be a thriving center of colonial medial enterprise. As Dr. McCarthy admitted many years later, any European who was even moderately ill bypassed the hospital and was sent back to Britain on the first available steamer.[109]

Because it was never meant to be a place of care for Europeans, the first colonial hospital in Accra was almost immediately neglected and underfunded, offering only the most basic of services. In 1896, a young English nurse recruited to work in Accra found the hospital to be in a dilapidated state:

> I was thunderstruck when I saw the hospital: the floor was clean, and that is all that could be said for it; the beds were such as an educated native would not sleep on in these days, very few bed-clothes, and what there were, all in rags, a few plates, knives, and forks, and I remember one man had brought in his own egg-cup. I was very much struck with the bare look, not only of the hospital, but all round, not a garden or tree to be seen, nothing but thick low bush, which I was told, and found afterwards, was full of snakes. I thought I had come to the most God-forsaken place on the earth.[110]

Supplies at the hospital were continuously short, to the degree that the nurses had to provide their own tea and sugar. Though the hospital did have a room for surgical services, it was not kept in good condition, and the surgical equipment was sometimes covered in rust.[111] One doctor even described the hospital as "primitive and disgusting."[112] The building's physical limitations were worsened by the low quality of the physicians working there. According to Principal Medical Officer Dr. Henderson, the hospital was only able to attract the "dregs of the profession"—doctors who had been unable to find work in England and often who had been dismissed from the West African Medical Services for "discreditable causes."[113]

But despite the limitations of the colonial hospital, the demand by African patients was steady, and by the 1890s the Medical Department felt compelled to add several more beds.[114] On average, Europeans were only using two beds at any given time, but the hospital was soon expanded to forty beds for Africans. No extant records show exactly who attended the hospital, so it is difficult to explain how demand for such a simple medical facility was sustained. One possibility is that the African merchant classes attended as a way to associate themselves with the medical practices of British elites, but considering the deplorable state of the facility, it is more likely that physicians made house calls for wealthy Africans. A second, more likely possibility is that African employees of the colonial government went to the hospital because they felt compelled to go there. In the late nineteenth century, there were hundreds of Gold Coast subjects working in the colonial government, employed as domestic laborers for colonial officials, and enlisted in the Gold Coast Constabulary. If they were absent from work because of illness, they were required to present records of their hospital attendance.[115] This argument is supported by the fact that the vast majority of patients at the hospital were males, who were far more likely to be working in the colonial service. Women had fewer direct contacts with the colonial establishment and were averse to seeking help from White male doctors, so they were much less likely to consider the colonial hospital as a therapeutic option. A third possibility is that African residents of Accra were taken to the hospital by force. For example, the diary of Kwaku Fri, a palm oil and rubber merchant, includes two cases of people who were injured in violent disputes and then taken to the hospital by police. These examples are supported by instances in the local court records that demonstrate that the police guided people in custody to the hospital, particularly in cases of trauma.[116] Yet a fourth possibility is that the beds in the hospital were filled with the destitute residents of Accra; according to colonial medical regulations, paupers were allowed to stay there for free.[117] Together, all of these factors may have led to a steady flow of African patients into the colonial hospital.

However, the expansion to forty beds also suggests that some African patients actually wanted to be there, seeing the colonial hospital as yet another option within the plurality of therapies in the city. Though most European medical techniques were of little use in the tropics, the hospital may have been a good option for procedures like the setting of bones, the surgical removal of foreign objects, and operations to deal with extreme cases of trauma. Unfortunately, the data are weak here, and it is not possible to make a strong assertion about the popularity of particular therapies at the hospital.

Though the patients at the colonial hospital were mostly African, only European physicians were eligible to work there.[118] One notable exception to this rule was Sierra Leone–born, European-trained Dr. John Farrell Easmon. Hired in 1885 as a personal physician to Governor Brandford Griffith, Easmon, as the only African doctor at the hospital, inspired a spike in attendance by African patients.[119] So successful was he that, after ten years of work in Accra, he famously visited London to lobby Dr. Charles Gage-Brown to build a tropical-medicine training facility for physicians in Accra. Gage-Brown, a medical adviser to Joseph Chamberlain in the Colonial Office, was impressed by Easmon, and he pushed forward the idea for several months, but his successor, Patrick Manson, changed course and decided to establish a school for tropical medicine in London, citing the added expense of training in the colonies.[120] Easmon's bold visit to the imperial capital offers a glimmer of what might have happened had Accra become a center for medical research, but it was not to be. As scholars of medical history in Africa have demonstrated, the eve of the twentieth century marked a turn for the worse for African physicians. The Colonial Office began to invest in centers for tropical-medicine research in England and Scotland instead of in the colonies, thereby excluding Black physicians from the West African Medical Services. This change in policy made Easmon the last of a generation of physicians dedicated to imperial service, as the racism inherent in colonial rule pushed new African medical graduates into private practice.

The career of Dr. Benjamin William Quartey-Papafio, a physician who entered the profession at the precise time that the color bar was enforced in the West African Medical Services, serves as a sharp contrast to that of Easmon. Born in Ussher Town and trained in Edinburgh, Quartey-Papafio had gained experience while training under Dr. McCarthy and expected to follow doctors like Easmon into the colonial service. To that end, Quartey-Papafio worked as a junior assistant in the colonial ranks while he petitioned for several years for promotion to colonial medical officer.[121] Sadly, he was consistently denied, with the argument that White patients would never accept the medical authority of a Black doctor.[122] Unlike in British India, where Indian-born physicians played a significant role in extending the reach of colonial medical hegemony, West African–born physicians were barred from the upper reaches of colonial medical power, limiting their influence in expanding Western medicine in Africa.[123]

Dr. Quartey-Papafio was frustrated but not deterred. When he realized that he could not advance in the ranks of the West African Medical Services, he resolved to establish a private medical practice, the first ever in Accra. By 1905, he had built a clinic on High Street, in the heart of the merchant district. As a snub to the colonial government, he emblazoned the provocative slogan *"Domi Abra"* above the door, a phrase that translates to "if you love me, come."[124] As a consolation for his rejection from the colonial service, Quartey-Papafio found that he had a near monopoly on private medicine in Accra.[125] It is difficult to argue that, in an era before arsenic injections, sulfa drugs, and penicillin, Quartey-Papafio's practice was driven by the efficacy of his cures. Considering his experience as a colonial surgeon, he may have attracted clients who needed specific surgical procedures that African healers could not provide, but this could have amounted to only a small part of his practice. It is more likely that he attracted clients from wealthy African families in Accra, many of whom were trained in Britain and sought to associate themselves with European healing practices. Considering that Europeans had been seeking help from African healers for centuries, it would not be surprising if White merchants and sailors continued this trend. But no matter the clientele, Dr. Quartey-Papafio was the first African physician to make European medicine a legitimate option within the pluralistic healing culture of the city.

When Quartey-Papafio set up his practice at the end of the nineteenth century, European merchants were still living along-side Africans in Ussher Town and James Town. For practical reasons, Europeans needed to work near their clients and employees, in offices around the surfboat landing and in buildings on High Street. Business was good, and they had no intention of leaving the city core. Nonetheless, the discourse of the filthy African city had begun to take hold, leading to suggestions that Europeans should be geographically separated from Africans. During a visit to Accra in 1852, William F. Daniell, a Scottish surgeon of the British Army Medical Staff, described the city as an unsanitary maze:

> With the exception of the main thoroughfare and a few open clearances at irregular intervals, the streets were necessarily narrow, tortuous, and intricate, the close proximity of the various domiciles producing a perplexing diversity of bypaths, that, in similitude, approached the dubious windings of some mysterious labyrinth. Formed by the contracted spaces between the opposite walls and projecting roofs, their due ventilation and cleanliness was more or less impeded; consequently, they always continued in a dirty condition, and were likewise subject to that fetid effluvia, generated by the accumulation of filth and other domestic refuse thrown out by their occupants, who, from a constitutional indolency or love of ease, were neither impressed with the necessity of adhering to any sanitary precautions, nor yet endeavoured to obtain the salubrity that would spring from the removal of such morbific agents.[126]

Daniell's verbose description of midcentury Accra was an early iteration of a new discourse of the filthy colonial city—a European imagining of a crowded bazaar that evoked fears of miasma and cholera. It also reinforced racial stereotypes, portraying Africans as either unaware of the squalor within which they lived or too lazy to deal with it. Daniell's cliché of the indolent African, and his depictions of Ussher Town as a cesspool, repeat themselves in remarks found in the journals of Henry Stanley, who visited the city in 1873 and described what he deemed the "filthy habits of the native."[127]

But like the European business classes, the colonial government initially showed little interest in separating the populations of Accra along racial lines. Instead, the Gold Coast Medical Department tried to avoid the political dangers of segregation by attempting to tidy things around the edges. Medical officers initially hoped that cleaning up open-air slaughterhouses, fish-smoking ovens, and open gutters would be easy fixes for the sanitary problem. Their first target was the Salaga Market in the heart of Ussher Town, which was deemed especially dangerous because it was swampy and prone to flooding.

As one medical officer noted in 1883, "There is a large accumulation of water just beyond the market, of the dirtiest and filthiest kind, in which pigs rejoice to wallow and natives to bathe . . . it is not surprising the natives get guinea worm when compelled to drink this semi-fluid."[128] But what the British saw as a cesspool was actually the neighborhood's only reservoir of drinking water for livestock. Though it may have bred mosquitoes, the inhabitants of Accra relied on it to sustain their animals during the dry season. In 1889, the Public Works Department finally declared the pond a health hazard, and the assistant surveyor sent in a team of laborers to fill it with debris from a recently demolished building. As the work began, a crowd gathered to protest. As the work progressed, the onlookers became increasingly unruly, and the assistant surveyor felt compelled to call out the Gold Coast Constabulary to allow his team to continue their work. When the crowd threatened to attack, the police held firm. After some pushing and shoving and some minor injuries, the people who instigated the riot were arrested. The situation had calmed down by the end of the day, and the hole was eventually filled in.[129]

Filling the pond at Salaga Market counted as a minor victory for colonial health authorities, but the ongoing resistance offered by Ussher Town residents discouraged further plans to improve sanitation in Accra. Finding it impossible to act directly, Governor Nathan hoped to pass the duty to a new city council via the Town's Ordinance Act of 1892, which devolved responsibility for sanitation to an urban council comprising three members of the African professional classes, three Europeans appointed directly by the governor, and three representatives named by local chiefs.[130] But the local representatives on the Town Council soon realized it was yet another attempt to impose new taxes on the residents of the city. In an audience with Governor Bradford Griffith in 1896, the Ga chiefs protested their minority representation on the council, informing him that they would not accept the imposition of new taxes when they were already supporting the colony through indirect tariffs on imports and exports.[131] The chiefs conceded that the city was in poor sanitary condition, but they pointed out that towns and villages in the interior remained much cleaner than those on the coast, arguing that the unhealthy living conditions of Accra were due to urban growth caused by the presence of the Europeans. Some of the Africans living in Accra had been to England were well aware that pipe-borne water and sewer systems had already been built in most cities in the metropole. For them, any notion of racial inclination toward cleanliness or filthiness would have seemed absurd when the sanitation situation in Accra was simply a matter of matching infrastructural investment to the scale of the population. The chiefs were therefore puzzled as to why the British did not want to make sanitary improvements in the colonial capital that they seemed to regard as an imperial possession. Unwisely, Governor Griffith ignored their concerns. Two years later, the first attempt to collect taxes caused a riot that had to be suppressed by the police, and for several years after this, the residents of Accra adopted a policy of noncompliance, refusing to pay their taxes.[132] The colonial government did accomplish some small feats, such as enhancing drainage and building latrines in Ussher Town and James Town and reducing the number of pigs living in the city, but little else changed. In 1900, an observer from the Liverpool School of Tropical Medicine continued the refrain that Accra was a "noisome and pestilential district."[133] Many African residents might have agreed with this assessment, but they would not have understood why the colonial government wasn't taking bold steps to fix the problem.

Official concern about public health in Accra faded until it was reignited again during a yellow fever outbreak between 1894 and 1896. The disease was hardly a widespread epidemic, causing fewer than ten deaths, but it was nevertheless terrifying for the White community, who felt helpless to combat it.[134] In other colonies, outbreaks of yellow fever had generated so much fear among colonial officials that they enacted segregation laws or demolished whole neighborhoods, as in the retreat to Hill Station in Sierra Leone and the "bataille des paillote" in Senegal.[135] In the Gold Coast, the same notions of racial hygiene were in place, but the government reaction was slow. Ironically, it was Dr. John Farrell Easmon, the colony's chief medical officer and the only African in a ranking position in the Medical Department, who stressed the need for segregation as a means of stopping the spread of the disease. Steeped in contemporary understandings of miasma, he described the old quarters of Accra as "a sink of filth"[136] and argued that White bodies had to be separated from any "native reservoirs" of disease because they were not racially adapted to the tropics. However, even in the face of epidemic yellow fever, Governors Maxwell and Hodgson demurred, believing that African residents would contest any efforts at segregation.

It was not until 1901, when Matthew Nathan arrived as the new governor of the colony, that the sanitary syndrome took hold again. Nathan was not known as an avid segregationist, but he quickly fell into step with the pattern of scapegoating Africans for poor sanitation, describing the old quarters of the city as a "virtual cesspool" inhabited by people who were "naturally dirty."[137] Feeling pressure from the terrified White minority of Accra, Nathan decided that keeping Europeans a healthy distance from African populations was the key to preserving the viability of a White ruling class in West Africa, and he began drawing up plans for a residential suburb for colonial officers and European merchants.[138] This was a convenient strategy for the new governor, who was loath to spend scarce resources on sanitation when it was so much easier to simply abandon the old city of Accra. To prevent infection from yellow fever–bearing mosquitoes, he established a quarter-mile sanitary cordon, the estimated flight range of a mosquito, between the White and Black populations of the city.[139] Just as in South Africa, where the government exiled Africans to suburbs because of the belief that they polluted cities with disease, Nathan employed racialized notions of sanitation to define healthy and unhealthy spaces. The difference in Accra was that segregation happened in reverse: the Africans stayed in their ancestral neighborhoods, while the Whites exiled themselves to the periphery of the city.[140]

As soon as the colonial office approved Nathan's proposal for a European reservation, the governor zoned a patch of land on high ground to the northeast of Ussher Town for two exclusively White neighborhoods, to be known as Victoriaborg and the Ridge.[141] It was not exactly a remote location, like the hill stations found in India or Sierra Leone. It was more like a slight incline, and anyone was allowed to come and go between two neighborhoods during the day. However, Africans were required to leave the European quarter by nightfall. On her first visit to the city, Decima Moore, the wife of the future governor of the colony,

Gordon Guggisberg, described the stark transition between the two parts of the newly segregated town:

> The native quarter, through which we first passed, was an unimposing ramshackle collection of weather-beaten white-washed houses and huts, with naked children playing about in front and often a man or woman sitting and working a sewing-machine in the doorways. Further on the broad red road was lined with traders' stores, some belonging to European firms and some to natives—the various signboards showing a most interesting and diverse variety of names, such as Miller Brothers, Swanzy's . . . The Basel Mission Store, and the Bank of British West Africa. . . . After running through the town for over half a mile our road led on some open plains and we entered Victoriaborg, the European Government quarter. We passed several large buildings—the Hospital Club, High Court, Secretariat, Treasury, and numerous cool looking bungalows occupied by Government officials.[142]

Moore's description of the transition between an African world of dilapidated buildings and a European landscape of colonial architecture vividly describes the way that Governor Nathan, within a matter of a few years, had transformed race into space.

When Governor Rodger arrived in 1903, he applauded the outgoing Nathan for his dedication to public health, celebrating the fact that the European death rate in the colony had been cut in half since the move from Accra to Victoriaborg.[143] But in hindsight, it is difficult to see how segregation actually improved the health of European employees. In the absence of passbooks and strict police control over the movement of people in the colony, Africans and Europeans continued to mingle, even in the evenings when the mosquitoes were out. It is more than likely that many Africans spent the night in the reservation and that many Europeans continued to stay overnight in their business lodgings. Nor did the presence of a ramshackle hospital help matters of health for Europeans. One might rather assert that the widespread availability of quinine did more to reduce the death rate in Accra than any other colonial venture.[144] If the medical regime of the new capital was an expression of bio-power, it was a feeble colonial version of what was happening in Europe and did not come close to the version of racial hygiene found in Southern or East Africa. Colonial medical practices and ideas had finally extended beyond the walls of the slave forts where they had been confined in the past, but they were far from pervasive. Resistance to the Town's Ordinance Act made it impossible to co-opt African urban residents into endeavors to sanitize the city, and the scuffle over filling the pond showed just how hard it was to send sanitary crews into the heart of Ussher Town. Ironically, the drive toward segregation exercised more control over Europeans than Africans. Although a discourse of racial hygiene implicated Africans as a reservoir of disease, the colonial government found that it was neither politically expedient nor financially prudent to implement a comprehensive regime of public health in Accra during the nineteenth century.

Interlude: The Bubonic Plague Epidemic of 1908

In 1907, dead rats started dropping from the grass roofs of buildings in Accra. Then livestock started to die mysteriously. By the end of the year, people were dying too, and rumors of poisoning were rampant.[145] The third pandemic of bubonic plague, which had killed approximately thirteen million people in China and India at the end of the nineteenth century, had finally arrived in West Africa.[146] At the time, no African or European therapy could cure the dreaded disease, and the fear of a calamity was palpable.

With Governor Rodger on furlough, the acting governor, Major H. Bryan of the Gold Coast Regiment, turned to the only physician in town who could coordinate a campaign to fight the disease: Dr. Quartey-Papafio. Despite prior grievances with the colonial regime, Quartey-Papafio agreed to help Bryan, probably out of a sense of loyalty to his city more than anything else. Dozens of people had already died, and panic was gripping the residents of Accra.[147] In January 1908, Major Bryan called a meeting of local dignitaries at Government House and soon found himself assailed by local chiefs demanding that he do something to halt the epidemic. Dr. Quartey-Papafio stepped forward to reassure the Ga leaders that the disease could be controlled, but only if they followed the orders of the government health officials. The chiefs were not convinced. They questioned Bryan about what sort of plague fighting tactics would be used. Since he did not yet have a plan, Bryan equivocated, telling them that such information could not be released until he received word from London. When they asked him if local African healers might be involved in the plague-fighting campaign, Dr. Quartey-Papafio again came to his aid, declaring that, since their own healers had no cure for the disease, they would not be of any use during the campaign.[148] On this point the colonial general and the African physician were in accord.

The meeting minutes explain that the chiefs left having "promised their loyal assistance," but their line of questioning indicates that they were concerned about the measures that Bryan might take to control the epidemic.[149] Their fears were not unfounded. Shortly after the meeting, Major Bryan formed a Sanitary Committee with the right to inspect any dwelling suspected to harbor plague, to demolish any house deemed infected, and to quarantine anyone who had contact with the disease.[150] The chiefs would no longer be consulted, and anyone who obstructed or interfered with the work of an appointed sanitary officer could be jailed or fined. The terror of the epidemic presented the colonial government with an unprecedented opportunity to transform the discourses of bio-power into practice.

When Major Bryan wired London to announce that the city was infected with bubonic plague, the secretary of state promptly dispatched their best plague fighter, Dr. William John

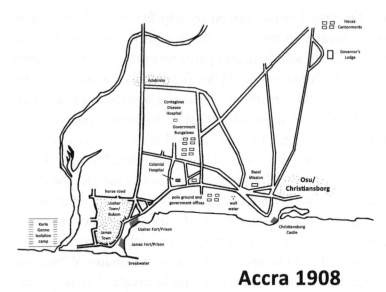

Accra 1908

Map 2.1. Map of Accra in 1908.

Ritchie Simpson. Simpson was a veteran of the British India Plague Commission, which had developed strategies to fight plague in Hong Kong and Calcutta. The commission had always been divided into two camps: biomedical experts who advocated for vaccination programs and public health reformers who argued for better sanitation. Simpson was a conservative member of the latter. He remained loyal to practices of quarantine and favored the demolition of infected neighborhoods. In 1901, while fighting plague in Cape Town, he had destroyed hundreds of infected dwellings and had isolated thousands of people in containment camps. The end result of his approach was the creation of African "locations" on marginal lands outside the city, an eerie precedent to the apartheid rule that would follow.[151]

After declaring victory over the plague in Cape Town, Simpson returned to London to write the *Treatise on Plague*, a field manual for colonial sanitation that contained a confusing mix of miasmatic and microbial etiologies. Simpson recognized that the bacteria that caused plague, *Yersinia pestis*, was transmitted by rat fleas, but he also argued that the disease could be spread through infected food, infected clothes, and cuts on the feet, betraying his pre-bacteriological beliefs about the putrefaction of decomposing matter in the soil.[152] Simpson did not necessarily distinguish between miasma and bacteria, because his practical concern was to take whatever measures necessary to prevent the spread of the disease. Notably absent from his book were methods for dealing with the complicated social issues that surrounded any plague-fighting campaign. For example, Simpson advocated burning infected dwellings to save the expense of fumigating them with sulfur, but he neglected to include advice about how to care for the people made homeless by such measures.[153]

Before Simpson arrived, the newly formed Sanitary Committee had already set to work fumigating infected houses and had attempted to demolish some dilapidated structures.[154] Their actions, however, were immediately halted by the threat of legal action by the owners. Failing to take control of the infected area, Major Bryan and Dr. Quartey-Papafio began to focus on isolating plague victims by conveying them under armed guard to the asylum in Victoriaborg, where they were forced to share space with mentally ill patients held in leg irons. Those who had made contact with the sick were also deemed contagious, so the police escorted them to a temporary isolation camp across the lagoon at Korle Gonno, on a piece of open land granted to the Sanitary Committee by Kojo Ababio, the chief of James Town. Isolating potential patients far from the urban core suited the Sanitary Committee, but Korle Gonno happened to be disputed territory. The chiefs of Ussher Town protested the actions of the wily Ababio, who had offered the land west of the lagoon as a means of making a claim on it for himself.[155] Tension over the contested land grew, and without enough police or sanitary officers, control over Korle Gonno was weak. Many so-called infected residents continued to sneak back into the town at night.[156]

When Simpson arrived in February, he brought with him a cargo hold full of plague-fighting equipment and a plan to demolish swathes of the old quarters of Accra. The Medical Department supported the initiative, hoping that with the help of Dr. Quartey-Papafio, they could win the support of the residents of Ussher Town.[157] Dr. Quartey-Papafio was born in Ussher Town, but Bryan and Simpson had overestimated his influence. When he led the Sanitary Committee into the neighborhood to destroy infected houses, the residents stoned him and forced his team to retreat. The colonial records claim that fetish priests spurred the people of Ussher Town to rebel, but the chiefs of Ussher Town, angered by the loss of Korle Gonno, may also have been complicit in the protests.[158] If it had been South Africa or French Africa, violent force might have been used to impose the rule of sanitation on the city, but at that point, Simpson paused. Rather than fight the locals, he waited for his order of twenty thousand doses of Haffkine's prophylactic to arrive. When it did, he began the largest mass inoculation campaign that British West Africa had ever seen.[159]

In May 1908, the Sanitary Committee opened four vaccination stations in the city with great fanfare. Simpson was the first to step onto the platform, brandishing a large needle filled with the serum, and Major Bryan and his wife were the first to be publicly injected. Dr. Quartey-Papafio and the Ga chiefs followed, taking the stand for their injections as a matter of public ceremony. Simpson must have been nervous at the time. During initial trials in India in 1902, Dr. Waldemar Haffkine's assistants had struggled to keep his serum pure, and the prophylactic had become contaminated with tetanus, resulting in the deaths of nineteen people.[160] To Simpson's relief, no one fell ill, and the residents of the city began to crowd the stations to receive the prophylaxis. Simpson would later state with pride that his team had inoculated over sixteen thousand people. This may have been an exaggeration, considering the population of the city stood at approximately fifteen thousand, but the numbers seemed to indicate that the inoculation campaign was a triumph for colonial medicine.[161]

Simpson believed that Haffkine's prophylactic was widely accepted because it prevented the spread of the disease, but this is hard to believe because the residents of Accra were not given enough time to see if it worked. It is more likely that the therapeutic act of piercing the skin was widely accepted simply because it was so similar to the ritual scarification that had always been used to inoculate patients against spiritual assault.[162] Furthermore, people in Accra may have understood Haffkine's prophylactic as a direct intervention against illnesses in the blood, a concept congruent with Ga etiological understandings of illnesses caused by spoiled or dirty internal fluids.[163] And finally, the practice of inoculation probably gained cultural momentum as the thing to do at the time. Getting the shot became normalized as part of the therapeutic culture of Accra, and Simpson noted that the demand for the prophylactic grew so dramatically that the Sanitary Committee established a new inoculation station where the well-heeled could pay two shillings to avoid the "'crush and delay" of the free stations. The Sanitary Committee inoculated approximately five hundred people at the pay-for-service station, making the bubonic plague epidemic a good example of how therapeutic choice could be a means of asserting one's social standing.[164] This is not, of course, to underestimate the fear of the plague that had spread through the city. It is also possible that people in Accra, White or Black, were so terrified of the disease that they would have accepted any medicine that promised immunity.

The apparent success of Simpson's inoculation campaign stands in sharp contrast to the failure of African healers to treat the plague. *Yersinia pestis* was not indigenous to West Africa, and therefore there was no specific African cure. African healers in the city

considered the plague so dangerous that they charged excep-
tionally high fees to treat it, making it popularly known as the
"one pound disease."[165] In one instance, a spirit medium marched
around the city beating a cowbell, declaring that she had made a
type of consecrated medicine to prevent the reoccurrence of the
plague. The next day, while distributing these medicinal charms
to Ga chiefs, she collapsed and died of the plague.[166] Not only
were healers dying from the disease, but they were also spreading
it. At some point during the epidemic, the plague appears to have
jumped from a bubonic stage, where persons could be infected
through the bite of the rat flea, to the pneumonic stage, where
persons could be infected via breath and sputum. There were several recorded cases of local healers dying from the disease within
a few days or less, which indicates that the illness had taken a
pneumonic form. Simpson feared that these healers would break
through the sanitary cordon, spreading the plague to all of the
towns and villages in the colony.

Yet as the year progressed, the number of cases began to dwindle. By December 1908, within almost a year of its arrival, Simpson declared Accra free of plague.[167] When the numbers were
compiled, 250 Africans had died, a number that a veteran like
Simpson would have regarded as negligible in comparison to his
previous battles against the disease.[168] And to Simpson's great de-
light, no Europeans were infected. Before he boarded a steamer
back to Liverpool, he once again tried to impress his ideas about
healthy living spaces upon the authorities of the Gold Coast, urg-
ing the Medical Department to demolish African dwellings and
build broad boulevards through Ussher Town and James Town.
The next year, the colonial government followed his advice by
increasing the Public Works budget for sanitary improvements,
which resulted in a brief flurry of activity that included the laying
of a few new streets, the construction of some rat-proof housing
at Korle Gonno and Adabraka, and some new equipment for the
Accra Laboratory.[169] The government also developed a long-term

plan for the construction of a reservoir to supply drinking water to the city, at the projected expense of £140,000. But there was never any plan to rebuild Accra. As Major Bryan, Dr. Quartey-Papafio, and the Sanitary Committee had learned, the residents of the city were not willing to go along with an urban plan that would displace them from their ancestral homes. Even the small amount of work completed after the plague epidemic required expensive compensation for people dislocated from Ussher Town, as well as the onerous construction of new dwellings on contested land. By the end of 1909, Simpson's dream of sanitizing the capital city had faded away, and Governor Rodger had already begun to divert colonial revenues toward the construction of a railroad to Kumasi.[170] Ga memories of the event faded quickly, remaining only in the talismanic presence of a medal of honor, given for loyal (and opportunistic) cooperation during the pandemic, in the house of former chief Kojo Ababio at Korle Gonno.[171] The sanitation syndrome, it seemed, had come and gone.

NOTES

1. Patterson, *Health in Colonial Ghana*, 30, 11; Addae, *Evolution of Modern Medicine*, 55.

2. Foucault, *History of Sexuality*, 1:140.

3. Bala, *Biomedicine as a Contested Site*, 2; Vaughan, *Curing Their Ills*; Swanson, "Sanitation Syndrome," 399; Butchart, *Anatomy of Power*, ix.

4. Gale, "Struggle against Disease"; Ryan Johnson, "West African Medical Staff."

5. Ronald Robinson, "European Imperialism and Indigenous Reactions in British West Africa, 1880–1914," in *Expansion and Reaction: Essays on European Expansion and Reaction in Asia and Africa*, ed. H. L. Wesseling (Leiden: Leiden University Press, 1978), 163.

6. Janzen, *Quest for Therapy*, xviii, 8–11.

7. Public Records and Archives Administration Department (PRAAD), SCT 2/4/12. May 5, 1877–May 28, 1879, 92.

8. PRAAD SCT 2/4/57. February 16, 1912–September 19, 1914. "Lutterodt vrs Amartefio," January 10, 1914, 115–16.

9. In another case, a man who had passed away was said to have taken "native medicines" from at least two healers. PRAAD SCT 2/4/1. January 6, 1857–May 15, 1861. May 21, 1858, 112–13.

10. PRAAD SCT 2/4/2. May 15, 1861–February 10, 1864. May 21, 1861, 16.

11. PRAAD SCT 2/4/18. September 29, 1892–January 15, 1894. "Afia Aba vrs Dodoo," October 10, 1892, 95–111.

12. PRAAD SCT 2/4/12. May 5, 1877–May 28, 1879. "Chief Labetia Allotey and Korkor vrs Police," October 12, 1877, 226; PRAAD SCT 2/4/25. March 25, 1897–August 30, 1897. "Ama Aku vrs Peter Martin Yoroahie (illeg.)," August 5, 1897, 577–79.

13. SCT 2/4/11. October 19, 1874, 125.

14. PRAAD SCT 2/4/2. May 15, 1861–February 10, 1864. May 15, 1861, 5–7.

15. PRAAD SCT 2/4/5. June 23, 1868–August 3, 1869, 453–55.

16. Field, *Religion and Medicine*, 161–84; Bentum, interview with the author, June 17, 2003; Tsofatse Thunder, interview with the author, June 6, 2006; Joyce Ayile Quaye, interview with the author, June 18, 2003.

17. PRAAD SCT 2/4/11. July 31, 1874–June 18, 1875. November 24, 1874, 177–79.

18. PRAAD SCT 2/4/2. May 15, 1861–February 10, 1864. May 15, 1861, 15; see also PRAAD SCT 2/4/2. May 15, 1861–February 10, 1864. March 31, 1862, 323.

19. PRAAD SCT 2/4/31. "Larson versus Bruce," May 10, 1900, 377.

20. Parker, "Witchcraft, Anti-witchcraft."

21. Daniell, "On the Ethnography of Akkrah," 13.

22. Daniell, "On the Ethnography of Akkrah," 13.

23. John Parker, "Mankraloi, Merchants & Mulattos: Carl Reindorf and the Politics of 'Race' in Early Colonial Accra," in *The Recovery of the West African Past: African Pastors and African History in the 19th Century, C. C. Reindorf and Samuel Johnson*, ed. Paul Jenkins (Basel: Baseler Africka Bibliographien, 1998), 41. Another case involving an abortifacient can be found in PRAAD SCT 2/4/18. July 28, 1891–September 28, 1892, 329–33.

24. Sakumo Wulomo, interview with the author, November 17, 2002.

25. SCT 2/4/31. "Larson versus Bruce," May 10, 1900, 369–98.

26. Another case of an herbalist defending himself in a colonial court can be found in PRAAD SCT 2/4/1. "Barker versus Annang," April 13, 1858, 98.

27. PRAAD SCT 2/4/10. October 22, 1872–July 31, 1874. "Theodore Willif versus John A. Swaniker," December 10, 1872, 85.

28. This estimate is made by comparing the CPI and the average daily wage as calculated on http://measuringworth.com/calculators /uscompare, a cliometric currency calculation service established by Lawrence H. Officer of the University of Illinois and Samuel H. Williamson of Miami University. The dollars were most likely Liberian dollars, which were pegged to the value of the US dollar.

29. PRAAD SCT 2/4/12. May 5, 1877–May 28, 1879. "The Queen against [illegible]," December 4, 1877, 361–62.

30. PRAAD SCT 2/4/12. May 5, 1877–May 28, 1879. "The Queen against [illegible]," December 4, 1877, 353. Even Commey's brother, who was also questioned during the trial, admitted that he did not know what sorts of medicines the *tsofatse* had used on his brother.

31. PRAAD SCT.2.4.12. May 5, 1877–May 28, 1879. "The Queen against [illegible]," 353, 356, 360–62. The original appeared clustered as one paragraph, without Q or A to distinguish between the responses. I have altered the passage to make it easier to read.

32. Hepper, *West African Herbaria*, 30.

33. Rømer, *Reliable Account of the Coast of Guinea*, 28, 171.

34. De Marees, *Gold Kingdom of Guinea*, 173.

35. Rømer, *Reliable Account of the Coast of Guinea*, 99.

36. Mary Esther Kropp Dakubu notes only a few contributions from Arabic to the Ga language, suggesting that terms like *shika* and *klamo* might have Arabic (perhaps via Mande) roots. Dakubu, *Korle Meets the Sea*, 141; Dakubu, *Ga-English Dictionary*, 81, 144.

37. Wisnes, *Letters on West Africa and the Slave Trade*, 132.

38. Pellow, "Power of Space," 424; Dupuis, *Journal of a Residence in Ashantee*, 72–75, 94–98, 178–80; see also Maier, "Nineteenth-Century Asante Medical Practices," 79; Silverman and Owusu-Ansah, "Presence of Islam," 325–39.

39. David Owusu-Ansah, "Prayers, Amulets and Healing," in *The History of Islam in Africa*, ed. Nehemia Levtzion and Randall L. Pouwels (Athens: Ohio University Press, 2000), 482.

40. Wilks, *Asante in the Nineteenth Century*, 257. For an example of a description of one of these amulets, see Taylor, "An Arabic Amulet."

41. "Copy of a Dispatch from Lieutenant-Colonel Purdon to the Earl of Bathurst, Colonial Records, no. 267," in *Records Relating to the Gold Coast Settlements from 1750 to 1874*, ed. J.J. Crooks (Dublin: Browne & Nolan, 1923), 232–33.

42. Owusu-Ansah, "Islamic Influence in a Forest Kingdom," 100.

43. Dakubu, *Korle Meets the Sea*, 134–35.

44. Spelling from Dakubu, *Ga-English Dictionary*, 76.

45. Odoom, "Document on Pioneers," 3; Sulemana Mumuni, "A Survey of Islamic Non-governmental Organizations in Accra," in *Social Welfare in Muslim Societies in Accra*, ed. Holger Weiss (Uppsala: Nordic Africa Institute, 2002), 140.

46. Mumuni, "Islamic Non-governmental Organizations," 141.

47. *Gold Coast Census*, 1891. Sulemana Mumuni notes that the first Ga man (Kwashi Solomon) converted to Islam around 1900; see "Islamic Non-governmental Organizations," 142.

48. Mumuni, "Islamic Non-governmental Organizations," 143.

49. Pellow, "Power of Space," 436. Stock notes that Hausa healers were found throughout West Africa and throughout the Sahel in the twentieth century, practicing therapies derived from the Quran (like *rubutu*—"slate washing") as well as minor surgery and divination. See Stock, "Traditional Healers in Rural Hausaland," 363–68; Abdalla, "Islamic Medicine and Its Influence," 89.

50. Peel, *Making of the Yoruba*, 198–99.

51. Amos and Ayesu, "'I Am Brazilian,'" 41.

52. *Governor Carstensen's Diary*.

53. Amos and Ayesu, "'I Am Brazilian,'" 45–46.

54. Pellow, "Muslim Segmentation," 419.

55. Adam Mohr, "Missionary Medicine," 435–36.

56. Mohr, "Missionary Medicine," 452.

57. Carl Christian Reindorf, *History of the Gold Coast*, 10, 13.

58. Carl Christian Reindorf, *History of the Gold Coast*, 15.

59. Jean Comaroff, "The Diseased Heart of Africa: Medicine, Colonialism, and the Black Body," in *Knowledge, Power, and Practice: The Anthropology of Medicine and Everyday Life*, ed. Shirley Lindenbaum and Margaret Lock (Berkeley: University of California Press, 1997); Comaroff and Comaroff, *Of Revelation and Revolution*; Landau, *Realm of the Word*; Hunt, *Colonial Lexicon*; Derek R. Peterson, "Gambling with God: Rethinking Religion in Colonial Central Kenya," in *The Invention of Religion: Rethinking Belief in Politics and History*, ed. Derek R. Peterson and Darren R. Walhof (New Brunswick, NJ: Rutgers University Press, 2002), 35–58.

60. Noel Smith, *Presbyterian Church of Ghana*, 55.

61. Wisnes, *Letters on West Africa and the Slave Trade*, 128.

62. Dakubu, *Ga-English Dictionary*, 94, 109.

63. By comparing and analyzing the sermons and publications of several famous charismatic pastors in the 1990s, Paul Gifford showed that references to increasing success and health were prominent, as were corresponding promises that the Holy Spirit could remove blockages. Gifford, *Ghana's New Christianity*, 46.

64. Meyer demonstrates the confusion wrought by debates about whether Jesus was an Ewe ancestral spirit. See Meyer, *Translating the Devil*, 78–79.

65. Zimmerman, *Grammatical Sketch*.

66. Jon Miller, *Missionary Zeal and Institutional Control*.

67. Peel, *Making of the Yoruba*, 222.

68. Basel Mission Archives, C-10.56.02, "The use of 'Salicylpulver' [Salicylic Acid = active ingredient in aspirin] as medicine for fever," MSS notes in German, author unknown, August 25, 1875.

69. Comaroff and Comaroff, *Of Revelation and Revolution*, 1:222; Allman, *Fashioning Africa*, 4–6; Joanne B. Eicher and Tonye V. Erekosima, "Why Do They Call It Kalabari? Cultural Authentication and the Demarcation of Ethnic Identity," in *Dress and Ethnicity: Change across Space and Time*, ed. Joanne B. Eicher (Washington, DC: Berg, 1995), 147–49; Akyeampong, *Drink, Power, and Cultural Change*, 44–45; van den Bersselaar, *King of Drinks*, 38–65.

70. Rocco, *Quinine*, 182.

71. Curtin, *Disease and Empire*, 21. There was a 30% mortality rate and an 80% morbidity rate from malaria.

72. Headrick, *Tools of Empire*, 68.

73. Curtin, *Disease and Empire*, 60–70.

74. Kemp, *Nine Years at the Gold Coast*, 37–40.

75. Rocco, *Quinine*, 250–80.

76. "Quininism," *Lancet* (January 13, 1838), 550–51.

77. Kemp, *Nine Years at the Gold Coast*, 37–40.

78. Dumett, "John Sarbah, the Elder"; Dumett, "African Merchants of the Gold Coast."

79. Chlorodyne was a mix of alcohol, chloroform, morphine, marijuana, and other trace vegetable elements. See Hale-White, *Materia Medica*, 280; Chlorodyne was recommended as an essential medicine for colonial officials in Great Britain, 43–45.

80. Burton and Cameron, *To the Gold Coast for Gold*, 231–32.

81. Warburg's Tincture contained rhubarb, saffron, fennel, myrrh, camphor, and angelica seeds, as well as nine grains of quinine added per ounce.

American Journal of Pharmacy 49 (1877): 269–71; Burton and Cameron, *To the Gold Coast for Gold*, 231–32.

82. Burton and Cameron, *To the Gold Coast for Gold*, 232.

83. Kemp, *Nine Years at the Gold Coast*, 37–40.

84. James Wilding, "Toxic Effects of Ten Grains of Antifebrin," *British Medical Journal* 2, no. 1498 (1889): 600–1.

85. DeCourse, *Archeology of Elmina*, 148; Stuart, *Dangerous Garden*, 67; *Gold Coast News*, April 25, 1885, in Dumett, "John Sarbah, the Elder," 673.

86. *Gold Coast News*, April 25, 1885, in Dumett, "John Sarbah, the Elder," 673.

87. Dover's Powder contained ipecacuanha and opium; Easton's Syrup was a mixture of strychnine, iron phosphate, and quinine; and Livingston Rouser was a recipe attributed to David Livingstone that probably contained quinine. See Ryan Johnson, "Tabloid Brand Medicine Chests"; *Extra Pharmacopoeia Martindale*, 1:812.

88. Kemp, *Nine Years at the Gold Coast*, 213–15, 223.

89. *Gold Coast Colony Blue Book* (Accra, Ghana: Government Printer, 1901)

90. Cardinall, *Gold Coast*, 158.

91. Kuczynski, *Demographic Survey*, 1:472.

92. Crellin, *Social History of Medicines*, 73.

93. Van den Bersselaar, *King of Drinks*, 179.

94. Van den Bersselaar, *King of Drinks*, 205.

95. Van den Bersselaar, *King of Drinks*, 205.

96. Dumett, "John Sarbah, the Elder," 673.

97. Jones-Quartey, "Gold Coast Press."

98. Newell, *Power to Name*, 44–61.

99. "Public Health Bill, 1875," 450; Swinson, *History of Public Health*, 71; Rosen, *History of Public Health*, 208.

100. Metcalfe, *Great Britain and Ghana*, 365, from speech by Earl of Carnarvon. House of Lords, May 12, 1874, reprinted in the *Times* (London), May 13, 1874.

101. Kuczynski, *Demographic Survey*, 365; Gale, "Struggle against Disease," 187.

102. Ngalamulume, "Keeping the City Clean"; Echenberg, *Black Death*.

103. Cherry, *Medical Services*, 41–49. See also, more generally, Foucault, *Birth of the Clinic*.

104. Swinson, *History of Public Health*, 67; Rosen, *History of Public Health*, 289; Foucault, *Birth of the Clinic*; Terry Johnson, *Health Professions*.

105. Echenberg, *Black Death*, 4.

106. *Korle Bu Hospital, 1923–1973,* 46.

107. For information concerning the Lutterodt family, see Tutu, "Asafoi," 100.

108. PRAAD ADM 5.4.12. "Gold Coast Hospital. Accra. Opening Ceremony by His Excellency Brig. Gen. Sir Frederick Gordon Guggisberg, K.C.M.G. D.S.O., R.E.," October 9, 1923, 5; *Korle Bu Hospital, 1923–1973,* 14.

109. American Colonization Society, *Liberia (Bulletin)* 1 (November 1892): 83.

110. "A Nurse Arriving on the Coast in the Good Old Days," an anecdote by an unnamed nurse (initials M. B.), in *Our Days on the Gold Coast,* Lady Clifford [Mrs. Henry de la Pasture, pseud.] (London: John Murray, 1919), 43.

111. Clifford, *Our Days on the Gold Coast,* 127.

112. Patterson, *Health in Colonial Ghana,* 19.

113. Kuczynski, *Demographic Survey,* 479.

114. *Korle Bu Hospital, 1923–1973,* 46.

115. Gold Coast Colony, *Gold Coast Handbook* (Accra, Ghana: Government Press, 1923), 350; Patterson, *Health in Colonial Ghana,* 19. Although there is no paper trail of "doctor's notes" from the early years of hospitals in the city, Twumasi conjectures that African employees were required to go to European hospitals to get health certificates to prove they were sick. See Twumasi, "Colonialism and International Health," 148.

116. Kilson, *Diary of Kwaku Niri,* 28, 36.

117. *Gold Coast Colony Blue Book* (Accra, Ghana: Government Printer, 1891), A12.

118. Clifford, *Our Days on the Gold Coast,* 127–28.

119. Patton, *Physicians, Colonial Racism,* 103; Patton, "Dr. John Farrell Easmon," 611.

120. Haynes, *Imperial Medicine,* 138–40.

121. For a biography of Dr. B. W. Quartey-Papafio, see Sampson, *Gold Coast Men of Affairs,* 202–5.

122. Terence Johnson, "Imperialism and the Professions," 288.

123. Arnold, *Colonizing the Body*; Bala, *Biomedicine as a Contested Site.*

124. Dr. Matthew Arnum Barnor, interview with the author, August 29, 2003. Dr. Quartey-Papafio wrote his slogan in Twi because the language was common in the city by that time and because he needed to attract new clients from outside the Ga community.

125. Patton, "Dr. John Farrell Easmon," 618.

126. Daniell, "On the Ethnography of Akkrah," 23.

127. Stanley and Prior, *Coomassie and Magdala*, 77–79.

128. *Gold Coast Colony Blue Book* (Accra, Ghana: Government Printer, 1883).

129. *Gold Coast Echo*, March 9, 1889, 3.

130. Samuel S. Quarcoopome, "Impact of Urbanization," 95–97; *Gold Coast Colony Blue Book* (Accra: Government Printer, 1908), L1, H2.

131. Gale, "Struggle against Disease," 195.

132. Gale, "Struggle against Disease," 196.

133. Patterson, "Health in Urban Ghana," 252.

134. Boyce, "Distribution and Prevalence."

135. Ngalamulume, "Keeping The City Clean," 190; Georg, *Pouvoir Colonial, Municipalites et Espaces Urbains*, 177–79.

136. Wright, *Politics of Design*, 266; Patterson, "Health in Urban Ghana," 252.

137. Gold Coast Government, *Annual Report on the Gold Coast* (1898), 27.

138. Boatens, *Geography of Ghana*, 5; Patterson, "Health in Urban Ghana," 252; Dumett, "Campaign against Malaria," 171. Nathan's opinions were in accord with those of S. R. Christophers and J. W. W. Stephens, two malariologists from the Liverpool School of Tropical Medicine, who had argued in 1900 that "to stamp out native malaria is at present chimerical, and every effort should rather be turned to the protection of Europeans." See Christophers and Stephens, "Destruction of Anopheles in Lagos," 19.

139. Dumett, "Campaign against Malaria," 171–72.

140. Butchart, *Anatomy of Power*, 128–29; Swanson, "Sanitation Syndrome," 399.

141. Boyle, *Diary of a Colonial Officer's Wife*, 152.

142. Moore and Guggisberg, *We Two in West Africa*, 45–46. This account is from 1908.

143. Gale, "Struggle against Disease," 198.

144. Gale, "Struggle against Disease," 198. By the turn of the century, the suggested prophylactic dose for quinine was four to five grains taken in tonic water, while the suggested cure was ten to thirty grains at once. See "Cinchona," in *Encyclopaedia Britannica*, 369–70.

145. Simpson, "Statement on the Outbreak of Plague," 606.

146. Echenberg, *Black Death*, 16.

147. Simpson, *Treatise on Plague*, 15.

148. PRAAD ADM 11/1/1747, "The Acting Governor to the Secretary of State," February 7, 1908, 24.

149. PRAAD ADM 11/1/1747, "The Acting Governor to the Secretary of State," February 7, 1908, 24.

150. PRAAD ADM 11/1/1747, Correspondence, Executive Council, Order in Council, January 11, 1908, 27–28; PRAAD Gold Coast Government, "Infectious Diseases Ordinance, 1908," *Government Gazette*, March 25, 1908, 273.

151. Van Heyningen, "Cape Town and the Plague of 1901," 72.

152. Simpson, *Treatise on Plague*, 381.

153. Simpson, *Treatise on Plague*, 360, 381.

154. PRAAD ADM 11/1/1747, "Executive Council. Memoranda of Action Taken," January 11, 1908, 29–30; PRAAD ADM 11/1/1747, "Acting Governor to Secretary of State. Enclosure 3," February 22, 1908, 87.

155. PRAAD ADM 11/1/1747. "Acting Governor to the Secretary of State," January 21 and February 22, 1908, 52. The British favored Ababio because he was literate (educated at the Methodist School) and because he supported the Asante Expedition of 1895–96 by providing 1,400 men as carriers. See Gocking, *Facing Two Ways*, 119.

156. PRAAD ADM 11/1/1747, "Acting Governor to the Secretary of State," March 16, 1908, 79.

157. Patterson, *Health in Colonial Ghana*, 48.

158. PRAAD ADM 11/1/1747, "Acting Governor to the Secretary of State," March 16, 1908, 79; PRAAD ADM 11/1/1747, "Medical Department Report," June 5, 1908, 153.

159. *Ordinances of the Gold Coast Colony*, 518; Ashitey, *Epidemiology of Disease Control in Ghana*, 4; Patterson, *Health in Colonial Ghana*, 70.

160. Ronald Ross, "Inoculation Accident at Mulkowal," 486.

161. Simpson, "Statement on the Outbreak of Plague," 608; PRAAD ADM 11/1/1747, "Acting Governor to the Secretary of State," February 22 and February 29, 1908, 57; PRAAD ADM 11/1/1747, "Third and Final Report of the Committee of Public Health," May 19, 1908, 169; PRAAD ADM 11/1/1747, "Minutes of a Meeting of the Committee of Public Health," April 17, 1908, 140.

162. Simpson, *Report on Plague in the Gold Coast*, 33–34.

163. Senah, *Money Be Man*, 161.

164. PRAAD ADM 11/1/1747, "Acting Governor to Secretary of State," February 29 and March 7, 1908, 58, 73.

165. Simpson, *Treatise on Plague*, 15.

166. PRAAD ADM 11/1/1747, "Meeting of the Committee of Public Health," July 30, 1908, 203. At least three other priests or healers were

known to have died, but no accurate statistics were taken. See PRAAD ADM 11/1/1747, "Report on the Fourth Outbreak of Plague in Accra," September 4, 1908, 228.

167. Simpson, "Statement on the Outbreak of Plague," 191.

168. Simpson, "Statement on the Outbreak of Plague," 191.

169. Kilson, *African Urban Kinsmen*, 8; *Gold Coast Colony Blue Book* (Accra: Government Printer, 1909), K3; Ashitey, *Epidemiology of Disease Control in Ghana*, 7.

170. Gold Coast Government, "Minutes of Legislative Council, June 6, 1908," *Government Gazette*, June 6, 1908, 515.

171. Kojo Ababio V. Korle Gonno, interview, Accra, Ghana, April 10, 1996.

THREE

THERAPEUTIC PLURALISM DURING
THE COCOA BOOM, 1908–1930s

AT THE START OF THE twentieth century, European demand
for cocoa increased dramatically, transforming the Gold Coast
into the wealthiest colony in tropical Africa.[1] The port city of
Accra, previously characterized as an "old-fashioned hap-hazard
sort-of-place," suddenly became a bustling transshipment point
for imports and exports, bringing in hundreds of workers from
around West Africa and from Europe.[2] The population grew exponentially, from a stagnant twenty thousand in 1910 to a vibrant
and diverse sixty thousand by the 1930s.[3] The changes wrought
by the cocoa boom emboldened government officials bent on imposing public health reforms, and in many respects medicine and
sanitation finally began to serve the British as a tool of colonization.[4] What had once been aspirational rhetoric in the reports
of medical officers was now normalized as a means of surveying
and controlling the biological processes of the subjects of the
Gold Coast. As in the settler colonies of Southern and East Africa, where an early movement toward the sanitation syndrome
began, and in French West Africa where new regimes of *mise en
valeur* were established on the basis of sanitary measures,[5] a new
type of bio-power was ascendant in British Africa, where the
will to control the subject population with measures of medical

coercion was now bulwarked by a higher degree of medical efficacy. No longer was Western medicine an external force to be imposed on the subject population; rather, the residents of Accra actually sought out some therapies offered by the colonial medical system because they promised cures that could not be found elsewhere.

However, telling the story of the expansion of colonial medical practices alone would obscure the depth of the changes occurring within other healing traditions during the cocoa boom. The world of African therapeutics still dominated, and details about the myriad of healing practices in the city were recorded in a series of studies by English anthropologist Margaret Field during the 1920s and 1930s. Field's comprehensive ethnography offers a wealth of detail about the daily lives of healers and patients as they sought out cures for both bodily and spiritual illness. Field tried to distill Ga healing culture down to a set of ethnic precepts, but at the same time she unwittingly offered evidence of the rapid change caused by the arrival of new healing traditions in the city.

Also in ascendance at this time were Christian and Islamic healing practices, though the sources describing their growth during this period are slim. The least well known, but perhaps the most dramatic, change in the healing culture of Accra during the early twentieth century occurred in the city's markets and shops. The rapid expansion of demand for patent medicines, or what became known in Ga as *blofo tsofa* (White man's medicine), created opportunities for patients to privately self-medicate or, if they chose, to define their medical selves in public by purchasing and consuming imported goods. So ubiquitous were patent medicines that they started to take on local meanings as patients appropriated them on local terms. Thus, despite the growing power of Western medicine, the residents of Accra remained largely free to seek out multiple forms of healing, sometimes combining seemingly incompatible disease etiologies and healing practices.

PLURALISM PAST AND PLURALISM PRESENT IN MARGARET FIELD'S *RELIGION AND MEDICINE OF THE GĀ PEOPLE*

Despite the immediate ravages of bubonic plague on the indigenous healing system, the epidemic of 1908 did little to displace domination of African healing cultures in Accra. Priests, spirit mediums, and herbalists continued to minister to most of the needs of the sick in the city, though their methods and backgrounds were becoming more diverse. The strongest evidence of the vibrancy of African healing comes from a broad study conducted by anthropologist Margaret Field, which showed that, even after centuries of contact with Europeans, the *wulomei*, *wontsemei*, and *tsofatsemei* of Accra were prospering by offering a wide variety of religious and health services. Field spent years searching for authentic African healing practices, and she enumerated a dogma of Ga healing precepts that is immensely valuable for understanding quests for therapy in the early twentieth century. However, in her effort to adhere to an antisyncretic approach, she inadvertently betrayed the composite nature of indigenous healing customs and hinted at the ways that patients were adopting ideas and practices from around West Africa and Europe.

Margaret Field moved to the Gold Coast in the late 1920s to take a position as an instructor at Achimota College, and during her time in Accra, she took an interest in Ga culture and language. She began to attend and record religious ceremonies along the coast, from Tema to Accra, and after several years of participating in the cultural life of Ga priests and healers, she returned to England to work on a dissertation at the London School of Economics (LSE). The result was her first monograph, *Religion and Medicine of the Gā People*, published in 1937. With her credentials in hand, she returned to Accra and received a promotion to the role of government anthropologist, succeeding R. S. Rattray, an anthropologist of the Asante who had trained at the LSE before her. Field followed her first publication with a more structuralist account of Ga society, the *Social Organization of the Gā People*, and wrote several articles and books about the Akan peoples to the north of the city, but she will always be best known for the rich description of the lives of the priests and healers in *Religion and Medicine of the Gā People*.

As a member of a new British school of anthropology that sought to describe non-Western cultures on their own terms, Margaret Field saw herself as following in the footsteps of esteemed scholars like Bronislaw Malinowski, Meyer Fortes, and E. E. Evans-Pritchard.[6] However, as a woman in a male-dominated field, she was subject to overt and jarring sexism. When Field published *Religion and Medicine* in 1937, Fortes and Evans-Pritchard dismissed the book as "amateur science," referring to the author as "Miss Field" rather than using her appropriate title of doctor. They also suggested that she had been too "independent" because she had not consulted enough with the major scholars in her discipline.[7] Nonetheless, she continued her quest to understand the non-Western mind, which she analyzed through the lens of the burgeoning discipline of psychology. Today, Margaret Field's ethnographies of the Ga might be dismissed for positioning Ga society within the trope of the ethnographic present, or for playing loosely with Freudian theories of personality, but at the time they were understood as progressive contributions to the social sciences. For historians today, they offer a trove of detail about health and healing in the colonial capital of Accra.[8]

Margaret Field stated clearly in her work that it was her goal to reveal the "invisible roots of life" of the Ga people.[9] This was her way of aligning her work with the broader project of anthropology in the early twentieth century, which was supposed to make sense of the particular cultural idioms of each ethnicity. But one might wonder if her informants were really forthcoming in a way that offered her the deep sort of knowledge she wanted. Considering that her work relied heavily on confidants from the village of Tema (to the east of Accra), one might ask whether much of Field's work is conjecture based on sparse sources.[10] But if we judge her work by comparing it to contemporaneous court records, Field's depiction of the African healing traditions of Accra was not a contrivance. Many of the practices she described—including the use of therapy management groups and the movement of patients between multiple healers—correlate directly with evidence brought forward by people in the colonial courtroom. Additionally, the use of spirit possession, animal sacrifice, libations of alcohol, inoculation with *ti*, trials-by-ordeal, and consecrated oath devices all appear anecdotally in trials during the same time that Field was doing her research.[11] In other words, Field's earnest assertion that African healing traditions were alive and well in Accra at the start of the twentieth century was absolutely true. Not only that, but Ga healing practices showed remarkable continuity with evidence from previous centuries.

But though Margaret Field remained fixed on revealing the underlying principles of Ga healing, she also understood that Ga healing culture was a composite of disease etiologies (including the hybrid Ga/Akan concepts of the body, the soul, and witchcraft); healing practices (including local practitioners and healers from distant regions); and material cultures (including local and imported herbs and charms).[12] She wanted to show how Ga religion and healing—or as she termed it, the "true *Ga* life"—ran "amazingly strong and deep," and to do so she spent much of her time demonstrating a cultural cohesion between Ga ritualists and their followers. But she also described Accra society as an "intricate tangle of fragments of tribes and families" who demonstrated respect for differences in one another's religious cultures.[13] This toleration, Field admitted, was correspondingly extended to "other people's medicines," both to professional healers and the average patient. One Ga healer who was particularly close to Field, a spirit medium named Boi Bi Boi, informed her that he had collected his healing powers from as far afield as Liberia, the

Ivory Coast, and Dahomey.[14] Field also described her encounters with many non-Ga healers who imported deities, trafficked in water spirits, made alliances with invisible dwarves, and practiced the occult art of conjuring.[15] In particular, Field highlighted the spread of Nana Tongo, a witch-finding deity from the Tongo Hills in the Northern Territories of the Gold Coast Colony. Pilgrims to the shrine of Nana Tongo could purchase the power of the deity for a hefty fee and relocate the witch-finding god to their own community.[16] It is somewhat ironic that, in her attempt to delineate the fundamental components of Ga religion, Field was compelled to describe the plurality of non-Ga deities, practices, and medicines present in the city.

In order to sustain her argument that the inhabitants of the city were imbued with a robust Ga cultural identity, Field overtly played down any mixing with Christian and Islamic ideas and practices. Islam is silenced entirely in her work, a surprising omission considering that the Muslim population numbered in the hundreds during her tenure on the Gold Coast, including a substantial minority of Ga Muslim converts. She also tried to argue that the isolation of the Basel Mission had left the Ga culture of Osu intact, but in other parts of the book, she leaked out evidence that Ga Christians were still very much involved in Ga healing practices.[17] Field stated that the Christians of Accra were inveterate polytheists, tolerating the existence of other deities and spirits. "A Ga Christian," according to Field, "may believe that the ways of the heathen gods are bad, but he does not believe that there are no heathen gods."[18] She also mentioned the case of a churchgoer who had an attack of hysteria and was later diagnosed by a Ga spirit medium as being possessed by a local god.[19] Field's attitude here is patronizing, as she denies African Christians the possibility of a Pauline conversion, but the implication is that African patients in Accra continued to hold a pluralistic attitude toward healing, even within Christian congregations.

As an anthropologist of the British school, Field tried to read through European influences on African culture as much as possible to root out the core of a Ga primordial identity, but, in doing so, she often revealed the changes wrought by colonialism. In one breath, she admitted that the activities of the Gold Coast Sanitation, Medical, and Health Departments were extensive enough to reach into the lives of most of the inhabitants of the city. In another, she denied that the principles of sanitation could be comprehensible to the Ga. To try to close this circle, Field argued that the activities of the Medical Department had changed Accra but that they were misunderstood by the Ga as the actions of a bungling new deity known as *"Gov'ment"*:

> Among the great invisible gods who hold Ga prosperity in their hands has come a new, great, invisible god of less calculable and less tolerant quality, namely 'Gov'ment'. From his fabulously wealthy, heavenly home across the water he sends his gifts and his emissaries. . . . He is not tolerant: he quite deliberately destroys the holy places and hinders the vital rites of older gods. He is illogical: he does not build the new town latrine in place of the old latrine, but in place of the sacred grove. He has little idea of right and wrong, and cannot tell the difference between good people and bad.[20]

Field does not cover the disputes between this new god of *"Gov'ment"* and the older deities of the town in detail, but they would have been evident in the work of latrine crews, gutter cleaners, market inspectors, and dogcatchers. She claimed that even the sanitary inspectors who searched for mosquito larvae in the compounds of urban residents were understood to be emissaries of this new god.

Did anyone in Accra really think of colonial officials as part of a new godly complex? Probably not. There is no evidence that *Gov'ment* was ever elevated to the status of a deity—no shrines, no possessed mediums, and no songs related to *Gov'ment* appear in the historical record. Moreover, Field contradicts herself by claiming that the "general attitude of the people towards the fundamental needs of life" was unchanged by colonial interventions.[21] As an example, she provided a vignette describing a fully qualified and experienced dresser at the Gold Coast Hospital who, in the morning, would diligently treat patients according to European medical standards and then in the evening meet the patient outside the hospital to "recommend to him a medicine-man of a village ten miles away."[22] She intended to portray the shallowness of colonial medicine and the depth of Ga healing culture, but the passage also reveals that the residents of Accra found it easy to move back and forth between European-derived and African-derived therapeutic frameworks.

Field also offered glimpses into how lay remedies and imported medicines were produced in the homes of people in Accra. Her section on "Herbs in the Home" was intended as a description of the local herbaria, and it did include information about the use of common herbs. However, what is most intriguing about this section of her book is that it refers to imported medical equipment and drugs. While talking about the application of herbal remedies, she briefly mentioned that "enemas are in great favor and give much pleasure—in fact no single imported article can have given more joy than the enema syringe."[23] The mention of the syringe was likely added simply to get a chuckle out of her readers, but it hints at how imported medical tools were being used in conjunction with traditional herbal remedies. Field also noted a growing market for patent medicines when, as an aside, she derided patients who spent "money on such things as 'Brain and Memory Pills'," a reference to dubious imported nostrums advertised in newspapers.[24] By poking fun at African patients, perhaps to the point of insult, she revealed that they were experimenting with therapies beyond the purview of established traditions. The group of consumers that she described may have been a minority in the city, but they were a growing one, and they represented a new generation of urbanites who were comfortable with the new material culture of imported medicines.

COLONIAL MEDICINE AND THE SPECTER OF BIO-POWER: SANITARY REFORMS FROM 1908 TO THE 1920S

Margaret Field infantilized her informants when she claimed that they saw the so-called *Gov'ment* as a powerful and intolerant god, but her comments nevertheless demonstrated that the force of colonial sanitation and medicine was reinvigorated during the interwar period. Funding for medical and public health reforms began to increase slowly after the First World War, and the Gold Coast government divided the Medical Department into three distinct branches: the medical branch (responsible for clinics and hospitals), the health branch (responsible for sanitation, vaccinations, and preventive measures), and the laboratory branch (responsible for scientific investigations, clinical and pathological tests, and postmortem examinations).[25] The work of the medical and laboratory branches was most evident at the new Gold Coast Hospital at Korle Bu (covered in the following chapter), but the health branch intervened more and more in the daily life of the inhabitants of Accra by bringing pipe-borne water to Ussher Town, funding the construction of new markets, imposing fees and licenses on daily activities in the city, and dispatching mosquito brigades into the private spaces of the residences of Accra. Backed by the police, the courts, laboratory scientists, some influential Ga chiefs, and many African lawyers and doctors, the health branch was the arm of colonial government that posed the greatest challenge to the pluralistic network of healing in the city because it threatened to cut off patients from their therapy management groups and guide them into colonial hospitals.

It is important to note that the Gold Coast government's increasing interest in medical and sanitary reforms should not be taken as ethical commitment to ameliorate the health of the

subject population. Rather, the change in policy had a direct correlation to three external factors: the effective standardization
of quinine, the growth of the European population, and ongoing
fears of yellow fever. By 1900, the Colonial Office had regular-
ized the daily intake of quinine for colonial officials at four to
five grains, to be taken as a tonic with a citric or carbonic acid to
activate the alkaloids in the dose. If the prophylaxis didn't work,
then a suggested curative amount of thirty grains was to be taken
all at once.[26] Once dosages were standardized and quinine was
offered at moderate prices at the colonial post office, death rates
for Europeans declined steadily and the European population
of Accra began to grow, rising to an all-time high of over one
thousand persons by 1920.[27] But even with the gains made against
malaria, Europeans in Accra continued to regard the city as an
unhealthy and dangerous place to live. Yellow fever was a con-
tinuing source of anxiety for the White population, because there
was no cure or vaccine for the disease. When a small epidemic in
1910 killed nine Europeans in the coastal town of Takoradi, the
African population of the Gold Coast was once again labeled as
a reservoir for the disease. In Accra, the Korle Lagoon was again
deemed a spawning ground for malaria larvae, and the newly
appointed governor Clifford started planning further segregation measures, which, once again, were supposed to include the
demolition and segregation of parts of Ussher Town.[28]

However, just as soon as the sanitation syndrome began to take
hold, it petered out again. By 1913, Governor Clifford had abandoned plans to rebuild the city, citing financial concerns. Clifford
had been ambivalent about segregation anyway, expressing the
opinion that evicting Africans from their homes on the pretext
of maintaining the health of a White minority was not justified
when colonial officials were well aware of the dangers of residing
in tropical Africa.[29] Clifford was also reluctant to challenge the
African elites of the city, who dismissed the fear of yellow fever
as "white man's humbug," claiming that because of childhood

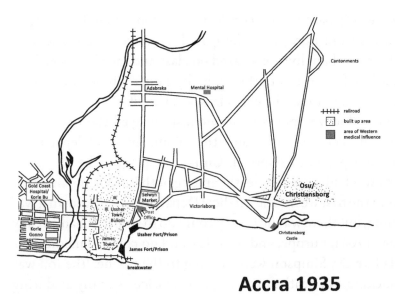

Map 3.1. Map of Accra in 1935.

immunity, Africans did not suffer from the disease.[30] Unlike the bubonic plague, yellow fever did not pose an imminent threat to both the colonizers and the colonized, so there was little chance of organizing a joint campaign to eliminate the disease from the colony, nor were there any imperial experts who could be called in to fight the illness at a time when the virus that caused it had not yet been isolated. Any hope of demolishing and rebuilding the city was further delayed by the First World War, when priorities were placed on marshaling resources for the war effort rather than on providing for sanitation and health. Unlike Senegal, where governors used the fear of contagion to pathologize the African body, or Brazzaville, where doctors used sleeping-sickness passports to divide the infected from the cured, or Cape Town, where politicians used notions of racial ecology to label Africans as a "social pest," segregation in Accra was undertheorized and generally deemed too expensive to impose. [31] In the absence of a firebrand racialist governor, and without a severe epidemic to spur racially based sanitary reforms, the movement to segregate Africans from Europeans dissipated. However, the foundation for future urban divisions based on class and race had been laid, as the northeastern suburbs gradually gained a reputation as the domestic domain of the elite classes of the city.[32]

The influenza epidemic of 1919 also delayed the rise of bio-power in Accra simply because the colonial medical department could not prevent its spread. Unlike the plague, the flu struck Accra suddenly, causing deaths among both Europeans and Africans in the first week. The Medical Department had known it was coming, but there was little they could do to stop it. It had already ravaged Asia, Europe, and America, and no colonial medical experts like Dr. Simpson were coming to the rescue. The toll was a shocking 655 deaths in Accra alone, twice as many as during the plague. However, there were no forced removals, no demolitions, and no inoculations. In fact, there were barely enough resources to bury the dead. Undeterred by their failures during the bubonic plague epidemic, African healers in the city set to work to fight the illness. A local newspaper recorded several new forms of herbal remedies that became available in the city during the epidemic, including an herb-pepper mixture used as a purgative and a type of powder (probably a *ti*) taken internally in a tincture of alcohol.[33] Nothing is known about the effectiveness of these cures, but it is unlikely that African remedies did anything but mollify the symptoms of the illness.

As stability and prosperity returned in 1919, government plans for a healthy capital began to take shape once again, this time under the leadership of a progressive governor who saw medicine as a keystone to future development in the Gold Coast. The Guggisberg years of the 1920s were a time of prosperity, a period that saw the construction of the railroad to Kumasi, the deepwater harbor at Takoradi, and the Prince of Wales College at Achimota.[34] Guggisberg also spent prodigiously on medical care because he equated a healthy workforce with a healthy colonial economy and because he believed that medicine was a gift that the colonizer could bestow on the colonized. In the years prior to his arrival, the governors of the colony had been obliged to limit their expenditures on health because of the modesty of export revenues and because of resistance from the residents of Accra, but in the 1920s, the exponential growth in cocoa export tariff revenue enabled Guggisberg to initiate an expansion of clinics and hospitals and the training of nurses and dispensers.[35] With the support of the new governor, it was conceivable that discourses of bio-power might finally align with the expansion of the three branches of the Medical Department in Accra.

One of Guggisberg's first actions as governor was an attempt to break the impasse between local African elites and the colonial government over sanitary reforms in the city. In 1919, he appointed a committee of local lawyers to review the performance of the Accra Town Council and mobilize them to participate in rebuilding the dilapidated quarters of Accra.[36] The African representatives on the Town Council saw an opportunity to parlay Guggisberg's overtures into political franchise. They delayed their response, and two years later they produced a report stating that the only way to get the residents of James Town and Ussher Town interested in sanitation would be to give all landowners of twenty-one years and older the vote and to allow ratepayers to elect a majority of African members to the council. Guggisberg ignored most of these demands. He had no intention of following recommendations for majority enfranchisement, but in 1924 he did concede to allowing a few additional men, drawn from the professional classes, to sit on the council, with a majority of the seats reserved for government officials. The paramount chiefs of James Town and Ussher Town and some African physicians in Accra supported the new Town Council, but the influential Nae and Korle priests dismissed the changes as an excuse to levy new taxes. The government of the Gold Coast had hoped that the newly constituted Town Council would result in a "political

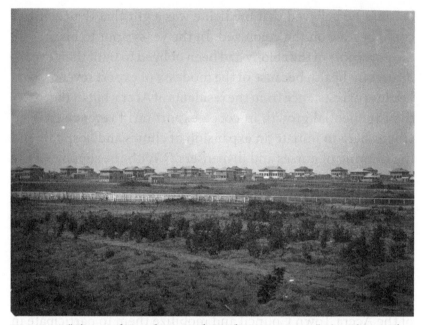

Figure 3.1. "The new bungalows on the Ridge, Accra, 1915." This photo offers a mosquito's view of the expanse of scrubland between the urban heart of Accra and the fenced-off "European Reservation." Governor Clifford was reluctant to continue the policies of segregation put in place by previous governors, arguing that those who came to the Gold Coast should be responsible for their own health. Nonetheless, the line of white bungalows on the distant horizon of the neighborhood known as the Ridge offers a stark impression of how sanitary segregation changed the built environment of Accra. (Source: Elizabeth de la Pasture (Lady Clifford), *Our Days on the Gold Coast: In Ashanti, in the Northern Territories, and the British Sphere of Occupation in Togoland* [London: J. Murray, 1919].)

sanitation" of unruly Ga leaders, enabling the Sanitation Department to conduct its work unimpeded, but the residents of Accra always regarded the council as an attempt to extend colonial rule over the city.[37]

Despite an initial lack of support, the new Town Council set to work creating a substantial base of revenues via the imposition of fees on daily activities. These tariffs were brought forward

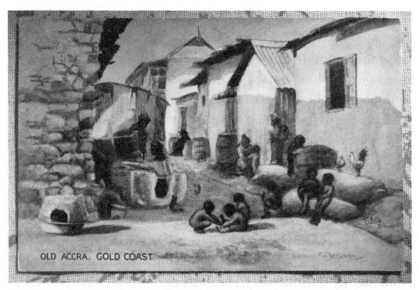

Figure 3.2. "Old Accra, Gold Coast." This is one of several postcards Chees-man painted for exhibition at the Wembley Exhibition in 1924, depicting a street in Accra with children playing and women busy smoking fish, later to be carried around the city for sale in steel pans (*bottom left*). Cheesman, who was employed by the Gold Coast government to chronicle daily life and development in the city, suggests in her postscript that this painting depicts a soon-to-be bygone era: "One of the squalid streets in old Accra which latter is steadily disappearing and giving way to broad highways and well-built dwell-ing houses." Viewed another way, this scene depicts the orderly urbanity of Ga women, smoking fish, drawing water from rain barrels, raising chickens, and caring for children, all in streets that have been swept clean. (Source: postcard by Edith Cheesman.)

incrementally in different parts of the city, in such a way as to normalize municipal administrations, and they proved to be an effective means of asserting control over sanitation in Accra.[38] The piecemeal collection of market rents, slaughterhouse fees, building fees, alcohol licenses, dog licenses, hawkers' licenses, and sanitary fines for harboring mosquito larvae brought in enough revenue to pay for the maintenance of drains, latrines, market stalls, and basic sanitary amenities. They also allowed for the reconstruction of both the Salaga Market and Makola (formerly known as Selwyn) Market, two key points in the distribution of foodstuffs in the city.[39] But the signature achievement of this short burst of sanitation-based tax collection was undoubtedly the arrival of a freshwater pipeline from the Densu River to the harbor, which allowed for the provision of clean water at pipe stands around the city. Surrounded by officials of the Medical Department, the governor opened the first tap in James Town, proudly declaring the success of the sanitation efforts of the Town Council and the Gold Coast Medical Department. Initially, locals were skeptical of the quality of the water, and the inaugural event was boycotted by local priests, who claimed that taboos prohibited them from drinking water that did not fall from the sky. Additionally, rumors began to spread that the water would cause barrenness in women. However, the arrival of the dry season spurred people to draw water from the taps, and eventually, the pipe stands were patronized by the general population.[40] A major health benefit from the introduction of pipe-borne water was a dramatic reduction in incidences of Guinea worm, a disease that had long been a source of pain and suffering in the city.[41] However, there is no evidence that this was a major factor in the acceptance of pipe-borne water in the city.

Both Governor Clifford and Governor Guggisberg made a concerted effort not to favor the European residential location with any special benefit from Town Council services, and gradually, the government began to abandon policies of segregation.[42] The city was still geographically divided by race, with Whites residing in Victoriaborg and the Ridge and Africans living in the old quarters, but Guggisberg eliminated any restrictions on the movement of Africans across the four-hundred-yard "neutral zone" between the two sectors of the city. Police still monitored the road between the two parts of the city at night, but with a different intent. The increase in the single, male, White population during the war and the cocoa boom had given rise to an

increasing number of sex workers in the city, and even though official segregation had ended, the government still felt compelled
to stop the movement of what was euphemistically known as
"black cargo" between the two neighborhoods.[43] Official segregation was no more, but intimate racial mixing continued to
be sanctioned. Once established spatially, the racial divisions of
Accra would prove difficult to undo.

The most controversial action taken by the Medical Department was the creation of the so-called mosquito brigades, a new
generation of sanitary inspectors hired by the Town Council
in the 1920s.[44] The position of inspector started at £72 per year,
a competitive salary that rose by increments of £4 per annum,
and offered the opportunity to advance through the ranks of the
colonial service.[45] Inspectors joined teams that operated like a
quasi police force with the duty of monitoring the sanitary habits
of the residents.[46] Many of them were born in Accra and spoke
Ga and Twi, but the residents of the city disliked them because
they had the right to enter compounds without the owner's permission and fine people for violations like improperly disposing
of rubbish or harboring mosquito larvae in water pots. Sanitary
inspectors were the closest point of contact with colonial authority for most inhabitants, and they were reviled for their intrusion
into the washing and cooking areas of compounds in the city,
which were gendered as women's spaces.[47] They even went so far
as to dump out precious water supplies or disturb women taking their baths.[48] One newspaper editor argued that mosquito-
larvae control measures were a "yellow fever bogey" invented
to create jobs for White medical officers.[49] Indeed, so many larvae violations were brought before the magistrates of the police
court in Accra that Ga speakers referred to it as the "Loloi [larva]
Court."[50] Dr. Nanka-Bruce, a member of the Aborigines' Rights
Protection Society and the only African physician on the Accra
Town Council, declared that the inspections were terrorizing
innocent people in Accra while at the same time neglecting to

punish Europeans harboring mosquito larvae in the "flower pots and ice chests" of Victoriaborg.[51] Even anthropologist Margaret Field protested, claiming that the inspections were tantamount to "religious persecution."[52] Indeed, there was at least one account of an inspector dipping his ladle into a sacred medicinal pot, a serious transgression that was met with indignation by members of the household he was inspecting.[53]

The house-to-house destruction of mosquito breeding grounds may have resulted in lower rates of malaria in the city, but the colonial government never offered any data to prove it, nor did they feel the need to.[54] The battle against malaria was never the primary motivation behind house-to-house searches for larvae anyway. The Sanitation Department had ordered the inspections with the hope of eliminating the presence of *Aedes aegypti*, the insect vector for yellow fever that posed such a risk to White employees. Destroying the larvae of *Anopheles gambiae*, the species that carried malaria, was just a welcome side effect of the campaign. Additionally, the inspections of private dwellings, in neighborhoods once considered off-limits to colonial officials, was a convenient way of tracking the activities of Africans in the city. This form of surveillance would later provide a means of collecting data on class, gender, property, and household composition, without the trouble of conducting official surveys. Marching through the alleys and compounds of Ussher Town and James Town with spray cans on their backs, the sanitary inspectors were the most recognizable agents of colonial bio-power in Accra.

Ironically, what really bothered the educated African elites of Accra was that the efforts made to sanitize the city did not come close to meeting British standards of urban sanitation. Dr. Nanka-Bruce was consistently critical of the piecemeal measures taken by the government. In a series of editorials, he noted that, despite its new construction, the Selwyn Market was surrounded by rubbish and in a poor sanitary state, and he called on the sanitary inspectors to monitor public spaces as closely as they monitored the domestic ones.[55] Of particular nuisance to Nanka-Bruce were the public latrines erected by the government, which he claimed were poorly built, foul smelling, and lacking in privacy.[56] He also pointed out that the city drains were completely dysfunctional—during the rainy season, the streets flooded because the gutters were clogged with human excrement and refuse, and during the dry season, they contained fetid pools of water that harbored mosquitoes.[57] Intermittent inspections, according to Nanka-Bruce, were simply not enough to keep the city in a healthy state, and he called on the colonial government to once again "consider breaking down and reconstructing the several congested areas in Accra."[58] Nanka-Bruce used discourses of bio-power to advocate for broad sanitary interventions into the lives of the colonized population, but the colonial government was more reticent, preferring to use the hysteria of the sanitation syndrome as a means of prioritizing the health of its own colonial officials.

During the 1920s and 1930s, the colonial police force, the courts, and the prison system also began to intervene in the healing culture of the city by guiding and coercing sick and injured subjects through a colonial network of institutions. This was particularly evident in the case of accidents involving physical trauma.[59] Patients who suffered from contusions, cuts, or broken bones were often rushed to physicians for surgery. For instance, in 1926, when a building inspector employed by the Town Council fell off the scaffolding of a mosque, he was treated by Dr. Macauley, a surgeon employed by the government.[60] In another case in the same year, police took a boy who fell from a tree to Dr. Nanka-Bruce's clinic to reset the bone.[61] And when the Gold Coast Hospital was built in 1924, police often rushed to the emergency room at Korle Bu. The growth of government operations meant that an increasing number of government employees and clients were drawn into the medical system.

An even larger category of injuries developed with the arrival of automobiles in the city.[62] In the previous century, an era of horse-drawn carriages, only one recorded carriage accident appears in the extant court records. The injured parties were tended to at home by African healers, without the involvement of police or surgeons.[63] But the high speeds of automobile collisions produced more dramatic cases of physical trauma than ever before.[64] When an accident occurred, the police sent the injured parties to the hospital and then filed reports, taking statements from the drivers and passengers.[65] These reports, which included the registration numbers of the automobiles, were used in court if anyone involved in the accident wanted to sue for damages.[66] Additionally, medical officers might be asked to file paperwork on injuries or, in the case of fatalities, sign a death certificate.[67] A legal paper trail thus developed, connecting the police and the courts to colonial medicine, as part of a larger network of colonial rule.

In the case of mental illness, the police arrested anyone suspected of violent insanity and sent them to the colonial asylum for assessment. The 1929 case of Ahudor, a customs clerk who was assaulted while walking with his wife, demonstrates how colonial medical control expressed itself in such cases. During a quarrel in the streets of Accra in 1929, Ahudor was struck over the head with a stick by a man named Akwei. Ahudor was knocked unconscious, and when he came to, his wife took him to a local surgeon, who examined him and ordered that he be sent to the hospital. He died later in the evening. The police imprisoned Akwei, and when he was brought before the magistrate, he was judged to be insane and sent to the mental hospital at Adabraka for a medical assessment.[68] In another case in the same year, a fight broke out at Selwyn Market between two Hausa-speaking vendors. In a rage, a woman named Masalachi struck the head of Mama Yadu against the wall of the market. The quarrel attracted the attention of the police, who arrived on the scene, arrested Masalachi, and sent her to the asylum to be "placed under medical observation."[69] Though the mental hospital offered little in the way of therapy, operating mainly as a place of confinement for dangerous patients, it fitted into a system within which colonial subjects involved in crimes could be isolated and observed by medical officers.[70] Victims of violence and people who were deemed mental patients became wards of the colonial medical system, thereby losing access to the therapy management groups that would normally arrange health care for them in the compounds of African healers.[71]

The police and the courts also began to intervene in the normally sacrosanct activities of the Ga priests if there was any sort of public disturbance at the major shrines. In the sensational Oyamia Case of 1926, a trial that the Accra public followed closely, a *woyoo* spirit medium was accused of coercing a person to stay at her shrine for ritual purposes. During the trial, the *woyoo* was possessed by a spirit and became so animated that the bailiffs had to hold her down to control the spasms. She was later convicted of "holding a person in pawn" and was sent to prison in James Fort.[72] And though the district commissioner of Accra was reluctant to suppress the activities of shrine priests, Ga spiritualists were sometimes helpless to stop state intervention into public disturbances. In 1927, when a riot broke out between two rival fishing villages on the Sakumo Lagoon, the police rushed in and arrested the instigators. The priest of Sakumo followed behind them, alleging that the police were usurping his religious and political authority because the two factions were supposed to report to him for mediation.[73] The police ignored the priest because colonial laws disallowed the use of any medicines deemed "noxious," forbade the act of putting people into fetish, and made illegal any sort of curse that fell under the category of defamation or slander.[74] The punishments could be severe, including fines starting at £25 and three months in prison. To maintain a peaceable relationship with inhabitants of the capital city, the British normally left African religious leaders and healers alone, but the threat of punishment was always present.

The sanitary interventions of the early twentieth century, when combined with the expansion of the powers of the police, the courts, the hospitals, and the prisons, amounted to a serious bid for hegemony by a medicalized colonial state. Through its various appendages, the Gold Coast government was finding new ways to transform the bodies of the sick into medical subjects of the state. This was colonial bio-power—an assertive form of state intervention that had the potential to cut the residents of Accra off from their therapy management groups and guide them down healing channels of exclusively European-derived therapies, posing a significant challenge to conventions of pluralistic healing in the city. However, there were real limits to how colonial medicine could alter the subjectivity of patients in Accra. As Field showed, the indigenous healing networks of Accra remained intact, and the therapy management groups that guided patients between healers remained in place, ascribing African meanings to their illness and embedding the agency of the patient within a caregiving collective. And as Nanka-Bruce demonstrated, there was so little government funding committed to the sanitary infrastructure that the Medical Department's interventions were ineffectual. The urban quarters of the city remained largely intact—there was almost no rebuilding of the old neighborhoods, no sewer construction, little investment in drains, and no attempt to directly challenge African healers. Colonial medicine was ascendant, but the pluralistic healing culture of the city seemed quite able to survive the challenges of the so-called *Gov'ment*.

AFRICAN-BORN PHYSICIANS IN THE
EARLY TWENTIETH CENTURY

In the early twentieth century, colonial medicine had a mostly White face. The vast majority of physicians and nurses were Britons, usually newly trained, seeking experience in the colonies and hoping to return home soon. As a physician who worked in the Gold Coast during the colonial era recalled, the colonial physician was a "puzzling figure for Africans": "He was usually a White male, a stranger who had to use an interpreter. He often asked impolite questions; demanded, for unknown reasons, samples of blood, urine, and feces; and sometimes cut open the bodies of the dead . . . some [of these men] were so disagreeable that people avoided them."[75] The cultural divide between White physicians and African patients was exacerbated by the fact that the Gold Coast Medical Department struggled to attract the best recruits from Britain.

But in the 1920s, a new cadre of African-born, British-trained physicians began to change African patients' perceptions of colonial medicine. As part of Guggisberg's initiative to Africanize the government service, he initiated the post of junior African medical officer, with a salary starting at £400 per year, a substantial pay packet for a colonial subject of the Gold Coast.[76] Though local physicians continued to rail at the limited opportunities for Africans at the higher ranks and the lower pay for African officials overall, the junior and middle ranks of the colonial service were nonetheless rapidly filling with educated Africans. Additionally, as the city grew, the possibilities for making a good living in private practice began to expand. Not only did being a doctor pay well, but it was also a high-status profession within colonial circles. A physician on the Gold Coast, whether White or Black, had access to the elite society that gathered at the prestigious Rodger and Accra Clubs and was also welcome at many official government functions.[77] By the 1920s, many schoolchildren were beginning to pronounce their desires to be doctors, deeming medicine to be an admirable profession.[78] A student at the Government Senior Boys' School in Accra even argued that "the value of the doctor's work is universally known."[79]

The most notable physician of early twentieth-century Accra was the aforementioned Dr. Frederick Victor Nanka-Bruce.[80] Born into a prominent James Town family, Nanka-Bruce was educated at the government school in Accra and was later apprenticed to a dispenser. He left Accra for medical school in Edinburgh in 1901 and returned to Accra six years later to take up temporary employment with the Medical Department, as part of a committee investigating infant mortality in the city.[81] Aware of the racism that continued to smolder within the West African Medical Service, Dr. Nanka-Bruce asserted his independence by staying politically active as a member of the Gold Coast Aborigines' Rights Protection Society, which led him to take up the role as the editor of the *Gold Coast Independent*.[82] Nanka-Bruce is the best known of the interwar cohort of African physicians, but he was soon joined by Dr. Van Hien, member of a merchant family from Osu; Drs. W. F. Renner Dove and Horace Dove, two sons of a prominent Sierra Leonean merchant from Ussher Town; and C. E. Reindorf, the son of Carl Christian Reindorf.[83] By 1923 the city contained six clinics run by African-born physicians, and they did not have to emblazon *Domi Abra* on their signs to attract clients; thanks to the growing population of wealthy African merchants and professionals in Accra, there were more than enough patients to sustain their practices.

Like the White doctors before them, African-born physicians were imbued with a strong belief in the efficacy of European medical techniques, and they regarded African healing traditions as an impediment to the improvement of health in the colony. By the late 1920s and 1930s, medical professionals had the advantage of being able to give quinine injections for malaria, arsenic injections for skin diseases, and surgical interventions for traumatic injuries, but otherwise, few techniques distinguished British-trained doctors from African healers. It was still the era before antibiotics, and physicians were well aware that they were competing with other therapeutic traditions. An inevitable question arises: If physicians did not have adequate healing techniques to supersede established indigenous healing practices, how did they manage to win the trust of patients? There are few sources available to answer this question, but one intriguing court case indicates how two worlds of healing managed to coexist in mutual tolerance.

In 1918, a teenage girl named Olivia, the daughter of a wealthy African merchant, fell sick at her home in Accra. Over the course of her illness, she was treated by two different practitioners. The first was Dr. Renner Dove, the son of a Sierra Leonean merchant who had trained in Britain and opened a medical practice in Accra.[84] He diagnosed Olivia with tuberculosis. The second practitioner was Merry Brew, an herbalist and spiritualist from the prominent Brew merchant family.[85] She diagnosed Olivia with a curse caused by witchcraft. When the girl died one year later, Dr. Dove's diagnosis was registered as the official cause of death, and Merry Brew had moved to Cape Coast, but Olivia's story did not end there. The late patient subsequently became the center of a malpractice suit that forms a useful a case study for observing how physicians, healers, patients, and therapy management groups interacted in the city.

When Olivia died, her mother, Dodaye, simply could not accept that she had lost her daughter to such a mundane cause as tuberculosis. Dodaye was convinced that Merry Brew had killed Olivia with some sort of devious therapy, so she marched through the streets of Accra, beating a cowbell and shouting out curses against her. Later, to further her case, Dodaye took Brew before a tribunal of the Ga chiefs, accusing her of spiritual malfeasance. Unfortunately, no records remain from the Ga traditional court, but it appears that Merry Brew was so offended by Dodaye's actions that she decided to sue Dodaye for defamation in a Gold Coast court.

When the trial in the colonial court began, Dodaye testified that her family had first called Dr. Dove to their house to cure Olivia, but while the physician was attending to the patient, Merry Brew arrived to inquire about Olivia's illness. After Dr. Dove left the room, Brew told Dodaye that Olivia's womb was being "eaten by witches" and claimed that she had a remedy that could fight off the attack.[86] Brew then left the house, and the family discussed whom they should employ to fight the illness. Though she was very sick, Olivia made it clear to her family that she wanted the services of Merry Brew as well as Dr. Dove, so Dodaye requested that Brew prepare a special consecrated healing draught composed of pieces of Olivia's red menstrual cloth mixed with some other personal items, burnt into a *ti*, and mixed with rum.[87] The potion was supposed to cleanse Olivia's reproductive system, but when Olivia drank the concoction she became sicker than before.[88] The treatment for witchcraft continued for a few more days, but Olivia's health still did not improve. Then suddenly, Merry Brew left for Cape Coast, seemingly to evade the consequences of the failing health of her patient.

On the witness stand, Merry Brew told the magistrate that she had a good reputation as a healer and that she made her living on the substantial fees that she charged for her services—an average of £4 per day, an excellent rate of pay for that time.[89] Her specialty was women's fertility problems, and she told the magistrate that before Dr. Dove had attended to Olivia, she had already been treating her, first with medicine for a venereal disease, and then later with a concoction to help her get pregnant. As the case progressed, it became clear that Olivia and her family had followed a double healing strategy as a therapy management group. They brought in Dr. Dove to directly treat Olivia's illness, which was either a lung infection or venereal disease, or maybe both. But they also sent for Merry Brew because they believed that their daughter had also been cursed by a fetish object that had been planted in their house by an enemy of the family.[90] Merry Brew told the magistrate that she neutralized the offending object with the same concoction of *ti* that she later gave to Olivia to drink. It was all part of a larger spiritual therapy that Brew claimed had already healed Olivia before she left for Cape Coast. She argued that the girl must have died from a new illness contracted when she traveled to the north of Accra for several days. On the strength of her defense, Merry Brew won her case, and Olivia's mother Dodaye was convicted of defamation.

Olivia's case shows that patients in Accra could find themselves caught between two therapeutic worlds. Dr. Dove was Olivia's family doctor in an official sense. He had tried earnestly to cure her lung disease, but in 1919, he had little to offer that would save her. Merry Brew seems to have waited patiently, accepting the work of Dr. Dove and actually delaying administration of her concoction until the girl had completed Dr. Dove's treatment. It is possible that Brew thought the two therapies would not mix well or that she wanted to avoid a conflict with a physician, but either way she demonstrated a tolerance for the existence of a completely different healing tradition. And as for Dr. Dove, there is no indication that he was aware of the alternative treatments, though he did meet Merry Brew at Olivia's house and might have suspected that she was treating the girl.[91] If he was aware that Olivia was being treated by an African healer, he might have felt the need to protest, but it would have been hard for him to do so without losing Olivia's family as clients. Dr. Dove would have known where he stood—he was a newcomer by comparison to Brew, a Western healer trying to find a niche among hundreds of other types of practitioners within the broader pluralistic healing networks of Accra.

CHRISTIAN HEALING, ISLAMIC HEALING, AND PATENT MEDICINES (*BLOFO TSOFA*)

Beyond African and Western therapies, the history of healing in the early twentieth century is severely limited by a lack of source materials, but there are signals that Christian healing, Islamic healing, and patent medicines were ascendant therapeutic traditions in Accra. Faith-healing movements in Christian communities outside of Accra were growing, and it is likely that they were growing in Accra too, though there is little direct evidence to show it. And there are almost no extant records to account for healing practices within the Islamic communities of the city, despite the fact that the Muslim population was a rapidly growing subsection of the urban population. More information is available about the growth in the patent medicine market (which became known as "white man's medicines," or *blofo tsofa*) during the 1920s and 1930s, but it comes from unconventional sources, like print advertising and oral history. Nonetheless, there is enough information to suggest that change was in the air for these soon-to-be prominent therapeutic traditions.

By 1920, the Christian community of Accra was composed almost exclusively of four denominations: Presbyterian, Roman Catholic, Methodist, and Anglican.[92] The largest of these was the Presbyterian Church, comprising the former Basel Mission enclaves whose property had been confiscated by the government during the First World War. The Christian community continued to grow, but only gradually. The conservative nature of the churches of Accra stands in contrast to revivalist movements that were happening in Nigeria. The Aladura ("praying people" in Yoruba) revivalist movement began at the start of the century and flourished during the influenza epidemic, when a group of Christian converts repudiated the use of colonial medicine and declared that they could use the power of the Holy Spirit to protect people from the disease. Soon afterward, faith-healing congregations began to spring up around the Gold Coast.

The earliest was the Faith Tabernacle Church, an offshoot of an American evangelical sect from Philadelphia, which broadcast its doctrine of faith healing via a periodical called the *Sword of the Spirit*.[93] The congregants of Faith Tabernacle firmly believed in divine healing, establishing "Faith Homes" as a place for flu sufferers to convalesce and pray.[94] The followers of the Faith Tabernacle Church sent home narratives about their victories over illness, some of which were reprinted in *Sword of the Spirit,* a type of feedback that inspired the rapid spread of the church, including the establishment of a branch in Accra. By 1926 there were more than one hundred Faith Tabernacle branches on the Gold Coast, but the congregations soon splintered over whether to use quinine pills to fight malaria, a practice that violated the church's prohibition against European medicines and its foundation of faith healing.[95] The church later dissolved, but a dedication to faith healing remained in the smaller churches of the colony.

By 1938, Faith Tabernacle in Accra had become the Christ's Apostolic Church, about which little is known except that ideas about the healing power of Jesus and the Holy Spirit would have been a core part of its dogma. Other revivalist churches included William Wade Harris's Twelve Apostolic Church, which had spread rapidly in the western part of the Gold Coast. Harris's ideas did, belatedly, spread to Accra, but they are not on record until 1953, when a splinter group from the Methodist Church established a small branch of the Twelve Apostolic Church in the city.[96] To the north, the prophet Samson Oppong, who claimed to be able to read the Bible from a handheld stone tablet, converted ten thousand people in the villages and towns of the Ashanti region, but this movement also seems to have had little impact in Accra.[97] Accra was surrounded by revivalist movements by the 1930s, and precepts of faith healing must have been known to Christians in Accra, but the city was hardly a center of evangelical fervor. Nevertheless, it is clear that a transition toward faith healing was about to take place.

Information about Islamic healing during the early twentieth century is also thin, but it suggests that substantial changes were taking place in the community. At the start of the century, the majority of Muslims in Accra lived just to the north of Ussher Town and were labeled as Hausa migrants in colonial records.[98] The city was growing so fast that, by the end of the 1930s, there were Muslim enclaves in suburbs such as Adabraka, Sabon Zongo, Nima, Kanda, and other small communities, leading all the way up the Odaw River to the market town of Madina.[99] Some of these communities were populated by new immigrant groups, like Sisala migrants from the northern regions of the Gold Coast, or Zabarima migrants from Niger.[100] Unfortunately, a lack of ethnographic work and a dearth of colonial records short-circuits our understanding about the healing practices within these enclaves.

Oddly, Muslim migrants do appear in colonial medical reports as research subjects at the Accra Laboratory. For instance, a particular strain of the disease isolated by Hideyo Noguchi in 1927 was named for a Muslim man who suffered from yellow fever, known only as Asibi in the medical reports.[101] How Noguchi found him is unknown, but we can guess that he worked in some capacity for the colonial government as a laborer, and was probably taken to the hospital when he was sick. In a similar case in 1931, a strain of relapsing fever spirochetes were taken from a Korle Bu Hospital patient named only as Aliferi, but again the medical documents contain only his first name and offer no details of his background.[102] We can again guess that he ended up at the hospital somehow, perhaps as a laborer, perhaps as a pauper, and was taken aside for special attention. What we do have as a specific fact is one passing mention from a research paper on relapsing fever that does prove Islamic apotropaics were used in the city. While delousing patients infected with the disease, Drs. Selwyn-Clarke, Le Fanu, and Ingram noted that amulets were "carried in great numbers by Hausas and Northern Territory tribesmen" for protection against illness.[103] All of this is to say that Muslim migrants found themselves caught up in the pluralistic healing network of the city, visiting Korle Bu while at the same time patronizing Islamic healers.

By contrast, patent medicines are quite visible in the historical record of the early twentieth century, as globally branded commodities with bold-print advertising campaigns in the newspapers of the Gold Coast. They were also part of a new generation of imported goods that was helping to generate a consumer society. In the 1920s, firms like the United Africa Company imported bicycles, cars, cloth, gin, toiletries, margarine, and many other goods into the city, and increasingly, Accra became a zone of display for foreign goods.[104] Patent medicines were a key component of this consumer trend, taking up the majority of ad placements in colonial newspapers.[105] Advertising helped to spur demand, and the value of drugs and medicines imported into the Gold Coast Colony grew exponentially, from £3,083 in 1891 to £142,115 in 1920, an increase of 600 percent in just thirty years.[106] No longer were patent medicines rare items brought to the city in the medicine chests of European travelers—by the 1920s, they were sold in major European-owned department stores, like Swanzy's, Kingsway, G. B. Ollivants, and the United African Company stores. They were also available in dozens of small chemist shops along Horse Road and High Street and at the market stalls in the Makola Market.[107] Moreover, there were no restrictions on the importation of proprietary medicines, likely because they offered a source of tariff revenue for the colonial government.

On the demand side, it is a little more difficult to pinpoint why patent medicines became so ubiquitous in Accra. In the United Kingdom, the popularity of patent medicines had begun to wane after the British Medical Association launched their "secret remedies" campaign in the 1910s, which questioned the medicinal value of patent medicines and revealed that they contained highly addictive compounds.[108] On the Gold Coast, medical authorities were also alarmed by the dangers of patent medicines. This official attitude was expressed by Dr. Nanka-Bruce, who derided the "pernicious custom of buying patent medicines," claiming that self-medicating with proprietary medicines distracted from the larger efforts to sanitize the city.[109] Margaret Field also commented on the presence of commodified medical products, claiming that gullible Africans were falling prey to medicine vendors who violated the "ancient ethics" of Ga healing.[110] But despite an official air of contempt for patent medicines, demand was high for *blofo tsofa*, which had become a distinct therapeutic option outside of colonial and African circles of healing power.

It is difficult to trace consumption patterns of patent medicines precisely, but the visibility of specific medicinal products in newspapers and in the memories of people living in Accra today indicate that patent medicines were widely consumed. As imported products, they arrived with their own unique healing properties and medicinal meanings, which were presented to the reading public via ads and labels. The emergence of what Karin Barber has called a "stratum of literates," a new class of government and commercial employees in West Africa, meant that there were hundreds, perhaps thousands, of residents reading about the promise that patent medicines offered.[111] And some patients using patent medicines may have internalized the maladies presented to them on the printed page, self-diagnosing with conditions like overwork, exhaustion, or neuralgia.[112] Historian of medicine Thomas Richards has claimed that patent medicines were "radically transitive remedies" that could generate an archetype of the colonial patient as self-healer, which in turn created an addiction to the identity-generating capacity of advertising.[113] This may have been the case for some sufferers in Accra, but newspaper ads did not always determine how the medicines were used. As patent medicines were worked into healing practices and daily rituals in Accra, they took on a new significance according to local "regimes of value" (to borrow a term from Arjun Appadurai).[114] Three medicines in particular, Atwood Bitters, Sloan's Liniment, and Woodward's Gripe Water, became immensely popular and filled a significant therapeutic role in Accra during the cocoa boom.

Atwood's Vegetable Physical Laxative Bitters, a combination of herbs and roots in a tincture of alcohol, was invented by Moses Atwood in Georgetown, Massachusetts, in 1840. Originally formulated as a cure-all for intestinal disorders, the product was so successful that Atwood patented the recipe. In 1877, the license was transferred to the Manhattan Medicine Company, which sold the product under the name of Atwood's Physical Jaundice Bitters until well into the twentieth century.[115] The medicine is still around today, but the license is held by JRB Enterprises Limited, a British company that wholesales patent medicines to Africa and India, where Atwood's Bitters is still popular. Atwood's is a widely recognized brand in Accra today and is still available in many of the city's chemist shops and pharmacies. Though expensive (triple the price of locally produced herbal laxatives), it continues to sell well because it is regarded not only as a strong laxative but also as a fertility medicine.[116] Atwood's Bitters, with its high alcohol content of 15 percent, is similar to locally manufactured herbal drinks, usually mixed with locally distilled gin, that are known to heal the womb after pregnancy and to generally increase fecundity. The demand for Atwood's Bitters in Accra during the colonial era can be understood as a product of "glocalization," an imported product that was invented in the United States, licensed in the United Kingdom, sold around the world, and imbued with new medicinal virtues in Accra.[117]

Sloan's Liniment (see fig. 3.3) offers a similar example. In the 1920s, the shops of Accra offered a number of patented emollients, but the most widely advertised was Sloan's Liniment. Invented by Earl Sawyer Sloan of Missouri, the liniment was originally a salve used to help horses recover from injuries, but it became popular in the United States and Europe for the aches and pains of arthritis and rheumatism.[118] James Michael Davidson has noted that Sloan's Liniment was left on burial mounds by African Americans in Texas; the reasons are unknown, but as a global medicine, the liniment seems to have taken on different meanings in

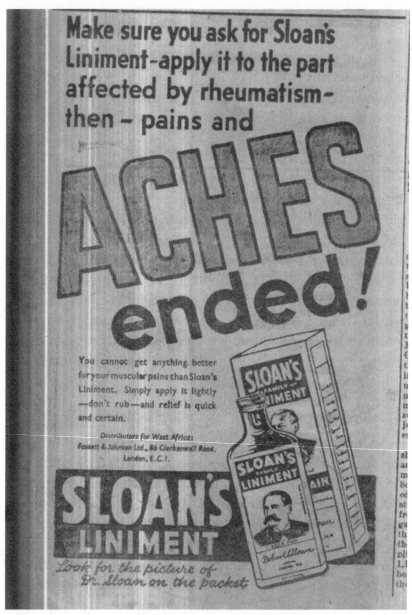

Figure 3.3. Sloan's Liniment. Sloan's was intended to relieve muscle pain, but it was used in a variety of other ways in Accra. The bold image of the inventor's face distinguished the product from other liniments, making it recognizable to illiterate consumers, who referred to it as the "old man" medicine. The advertisement also explicitly refers to West Africa, though it may have been adapted from an advertisement used for other markets. (Source: *Gold Coast Observer*, September 12, 1947, 238.)

different locales. On the Gold Coast, Sloan's was the most widely advertised liniment, and it had a ready market in a place where skin creams were commonly used to prevent chapping during the dry season. Sloan's garnered the nickname "old man" (said in Ga as *numo*) because of the image of the mustachioed Dr. Sloan on the label, and the liniment was known for its ability to penetrate the skin to quicken the setting of broken bones.[119] Sloan's was also diluted in water and mixed with local herbs to be taken internally as a blood tonic, once again to help mothers to "heal the sores in the womb" after childbirth.[120] In other cases it was diluted in warm water for use as a vaginal douche or an enema.[121] Like Atwood Bitters, people in Accra disconnected Sloan's Liniment from its Western meanings and gave it new uses in dealing with the health concerns of people living in Accra.[122]

Another medicine that sold well in the city in the early twentieth century was Woodward's Gripe Water, a tonic for babies with colic. Formulated by William Woodward of Stamford, Lincolnshire, in 1851, Woodward's Gripe Water was a tincture of up to 9 percent alcohol mixed together with sucrose, dill seed oil, and bicarbonate of soda to soothe a baby's stomach.[123] Woodward registered his trademark in 1876 and began to sell his medicine to the public in small quantities and to the children's wards of hospitals by the gallon. In the late nineteenth century, the medicine traveled around the world in the luggage of the wives of British servicemen, and Woodward advertised his product more broadly as a tonic for the children of the colonies. One advertisement showed images of cavalry and battleships, branding the Gripe Water as a guardian of infants around the British Empire.[124] Though Woodward probably envisioned his Gripe Water as a means of soothing English babies, it was also widely used by mothers in Accra as a pacifier. But unlike Atwood's and Sloan's, its practical use didn't change. Woodward's worked in Accra as it did around the rest of the British Empire—as a medicine to soothe colic.

Advertisements for Atwood's Bitters, Sloan's Liniment, and Woodward's Gripe Water were published again and again throughout the first half of the twentieth century, with little alteration. All of these advertisements, with the exception of one for Atwood's Bitters, were actually crafted for the intended target of White colonial officials, miners, merchants, and missionaries living around the empire, rather than directly to the West African market. Considering the growth of the African market for patent medicines and other consumer goods, it is odd that no advertising campaigns directly targeted African consumers. During the same time period in India, locally manufactured bottled nostrums did challenge the dominance of patent medicines, so importers were obliged to advertise and label their products with local languages and use local imagery to indigenize their products.[125] In order to compete with Indian products like Babuline Gripe Water, advertisers of Woodward's Gripe Water used Hindu images of gods like Krishna to embed their commodities within a local network of symbols. And in Uganda, some advertisers translated their copy into Luganda, as in the case of Zam Buk ointment and Dr. Ross's Vermifuge, two medicines that were also available on the Gold Coast.[126] But in Accra there were no local manufacturers of branded patented medicines to compete with, nor had the local languages of Ga and Twi become a significant part of print media culture. Since education in the city was conducted in English, using imported ads from the United Kingdom was still the best way to reach customers in Accra.

Even though advertisers did not substantially alter their print campaigns to target West Africans, patent medicines captured the imagination of the patients of Accra. Patients in Accra found that, despite their dubious reputation in the United Kingdom, some patent medicines had genuine value as palliative treatments for common illnesses. They also imbued them with new values, like fertility.[127] What's more, these medicines were readily available and cheap. Patients could find patent medicines almost anywhere in the city, at a price that was only a little more expensive than local herbal tonics and a lot cheaper than costly African rituals or exorbitant physician fees.[128] Moreover, patients could individually choose how they wanted to use patent medicines. They could consume them privately, an option invaluable to sufferers of venereal disease, for example. Or they could take the medicines publicly, as a means of associating themselves with the aspirational consumption patterns of Europeans and African colonial elites.[129] As the twentieth century progressed, patent medicines became essential tools in an expanding kit of self-medication, with the added advantage of offering a way to adopt the independent lifestyle of a modern colonial subject.

Interlude: Gordon Guggisberg and the Methods of Modern Medicine

On October 9, 1923, Gordon Guggisberg left Christiansborg Castle in a small motorcade for a trip to the grounds of the brand-new Gold Coast Hospital. He passed the bungalows of the European Reservation and drove along the crowded horse road that skirted Ussher Town and James Town. The cars then crossed the bridge over Korle Lagoon to arrive at a broad gulley of cleared land known as Korle Bu. When he stepped out of his car, a brass band struck up the tune *"Awole Gorgi, Gorgi No. 1 Hossey"* (All Hail Georgie, Georgie, Number One Horsey!)—a playful lyrical tribute to the paternalistic charisma of the governor. Surrounded by Medical Department officials, British-trained African doctors, and Ga chiefs, Guggisberg took the podium in front of the brand-new outpatient ward and began to speak. He declared that the Gold Coast Colony had made tremendous progress in recent years but that it remained underpopulated.[130] After a long period of stagnation and warfare, he argued, the Gold Coast needed to use the "methods of modern medicine" to revitalize its population and secure a prosperous future.[131] The new colonial hospital,

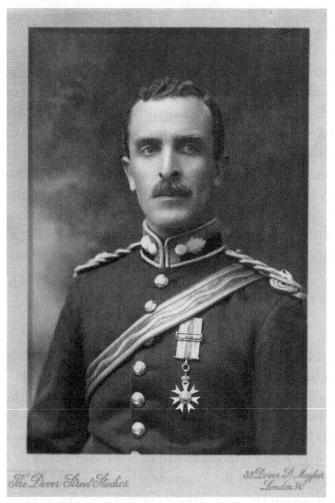

Figure 3.4. Governor Guggisberg official portrait (circa 1921), self-portrait, and statue in front of Korle Bu Teaching Hospital (1922). Leading the Gold Coast through a period of unprecedented prosperity, Frederick Gordon Guggisberg exuded confidence and financed major infrastructure projects, such as Achimota College and Takoradi Harbour, on the Gold Coast. Guggisberg believed that economic progress depended on the health of the working population, and his health reforms expanded colonial medical care in Accra, epitomized by the construction of the Gold Coast Hospital at Korle Bu. He remains an icon of colonial medicine in Accra—his name has been given to the major thoroughfare that runs from Accra across the lagoon to the hospital, and his statue stands in front of the historic outpatient ward, the first building erected on the Korle Bu campus. (Source: Wikipedia.)

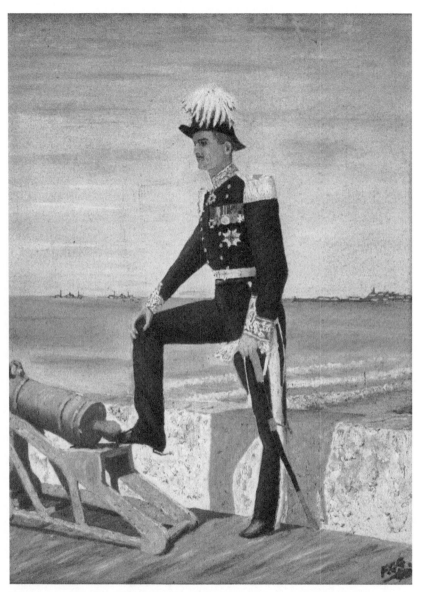

Figure 3.4. *Continued*

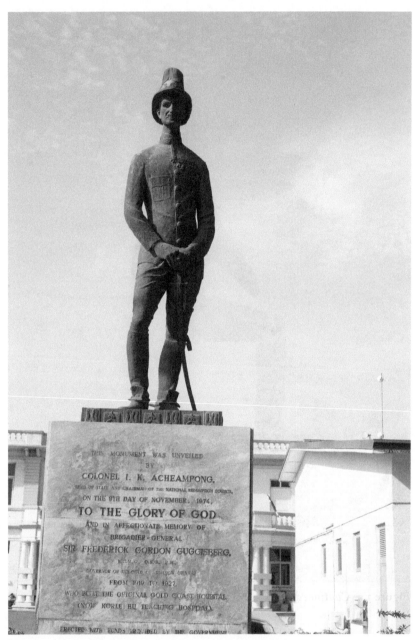

Figure 3.4. *Continued*

he declared, was more than just an institution; it was a promise from Britain to care for "the native peoples who have entrusted themselves to her charge."[132] For the first time in the history of the Gold Coast, a governor was able to articulate a coherent, albeit paternalistic, vision for European-derived medical care in the colony.[133]

Guggisberg's soaring rhetoric might have seemed fresh on that particular day in 1923, but the words were secondhand, borrowed from the "dual mandate" of colonialism established by Frederick Lugard in Nigeria.[134] According to Lugard, the expansion of British economic interests in Africa had to be predicated on the spread of "civilization," which included the provision of European medicine.[135] As governor of Nigeria, Lugard stated in 1919, "The white man was at first engaged in consolidating his own position, and making the tropics more healthy for Europeans engaged in their development. He has now accepted the principle that they must be made more healthy for the native population."[136] Indeed, the construction of the Gold Coast Hospital, though now closely associated with Guggisberg, was actually part of a much larger British dream of a building a robust West African economy with a ready supply of healthy workers.

It should also be noted that, though Guggisberg did become the champion of a "great African Hospital" for the Gold Coast, it wasn't really his idea.[137] Many governors before him had wanted to build a new hospital, and Guggisberg's immediate predecessor, Governor Clifford, had commissioned a set of blueprints before Guggisberg arrived, entrusting the project to his personal physician, Cecil Le Fanu, former public health officer in Navrongo. With Clifford's encouragement, Le Fanu set to work designing the layout of the hospital, but the project remained on hold during the war. When Guggisberg arrived on the Gold Coast in 1919, Le Fanu remained as the governor's physician, and he likely advocated for the completion of the hospital project.

Strangely, despite Le Fanu's desire to create an inclusive hospital that served everyone regardless of race, his role at the institution has been largely forgotten.[138]

Guggisberg arrived in Accra during the most prosperous era in the history of the city, and just in time to take credit for the erection of the new hospital, but he does deserve some recognition for the progressive direction that the hospital took during its early years. Initially, the Gold Coast government had considered implementing a French colonial model of training, one that placed surgical and technical duties in the hands of White doctors and White technicians, leaving menial labor to a large class of low-paid "native dressers."[139] While mulling over the idea in 1921, Guggisberg decided to send Dr. Arthur O'Brien to Dakar, in an effort to gain insights from advances at French colonial hospitals. O'Brien returned with a negative view of the French model, encouraging Guggisberg to reject the proposed two-tier, racially based approach and replace it with a Fabian vision of medical care that combined the proficiency of middle-class voluntary hospitals with the universality of working-class infirmaries.[140] It was at that point that Guggisberg decided to make the Gold Coast Hospital a training ground for African doctors, nurses, dispensers, sanitary inspectors, and laboratory technicians. He assumed that these local medical professionals would be supervised initially by White physicians, but hoped that African graduates would eventually return with medical degrees from Britain to administer the institution.[141] Guggisberg wanted the Gold Coast Hospital to serve everyone in the colony, regardless of color, and to be operated eventually entirely by the subjects of the Gold Coast. Not surprisingly, the governor's efforts were greeted with warmth and enthusiasm by the African elites of Accra, particularly the British-trained African doctors of the city, who had for so long been excluded from participation in the colonial medical system.[142] The hospital soon became home to a burgeoning medical subculture propagated by Africans, who filled positions as nurses, doctors, and technicians. Though some patients were reluctant to submit to the new types of therapies offered at the hospital, many patients in Accra developed a fondness for the institution. In a few short years, the hospital took on the simple Ga moniker of its geographic location, Korle Bu. It had been officially adopted as a new setting for healing in the city.

NOTES

1. Fage, *Introduction to the History of West Africa*, 194; Stearns and Langer, *Encyclopedia of World History*, 795.

2. Macmillan, *Red Book of West Africa*, 173; Dickson, "Evolution of Seaports in Ghana," 109; Hambly, "Review of M. J. Field," 312; Field, *Religion and Medicine*, 2.

3. Acquah, *Accra Survey*, 31.

4. MacLeod and Lewis, *Disease, Medicine, and Empire*, x.

5. Conklin, *Mission to Civilize*.

6. Barth, et al., *One Discipline, Four Ways*, 22.

7. Meyer Fortes, "Review of Field"; E. E. Evans-Pritchard, Review of *Religion and Medicine*.

8. Field, *Religion and Medicine*, v.

9. Field, *Religion and Medicine*, 134.

10. Parker, *Making the Town*, 17.

11. Field, *Religion and Medicine*, 72, 90, 95, 101, 131, 138. See also PRAAD SCT 2/4/57, "Lutterodt vrs Amartefio," February 16, 1912–September 19, 1914, 115–16; PRAAD SCT 2/4/53, "Kojo Ababio IV versus T.R. Quartey," August 31, 1912–February 13, 1913, October 1, 1912, 238; PRAAD SCT 2/4/51, February 16, 1912–September 19, 1914, May 13, 1912, 180; PRAAD SCT 2/4/50, September 21, 1911–April 12, 1912, "Kobina Jasi versus Kofi Tchum," November 16, 1911, 268.

12. Field, *Religion and Medicine*: on disease etiologies 92–96, 137; on healing practices 77–78, 123–30; on material cultures 37, 114, 120, 123–24, 131, 140.

13. Field, *Religion and Medicine*, 3.

14. Field, *Social Organization of the Gā People*, 104.

15. Field, *Religion and Medicine*, 129–30, 138–41.

16. Allman and Parker, *Tongnaab*, 19; Field, *Religion and Medicine*, 138.

17. Field, *Religion and Medicine*, 132.

18. Field, *Religion and Medicine*, 132.

19. Field, *Religion and Medicine*, 101.

20. Field, *Religion and Medicine*, 132.

21. Field, *Religion and Medicine*, 132.

22. Field, *Religion and Medicine*, 134.

23. Field, *Religion and Medicine*, 130.

24. Field, *Religion and Medicine*, 133n1.

25. Patterson, *Health in Colonial Ghana*, 11.

26. "Quinine," *Encyclopaedia Britannica*, 758. (15 grains = 1 gram).

27. Macmillan, *Red Book of West Africa*, 165; Patterson, *Health in Colonial Ghana*, 36.

28. Addae, *Evolution of Modern Medicine*, 370–71.

29. Addae, *Evolution of Modern Medicine*, 43.

30. *Gold Coast Leader*, 12–26 (August 1911), 3.

31. Ngalamulume, "Keeping the City Clean," 189; Neill, *Networks in Tropical Medicine*, 104; Swanson, "Sanitation Syndrome," 391.

32. Pierre, *Predicament of Blackness*, 27–31.

33. Patterson, "Influenza Epidemic of 1918–19," 1.

34. Cardinall, *Gold Coast*, 46.

35. *Korle Bu Hospital, 1923–1973*, 14. The Gold Coast spent significantly more on sanitation than did other colonies, such as Nigeria and Kenya, where the medical budget averaged around 7 percent during the 1920s. Arthur E. Horn, "Control of Disease in Tropical Africa: Part I," 24.

36. Akyeampong, "Boxing in Accra," 44.

37. *Accra Town Council Minutes*, September 13, 1926; *Gold Coast Independent*, October 30, 1926, 1316. For more information about resistance to the Town's Ordinance Act, see Parker, *Making the Town*, 222–27; Gocking, *History of Ghana*, 52–54.

38. Acquah, *Accra Survey*, 26.

39. Gold Coast Colony, *Report on the Medical Department*, 21.

40. Field, *Religion and Medicine*, 131–32; Patterson, "Health in Urban Ghana," 253.

41. Patterson, "Health in Urban Ghana," 263; Macfie, "Intravenous Injection," 654–55.

42. Addae, *Evolution of Modern Medicine*, 43.

43. Newell and Gadzekpo, *Selected Writings*, 90; Patterson, "Health in Urban Ghana," 255.

44. Addae, *Evolution of Modern Medicine*, 129.

45. Gold Coast Government, *Civil Service List* (Accra: Government Press, 1917), 173; PRAAD Accra Town Council, *Estimates of Revenue and Expenditure* (1931–32), 6.

46. *Gold Coast Independent*, February 5, 1927, 173.

47. Parker, *Making the Town*, 199.

48. Patterson, *Health in Colonial Ghana*, 40.

49. Patterson, *Health in Colonial Ghana*, 40.

50. *Gold Coast Independent*, November 24, 1928, 1106; Parker, *Making the Town*, 199.

51. *Gold Coast Independent*, May 20, 1939, 471; *Gold Coast Independent*, July 24, 1926, 899.

52. Field, *Religion and Medicine*, 132n1.

53. "The Sanitary Inspector's Ladle," *Gold Coast Nation*, June 15, 1916, 1379.

54. Patterson, *Health in Colonial Ghana*, 40; Scott, *Epidemic Disease in Ghana*, 42; Addae, *Evolution of Medicine*, 128.

55. *Gold Coast Independent*, September 4, 1926, 1060–63; *Gold Coast Independent*, January 26. 1929, 113.

56. *Gold Coast Independent*, December 15, 1934, 1190; *Gold Coast Independent*, July 24, 1926, 802.

57. *Gold Coast Independent*, September 4, 1926, 1063; *Gold Coast Independent*, July 23, 1926, 805; *Gold Coast Independent*, July 24, 1926, 802; *Gold Coast Independent*, September 25, 1926, 1156; Patterson, "Health in Urban Ghana," 256.

58. *Gold Coast Independent*, January 26, 1929, 114.

59. Patterson, *Health in Colonial Ghana*, 82 and table 28. Patterson shows that accident victims in the colony as a whole made up more than 10 percent of all hospital cases during some years in the 1920s.

60. *Gold Coast Independent*, October 2, 1926, 1185.

61. "Accident at a Faanaa Village," *Gold Coast Independent*, December 25, 1926, 1639; for another example, see PRAAD SCT 2/4/57. February 16, 1912–September 19, 1940, 191–220.

62. Arn, "Third World Urbanization," 430.

63. PRAAD SCT 2/4/25, "A.F. Lokko versus Connell," March 25, 1897–August 30, 1897, April 27, 1897, 130–33.

64. Automobile imports to the colony grew from 283 in 1921 to over 2,000 in 1929. Cardinall, *Gold Coast*, 107.

65. For accounts of automobile accidents in the newspapers, see *Gold Coast Independent*, December 18, 1926, 1606; *Gold Coast Independent*,

March 2, 1929, 271; *Gold Coast Independent*, January 8, 1927; for cases from court records in the 1930s and 40s, see PRAAD RG 16/2/23, "J.O. Tettey for Adjaye Quarcoo v Cobblah, 26/10/36, 498–505; PRAAD RG16.2.31, "Tettey vs Osamfo Adorkor," 12/20/49, 192; PRAAD RG 16.2.18, "Wazil Hausa versus Belenyah," 12/4/45, 303–4.

66. For an example of a civil case involving a car accident, see PRAAD ADM 23/9/36, "J.B. Blankson v. J.W. Quarshie," 317–18.

67. Clifford, *Our Days on the Gold Coast*, 29.

68. *Gold Coast Independent*, January 12, 1929, 79.

69. *Gold Coast Independent*, January 12, 1929, 82.

70. Forster, "Short Psychiatric Review of Ghana," 28.

71. Field, *Social Organization of the Gã People*, 105.

72. *Gold Coast Independent*, October 16, 1926, 1254.

73. *Gold Coast Independent*, March 26, 1927, 399.

74. *Gold Coast Independent*, January 15, 1926, 75.

75. Patterson, *Health in Colonial Ghana*, 15.

76. Kimble, *Political History of Ghana*, 109.

77. Clifford, *Our Days on the Gold Coast*, 56; Prais, "Imperial Travelers," 22.

78. Clifford, *Our Days on the Gold Coast*, 223–45.

79. Clifford, *Our Days on the Gold Coast*, 223.

80. Sampson, *Gold Coast Men of Affairs*, 179.

81. Addae, *Evolution of Modern Medicine*, 227.

82. Sampson, *Gold Coast Men of Affairs*, 178–80.

83. Gold Coast Colony, *Gold Coast Handbook* (Accra: Government Press, 1923), 596–97.

84. Patton, *Physicians, Colonial Racism*, 156–57; *Marcus Garvey and Universal Negro Improvement Association Papers*, 53n1.

85. The Brew family was prominent in the history of Anamaboe and Cape Coast. See Sparks, *Where the Negroes Are Masters*.

86. PRAAD SCT 2/4/69, "Merry Brew versus Doday," May 17, 1918–November 14, 1919, October 10, 1919, 546.

87. A "shame cloth" is known as *bue* in Ga and is traditionally worn during menstruation, a time when women who follow the taboos of the local shrines must observe proscriptions regarding their movement through religious sites and their contact with religious officials. This composite medicine is similar to forms of *ti* found in Accra today.

88. PRAAD SCT 2/4/69, "Merry Brew versus Doday," May 17, 1918–November 14, 1919, October 10, 1919, 546.

89. PRAAD SCT 2/4/69, "Merry Brew versus Doday," May 17, 1918–November 14, 1919, October 10, 1919, 548.

90. PRAAD SCT 2/4/69, "Merry Brew versus Doday," May 17, 1918–November 14, 1919, October 10, 1919, 549.

91. PRAAD SCT 2/4/69, "Merry Brew versus Doday," May 17, 1918–November 14, 1919, October 10, 1919, 546.

92. Noel Smith, *Presbyterian Church of Ghana*, 140–41.

93. Mohr, "Capitalism, Chaos, and Christian Healing," 71.

94. Mohr, "Capitalism, Chaos, and Christian Healing," 70.

95. Allan Anderson, *Introduction to Pentecostalism*, 117.

96. Acquah, *Accra Survey*, 148; Baeta, *Prophetism in Ghana*, 21; Haliburton, *Prophet Harris*, plate after 202.

97. Kofi Asare Opuku, "A Brief History of Independent Church Movements in Ghana since 1862," in *The Rise of Independent Churches in Ghana* (Accra: Asempa, 1990), 17; Gerald H. Anderson, *Biographical Dictionary of Christian Missions*, 506–7.

98. Selwyn-Clarke, Le Fanu, and Ingram, "Relapsing Fever," 390.

99. Mumuni, "A Survey of Islamic Non-governmental Organizations," 139.

100. Scott, *Epidemic Disease in Ghana*, 128.

101. Scott, *Epidemic Disease in Ghana*, 32–33.

102. Russell, "Experimental Relapsing Fever," 36.

103. Selwyn-Clarke, Le Fanu, and Ingram, "Relapsing Fever," 425.

104. Prais, *Imperial Travelers*, 141–43; van den Bersselaar, *King of Drinks*, 215; Dwight, Malefyt, and Moeran, *Advertising Cultures*, 41. Thomas Richards commented that the discourse of colonization produced by explorers like Henry Morton Stanley conceived of Africans in terms of their relationships to exports and imports; see Richards, *Commodity Culture of Victorian England*, 123.

105. Senah, *Money Be Man*, 120.

106. *Gold Coast Colony Blue Books* (Accra, Ghana: Government Printer, 1891, 1920).

107. Macmillan, *Red Book of West Africa*, 173.

108. British Medical Association, *Secret Remedies*; British Medical Association, *More Secret Remedies*; Cramp, *Nostrums and Quackery*; Loeb, "Doctors and Patent Medicines," 411.

109. *Gold Coast Independent*, November 6, 1926, 1357.

110. Field, *Religion and Medicine*, 133.

111. Barber, *Africa's Hidden Histories*, 8. For more information on literacy rates, see T. David Williams, "Sir Gordon Guggisberg," 305; Agyemang, *Century with Boys*, 92.

112. *Gold Coast Independent*, Saturday, July 1, 1922.

113. Richards, *Commodity Culture of Victorian England*, 195, 202–3.

114. Appadurai, *Social Life of Things*, 21, 50.

115. US Supreme Court, *Manhattan Medicine Co. v. Wood*, 108.

116. Hannah Ofusu, interview with the author, June 20, 2006; Ama Wiafe, interview with the author, June 20, 2006.

117. *Glocalization* is a term derived from the business jargon of the 1990s and was later popularized by sociologists Roland Robertson, Keith Hampton, and Barry Wellman. Barry Wellman, "Little Boxes, Glocalization, and Networked Individualism," in *Digital Cities II*, ed. Makoto Tanabe, Peter van den Besselaar and Toru Ishida (Berlin: Springer, 2002), 11–25; Wellman and Hampton, "Living Networked On and Offline," 648–54.

118. Davidson, *Mediating Race and Class*.

119. Sister Mary, interview with the author, June 13, 2006; Dmitri van den Bersselaar has shown how gin brands became indigenized with truncated names that represented images on the labels, like "bird" and "money" gin. European marketers were aware of these local names, and they flooded the market with similar-looking products to take advantage of prior brand recognition. Van den Bersselaar, *King of Drinks*, 11–53.

120. Hannah Ofusu, interview with the author, June 11, 2006; Felicia Lamptey, interview with the author, June 10, 2006.

121. Augustina Quaye, interview with the author, June 20, 2006; Ama Wiafe, interview with the author, June 20, 2006.

122. Kojo Senah records Sloan's Liniment as one of the commonly used medical antiseptics in Bortianor in the 1990s. Senah, *Money Be Man*, 120, 124.

123. Blumenthal, "Gripe Water Story," 172–73; Tanner, *Index of Diseases and Their Treatment*, 155; Dobson, "Malaria in England."

124. Blumenthal, "Gripe Water Story," 173.

125. Kajri Jain, "New Visual Technologies in the Bazaar: Reterritorialisation of the Sacred in Popular Print Culture," in *Sarai Reader (2003): Shaping Technologies*, ed. Jeebesh Bagchi, Monica Narula, Shuddhabrata Sengupta, Geert Lovink, and Marleen Stikker (Sarai Media Lab, Autonomedia), 49.

126. *Matalisi* [Messenger], December 14, 1924, 10; *Ebifa Mu Uganda* [News from Uganda], September 1937, frontispiece.

127. Gesler, "Illness and Health Practitioner Use," 27.

128. Gesler, "Illness and Health Practitioner Use," 29; Senah, *Money Be Man*, 160. Senah also notes that store-bought medicines usually have longer shelf lives than the average local herbal remedy.

129. Benjamin Orlove and Arnold J. Bauer, "Giving Importance to Imports," in *The Allure of the Foreign: Imported Goods in Postcolonial Latin America*, ed. Benjamin Orlove (Ann Arbor: University of Michigan Press, 1997), 18.

130. ADM 11/1/850, "Letter from the Acting Secretary for Native Affairs to the Colonial Secretary," S.N.A. 36/1923 Special Warrant for £448.9.6, January 30, 1924; ADM 11/1/850, "Memorandum from the Secretary of Native Affairs to the District Commissioner, Accra," S.N.A. 36/23 October 6, 1923.

131. *Korle Bu Hospital, 1923–1973*, 15, 36, 38.

132. Taken from a quote from the back of a postcard entitled "A Ward in the Hospital for Africans, Accra, Gold Coast," in the Smyly Gold Coast [i.e., Ghana] Collection, 1911–1929, Cambridge University Library: Royal Commonwealth Society Library, GBR/0115/Y30448L, selected postcards of the Gold Coast [i.e., Ghana], West Africa 1924: series II, PC Gold Coast/7-11, 1924.

133. *Korle Bu Hospital, 1923–1973*, 36.

134. For examples of Lugard's reliance on the triumph of medicine in Africa, see Lugard, *Dual Mandate in British Tropical Africa*, 144, 151–54.

135. Desai, *Subject to Colonialism*, 2, from Lugard, *Dual Mandate*, 94–95.

136. Lugard, *Dual Mandate*, 92–93. Lugard footnotes this passage as the words of Colonel Amery of the Colonial Office in 1919.

137. Addae, *Evolution of Modern Medicine*, 68.

138. Addae, *Evolution of Modern Medicine*, 68; James Le Fanu, "Cecil Le Fanu: A Doctor and a Gentleman," August 9, 1998, http://www.lefanus-online.org/profiles.html#178.

139. Patton, *Physicians, Colonial Racism*, 157–58.

140. For a brief history of the creation of the Ministry of Health and the growing coordination of class-based hospital systems in London, see Rivett, *Development of the London Hospital System*, 184.

141. Patterson, *Health in Colonial Ghana*, 16–17.

142. Wraith, *Guggisberg*, 240; Patterson, *Health in Colonial Ghana*, 18.

FOUR

COLONIAL MEDICAL CULTURE
AT KORLE BU, 1923–1945

WHEN THE GOLD COAST HOSPITAL opened in 1923, its success was not guaranteed. European medical culture had been present in Accra for centuries but had achieved little more than niche status as a minority therapeutic alternative. The former colonial hospital bungalow had been a modest success, but in a vibrant therapeutic marketplace, there was no reason to believe that African patients would flock to a new colonial institution. But from Governor Guggisberg's perspective the hospital had to succeed if he was to sustain his progressive agenda to modernize the Gold Coast. He believed that both the colony, with an estimated population of 2.3 million, and the capital city, with a population estimated at 44,000 (including 3,000 Europeans), were underpopulated and growing at too sluggish a rate to sustain an important role within the imperial economy.[1] The new institution promised to increase the general health of workers in the Gold Coast and, by extension, grow both the population and the economy, a necessity in order to expand railway, mining, and agricultural projects. It also saw the hospital as a fulfillment of a pledge: medical treatment as advanced as any provided in Britain, to anyone in the colony, whether White or Black.

As it turned out, the African residents of Accra did embrace the new institution, but not for the reasons Guggisberg and the

Medical Department expected. As in the missionary dispensaries and the old colonial hospital, most of the action at Korle Bu took place at the outpatient ward, where patients sought out pills and injections for yaws, syphilis, gonorrhea, and malaria. In other words, quick fixes drove the increasing demand for colonial medicine. Patients were less interested in long stays at Korle Bu, but the new institution was designed in such a way that once they arrived on the hospital campus, they sometimes found themselves drawn in by new forms of colonial bio-power. The spatial design of the new hospital allowed physicians to line up patients, separate them from their therapy management groups, control their movement through buildings, aggregate them with patients with similar illnesses, and place them under constant surveillance. This meant that patients who may have stopped by Korle Bu hoping for an easy cure sometimes found themselves enmeshed within a set of "material coercions" (as Foucault would put it) that transformed them, quite suddenly, into subjects of a new type of colonial medical regime.[2]

Concurrently, the new hospital opened up new avenues of distinction for the aspirant, professional medical classes of Accra. For decades, Western-trained African physicians had struggled for recognition within the West African Medical Services, but at Korle Bu they suddenly found themselves working side by side with White doctors and mingling with White colonial elites in a way that they never had before. Nurses too were able to learn techniques of specialized care, a major advance from the basic work they did at the old colonial hospital. And by working with new machinery, dispensers and technicians also found room to expand their professional expertise. This new cadre of professionals continued to suffer the indignities of racism and exclusion, but they endured such experiences as a rite of passage, hoping that they might one day take leadership roles at the new institution.

The culture of colonial medicine also spread beyond the hospital campus during the 1920s and 1930s, through a network of

maternity clinics where women doctors and nurses taught a public form of medicalized parenting known as mothercraft.[3] One
notable agent in the cultural transformation of maternal care was
Cicely Williams, a physician best known for naming *kwashiorkor*,
a debilitating childhood nutritional deficiency that was common
in the city. During her term at Korle Bu, she sought to bridge linguistic gaps between the patients and doctors, helping to weave
Korle Bu and its satellite clinics into a network of maternity care
facilities. Williams, along with dozens of other British and African physicians and nurses, built a successful counterculture of
midwifery and mothering, challenging long-established traditions of Ga infant and maternal care.

WESTERN MEDICAL SUCCESS AT
KORLE BU: AN EVALUATION

When it opened in 1923, Korle Bu was the largest hospital in West
Africa, with over two hundred beds for inpatients and a large outpatient ward to serve people from around the colony.[4] Fees were
modest, or waived entirely for those who could not pay. Imported
medicines were also readily available at reasonable prices, and
the large dispensary kept in stock the latest European pharmaceuticals and supplies. Korle Bu became a full-service medical
institution, offering therapies for everything from coughs and
colds to thoracic surgery, and the patient registers are replete with
hundreds of different ailments that sufferers brought to the hospital in the hope of a cure. In fact, in many ways, Korle Bu did live
up to Guggisberg's vision of the model hospital in West Africa.
The dingy old colonial hospital on High Street became a distant
memory as Korle Bu became known throughout the colony and
the region as a center for colonial medical care.

On the surface, patient demand seemed to indicate that Korle
Bu was a spectacular success. In 1924, the doctors and nurses of
the new hospital treated a total of fifteen hundred inpatients, and

over a decade later, by 1938, this had more than doubled to almost four thousand per year. Outpatient demand also grew rapidly, reaching 11,283 in 1926–27 and 17,903 in 1938.[5] By the 1930s, the hospital was crowded to the point of overcapacity but could not be expanded because of retrenchment of government spending during the depression.[6] However, the statistical success of Korle Bu deserves some scrutiny. When the outpatient numbers are compared with dispensary attendance in other parts of the colony, they do not seem quite so dramatic. For example, in 1927–28 Korle Bu saw around 14,000 outpatients, a very large number in comparison to the old hospital but only about one-tenth of the 120,000 patients seen at clinics around the colony.[7] Smaller dispensaries in remote regions of the colony often attracted more patients than Korle Bu, exemplified by the Upper West Region, where a single Catholic mission saw more than 30,000 outpatients annually for the treatment of yaws, malaria, trypanosomiasis, and other illnesses during the 1930s.[8] Nor was attendance at Korle Bu dramatic when compared with hospitals in Nigeria and Uganda, whose patient numbers also rose significantly during the 1920s.[9] In fact, much of the success in attracting patients can be attributed to the exponentially expanding urban population of the city and the colony.

Moreover, the popularity of Korle Bu cannot be attributed broadly to Guggisberg's "methods of modern medicine" but rather should be attributed to a handful of specific injections that were popular not just in Africa but around the world. Patients came to Korle Bu for things like neoarsenobillon for yaws and neosalvarsan for syphilis and gonorrhea, chemical treatments that they found superior to local herbs.[10] Ga healers could treat ulcerations on the skin caused by these diseases, usually by bathing sores with herbal infusions, then dressing the lesions with pepper, copper sulfate dust, and palm oil, but such therapies could be both tedious and expensive.[11] Patients came to prefer the rapid action of injections of arsenical compounds into the gluteus maximus—which colonial doctors referred to as "bum-punching"—because their effects were observable within a matter of days.[12] Injections of quinine sulfate for severe cases of malaria were also popular, making it the third most common illness treated at the Gold Coast Hospital. Treatments for injuries, bronchitis, conjunctivitis, and constipation were also common in the hospital records, although to a far lesser degree.[13] Other treatments at Korle Bu were statistically insignificant because they were divided among dozens of different ailments and given to a relatively small number of people.

The demand for so-called bum-punching may have surprised doctors at Korle Bu, but African patients lined up for injections for several reasons.[14] First, for centuries, healers in Accra had been making cuts on their patients' skin and rubbing them with inoculants. Africans might have seen the injections given at the outpatient ward at Korle Bu as a therapy that ran parallel to the ritual incisions that they were already familiar with. Moreover, the popularity, and apparent success, of injections with Haffkine's prophylactic during the bubonic plague campaign in 1908 had already established a precedence for demand for European-derived inoculants.[15] Additionally, it must have helped that many African doctors and nurses were giving the injections. It is said that when C. E. Reindorf (son of Carl Christian Reindorf) became the director of the Venereal Disease Clinic in 1920, the number of patients seeking treatment for syphilis and gonorrhea rapidly increased.[16] Finally, and most importantly, the cures offered at Korle Bu worked quickly. Though painful, injections of the latest chemical formulae could, within days, halt the progress of diseases that caused sexual dysfunction, bodily disfigurement, or death.

Although they favored the bustling outpatient ward, patients were not as enthusiastic about filling the beds of the Gold Coast Hospital. By the 1920s, patients in Britain had come to accept that suffering from an acute illness might require a stay at a hospital, but this was not necessarily the case in Accra.[17] The resident medical officer at the time, Dr. Selwyn-Clarke, noted that the Africans in the city did not "take kindly to hospital treatment," adding that they only submitted after being pressured to do so and that they were eager to be discharged as soon as possible.[18] While inpatient numbers did rise, reaching over two hundred bed stays per day, most of these patients would have had severe malaria or other ailments that did not require them to go under the knife. Indeed, it was often the power of colonial medical authority that detained colonial subjects at Korle Bu, rather than patient demand.

The celebration of Korle Bu as a center for medical research also requires some qualification. Since the rise of institutional racism within imperial circles, the colonies of European empires had been sidelined in the search for the cure for tropical diseases, despite their proximity to pathogens. When Easmon was refused funding in the 1880s, it seemed that the dream of participating in the new field of tropical medicine had faded away—not just on the Gold Coast but around West Africa.[19] However, the relocation of the Accra Laboratory to the Korle Bu campus in 1923 offered some hope that the new institution would become home to a new wave of medical research. The new Accra Medical Research Institute offered far more space and equipment than the laboratory in a bungalow at Victoriaborg. Scientists working at Korle Bu now had access to a pathology lab, an incubator room, cages for testing drugs on animals, and a mosquito-proof house for research on insect-borne illnesses. With these facilities, they managed to publish several papers on the transmission of malaria, trypanosomiasis, and relapsing fever. The institute is perhaps best known for a short burst of research on yellow fever, funded by the Rockefeller Institute in 1927, during which two luminaries in the global medical research field, William Alexander Young and Hideyo Noguchi, worked on the hospital campus. At one point in 1927, Noguchi had almost eight hundred monkeys and apes jammed into a menagerie of cages, to be used to test vaccines for yellow fever. During these heady days of intensive research, patients on the hospital campus recalled hearing Noguchi screaming in anger when his experiments did not go as planned.[20] Sadly, tragedy struck in January 1928, when laboratory mistakes resulted in the infection of both Young and Noguchi.[21] After their deaths, the employees of the Medical Department sanitized the laboratory, culled the monkeys, and closed down the Rockefeller facility, effectively halting medical research until after the Great Depression and the Second World War.[22] It should also be added that the Gold Coast government had never intended that the Accra Medical Research Institute would be a site for African scientists to conduct basic research on a broad spectrum of maladies. As the focus on yellow fever suggests, the laboratory at Korle Bu had a pragmatic purpose: to find cures for the tropical diseases that endangered colonial officials or that hindered the productivity of the colonial labor force.

The dream of turning the Gold Coast Hospital into a center for medical training also fell well short of Guggisberg's dream. The construction of the new institution reignited the hope that Accra could be a center for medical teaching, but the governors of other British West African colonies refused to allow training to be centralized at the Gold Coast. Plans for a teaching hospital were postponed for years and officially canceled by the colonial office in 1931, to be replaced only with the continuation of a modest scholarship program for Africans to train as physicians in the United Kingdom.[23] An apprenticeship program for nurses was initiated at Korle Bu in 1927, but a similar program for dispensers was delayed for several years, until Governor Slater managed to allocate funding in 1931. Although Korle Bu remained an important training ground for Africans returning from the United Kingdom with medical certificates and degrees, it was not until 1964, long after Ghanaian independence, that the Korle Bu name would merit the name of "Teaching Hospital."[24]

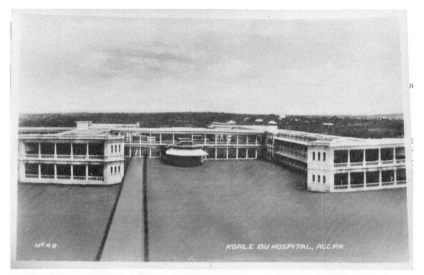

Figure 4.1. Rear views of the Gold Coast Hospital, with laundry department in the foreground, circa 1940. The white bedsheets in fig. 4.1b are spread out to dry in the hot sun outside the laundry department, where men and women are working in a shady breezeway. Also evident is the power pole, which brought electricity from a generator on the campus to provide power for the machinery and lights in the hospital. The gazebo (*left*) served as the staff cafeteria, and in the distance, beyond a lightly inhabited and leafy cordon sanitaire, the crowded houses of Ussher Town are just barely visible. (Source: *Guardian* online, "Accra a Century Ago: Life in Ghana before Independence—in Pictures," March 7, 2017.)

COLONIAL BIO-POWER AT KORLE BU

Quick cures drew patients to Korle Bu, but they can't account entirely for the overall success of the institution. There were other factors at work. The same sorts of incentives and directives that had channeled patients toward the old colonial hospital were still in place, and their influence continued to grow. Colonial subjects working in Accra, whether in the army, the police force, schools, government service, or a European firm, may have been expected to seek treatment at Korle Bu when they were ill. Thus, the expansion of the colonial government

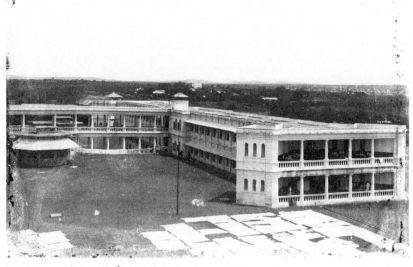

Figure 4.1. *Continued*

and economy meant the expansion of the number of patients beholden to a colonial medical gaze. Once a patient had made the journey across the bridge to the hospital campus, they could find themselves transformed from a colonial subject into a medical subject.

In the 1920s, a patient who chose to patronize an African healer would arrive at a compound with their retinue of family and friends and present themselves as a patient for rituals that they hoped would result in bodily and spiritual health. Visiting a clinic owned by an African physician was similar, in that a patient could choose to see them or request that the physician visit their home. Korle Bu was different. Patients who entered the wards of the Gold Coast Hospital had to leave their therapy management groups outside the doors. Patient submitted themselves autonomously to the authority of European medicine, allowing their bodies to be cleansed, dressed, and placed in beds, row on row, sleeping with strangers, in the long wards of the new hospital.

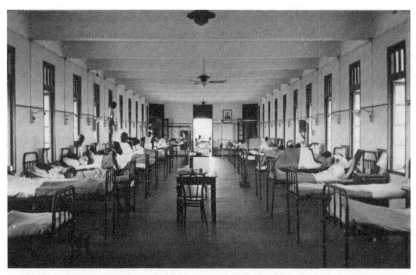

Figure 4.2. A ward of the Gold Coast Hospital, with a nursing station and a portrait of King George. Constructed according to the Nightingale model, the wards of Korle Bu were built to facilitate the flow of air. Also evident is a hierarchical medical gaze; patients were monitored from the nurses' station in the center of the ward and were under constant surveillance by the eyes of King George. The therapy management groups that normally accompanied patients were restricted to visiting hours only. (Source: Basel Mission archive photo, ref #: QD-30.102.0002.)

Rather than choosing to healer-hop, they were placed in a position where the healers did the hopping, as doctors, nurses, and technicians moved from patient to patient. In this way, the Gold Coast Hospital concretely represented a transition from patient care embedded within kin and culture to the treatment of abstracted, medicalized bodies.

Korle Bu's layout formed an elaborate stage for the a patient's encounter with colonial medicine. A sick person arrived at the front door and made a series of quick transitions into medical subjecthood. Anyone admitted had to pass through an ablution block of water taps and washbasins, where they were bathed and disinfected before they were given a bed. The hospital was laid out in an H-shape, an inherited legacy of medical architecture adapted to the African tropics with sweeping multistory edifices supported by neoclassical columns and long hallways with open wings designed to allow salubrious breezes to flow in and out of the building.[25] Patients were taken into "Nightingale wards," which allowed for both adequate spacing between sick bodies and the hierarchical surveillance of patients.[26] Portions of the hospital were designated as isolation wards, with patients categorized according to their degree of infectiousness. Some areas were entirely aseptic, such as the surgery wards, where patients brought in for operations were stripped of all clothing except for their hospital gowns. Under no circumstances were patients allowed to bring amulets or any other consecrated charms into the operating room.[27] Though they may not have realized it, the patients of Korle Bu found themselves embedded within European medical history, in buildings that reflected Joseph Lister's principles of sterilization, Florence Nightingale's patterns of patient spacing, and Sir William John Ritchie Simpson's obsession with light and ventilation.[28]

The hospital was also designed to effectively separate human bodies from bodily fluids, soiled clothing, and cadavers. The former colonial hospital had rudimentary outdoor latrines and baths, but Korle Bu had running water and toilets inside the building.[29] Human waste was disposed of in a way that was novel for most inhabitants of the city: it was flushed down the drain. Initially, many of the employees were uncomfortable using indoor bathrooms because they lacked privacy, but eventually, the employees adapted to the convenience of toilets, and as a joke, they intimidated patients by threatening "to flush them down the toilet" if they misbehaved.[30] At the old hospital, nurses washed sheets and bedclothes by hand, but at Korle Bu this job was delegated to a team of women trained to use electric laundry machines and a disinfecting machine in the boiler room. The handling of cadavers also differed at Korle Bu. The typical mortuary practices of African residents in the city included dressing the body for presentation in the home, then transporting it outside the city for burial in government-approved graveyards, all within one or two days.[31] When the mortuary building was inaugurated at Korle Bu, dead bodies could be removed from the scene of death immediately and taken by motor hearse to the hospital for refrigeration. Cadavers could also be kept aside for postmortem inspection if they were thought to have any value for research. Coffin stores began to pop up next to the mortuary, so family members could take their deceased relatives back to their homes in caskets.[32]

Korle Bu could be a terrifying place for patients, who were often unsettled by medical equipment and procedures. The sight of iron lungs, gas canisters, and hypodermic needles would have been discomfiting to most patients, and the use of anesthetics inspired a great deal of trepidation. D. H. Reindorf, a member of the prominent Ga family and an anesthetist at Korle Bu, recalled that he was both honored and feared as a member of the surgical team: "I was for a considerable period the sole Anaesthetist and when going from the Dispensary to the Theatre with pomp and parade, all my admirers and patients, ready for the operation, cheered me by saying 'OKUM NIPA' was coming: meaning I put people to sleep or literally killed them temporarily."[33]

Reindorf's nickname demonstrates the anxiety and reverence that patients had for those given the authority to render someone unconscious. Although the hospital's technology granted employees healing power over their fellow subjects, the patients at Korle Bu were understandably unnerved by the control they asserted over states of consciousness. In other parts of Africa, the use of anesthesia also challenged the building of trust in Western medicine, leading to rumors of vampirism and zombiism.[34] No such rumors are extant in records, but patient ambivalence was clear.

Surgery was also contested at Korle Bu. Although African healers in Accra did have some painful therapies, such as slicing the skin to rub in dry powders, radically intrusive surgical acts such as opening the chest cavity were exclusive to colonial medical practice. In order to convince a patient to be put to sleep and opened up, surgeons at Korle Bu had to master the art of bedside manner. When Dr. Nanka-Bruce reminisced about his first few years at Korle Bu, he recalled that encouraging a patient to submit to an operation was a time-consuming process. When he returned from Edinburgh he was shocked to find that it would take "hours, and even days, to beg and coax a would-be patient to submit to an operation for his own benefit."[35] Even though surgical procedures for "indigents" (as African subjects of the Gold Coast were known in hospital records) were conducted free of charge, not all attempts to convince patients to go under the knife were successful.[36] As one nurse recalled, patients often "disappeared from the hospital on the eve of their operations."[37] Surgeons at Korle Bu did have a steady supply of trauma victims who were brought to the hospital after accidents, but voluntary surgery was a hard sell. In a setting like Accra, where internal medicine was a new practice, it is understandable that some patients would forgo surgery if the terror of treatment outweighed the promise of a cure.

Perhaps the greatest expression of colonial bio-power at Korle Bu was the way parents offered up unwanted children to the colonial state, allowing the staff of the hospital to raise and name the foundlings. During the interwar period, many children ended up at the hospital after being abandoned on land owned by the colonial government, like the railway station in Accra or the golf course on the grounds of Korle Bu. Others were simply left at the hospital and never picked up by their parents.[38] These children became wards of the Gold Coast government, and they were nursed, cared for, and raised by the doctors and nurses at Korle Bu. Two examples loom large in the memories of the nurses who worked at the hospital during the interwar period. The first is Grace Ward, a baby born to a woman from the Northern Territories who died in childbirth at the hospital sometime in the 1930s. The child was initially given the name Grace O'Brien, in homage to the first woman medical officer, Grace Summerhayes, and the first chief medical officer, Arthur O'Brien, but was later officially renamed Grace Ward because she had become a ward of Korle Bu Hospital. Grace grew up at Korle Bu and worked as an assistant to the nurses until she was old enough to be sent to board at Achimota College.[39] A second example was a seven-year-old boy known as Akesie, who was brought to the hospital with sarcoma of the neck. The prospect of surgery terrified his parents, so they abandoned the boy to his fate. As a former nurse, Mrs. Mould, recalled, Akesie survived a tracheostomy operation and grew up in the hospital, eventually working as an assistant to the nurses and patients.[40] In the absence of an institution like Korle Bu, a child such as Akesie might have been passed to a priest of a local shrine for protection, where he would have grown up as a servant of a deity, but within the newly medicalized colony, the staff at Korle Bu found themselves in charge of the very lives of the child subjects of the Gold Coast.

The Gold Coast Hospital offered a type of patient experience that was completely unique in the history of Accra. As soon as a sick person and their loved ones entered the hospital, they had to put their trust entirely in the hands of medical experts, and they were unable to contribute their opinions to the progress of the therapy. One can imagine how disorienting it might have been to be taken from one's family, washed down by a nurse in the ablution room, dressed in a hospital gown, and asked to lie on a bed, beneath the whir of the ceiling fans, listening to a nurse playing jazz on the ward piano. One can also imagine how disconcerting it might have been to hear the clicking of the X-ray machine, feel the heat of the surgery lights, or be imprisoned inside an iron lung. Becoming a patient at Korle Bu was much more than picking and choosing between therapists in Accra. Submitting to the role of patient inside the hospital meant an effacement of one's cultural self and a bodily submission to the colonial medical gaze. Though a stay at the hospital might have been temporary, it involved separation from the pluralistic healing networks that patients normally relied on. Korle Bu brought patients in Accra the closest they had ever come to medical subjecthood within the new, medically focused colonial regime.

PROFESSIONAL DISTINCTION AT KORLE BU

Many factors increased patient demand at Korle Bu, but the most important reason for the long-term success of the Gold Coast Hospital was that it satisfied the aspirations of the burgeoning African middle classes of Gold Coast. There had always been an African merchant elite in the colonial capital, but during the prosperous era of the cocoa boom, the number of professionals and businesspeople expanded rapidly. The aspirant classes, and their children, sought to appropriate at least some of the levers of power within the colonial state, and the campus of Korle Bu offered a place where colonial subjects could acquire cultural capital by appropriating the tastes and pastimes of their colonial supervisors. Africans employed at the new hospital were still subject to the dictates of White medical authorities, and they were never allowed to supervise White employees, but as a cohort of medical workers at a brand-new institution, they saw themselves as part of a modern workplace that allowed them to distinguish themselves within colonial society. A deep camaraderie emerged among the first generation of employees at Korle Bu, as they forged professional bonds through the shared work of caring for patients and emotional bonds by enduring the indignities of racist colonial rule.

When the Gold Coast Hospital opened, the colony was desperately short of trained nurses. In the 1920s, the economy was booming, and most women could make more money trading in the market than they could working in a hospital.[41] The monthly wages at Korle Bu were low, ranging from three to five pounds, but the benefit of working at the hospital was not always measured in financial terms.[42] Unlike in South Africa, where nurses were recruited from Anglican and Roman Catholic sisterhoods, the bulk of new recruits at Korle Bu were literate graduates from government schools, young women who hoped to elevate their social status by seeking professional fulfillment outside the traditional commercial activities of market women in Accra.[43] The opening of the hospital created a brief window of opportunity for aspiring nurses because demand for personnel was so high they were admitted "purely on their own willingness to train."[44] They were not required to take any courses or examinations, and they were expected to learn on the job.[45]

Mrs. Quartey-Papafio-Coker, a former nurse at Korle Bu, recalled how, one day, she simply took a walk over the bridge over the Korle Lagoon to take on her new career: "[My cousin said that] if I accompanied her to the Gold Coast Hospital, I would be employed almost instantly. So I accompanied her, walking from Faase Quarter in Accra to Korle Bu where a brief interview took place. I was led away into a waiting room and after a little while a lady came and looked at me from head to toe, took a few measurements and . . . brought me some uniforms. I had become a nurse-in-training."[46]

Within the medical workforce of the Gold Coast Colony, the new nurses of Accra took on the nickname *kolebu awula*, or "hospital ladies"—a moniker of femininity and respect for the daughters of the elite families of Accra.[47]

Korle Bu also created opportunities for men who aspired to become physicians. In the 1910s, the restrictions on employment in government hospitals had been eased slightly, but by 1912 only

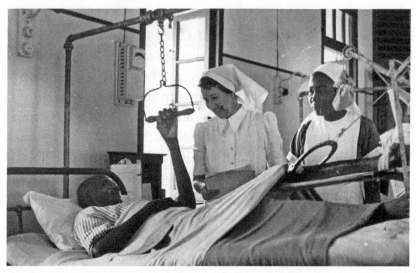

Figure 4.3. The matron of the Gold Coast Hospital, Miss M. A. Henry, stops to chat with a patient, circa 1945. Authority at Korle Bu was always held by White employees. This photo offers a contrast between the smile of the supervisor (*left*) and the pursed lips of her unnamed Black nursing assistant (*right*). The uniforms of the two women indicate their rank among the nursing sisters of the hospital. (Source: Basel Mission archive photo, ref #: QD-30.102.0003.)

8 of the 214 physicians in the West African Medical Service were African. For decades, barriers to entry discouraged young male graduates from entering medicine, forcing them to choose careers in business or law instead, but when the Gold Coast Hospital opened, aspiring physicians hoped that an egalitarian institution would end the racism that had plagued the medical services of West Africa in the past.[48] Prior to the opening of Korle Bu, the governor had already created a new position of junior African medical officer, which allowed newly trained African doctors to work at colonial medical facilities until they gained enough experience to become full-fledged medical officers. African doctors initially protested this new rank, arguing that it was just another way of keeping Africans out of administrative roles in the

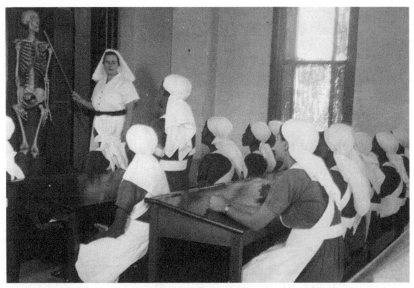

Figure 4.4. African nurses are trained in every branch of medicine and surgery at the Gold Coast Hospital, Accra. Here is a class of students at a lecture by Senior Sister Mutton, circa 1940s. Instruction in nursing at Korle Bu was led entirely by British colonial medical staff. African nurses were the rank and file of the institution, and they understood that they would never be able to inherit the role of matron. (Source: Basel Mission archive photo, ref #: QD-30.102.0007.)

Medical Department. However, the junior officer role was well paid at £400 per annum. More importantly, it offered opportunity to work at Korle Bu. As soon as the institution opened, its chief medical officer, Dr. O'Brien, appointed three junior African medical officers.[49] In 1926, Guggisberg further demonstrated his commitment to placing African physicians in positions of authority when he posted Dr. E. Tagoe (who had trained at Korle Bu) to supervise a hospital in Dunkwa, a mining town in the Western Region of the colony, despite vigorous protests from the White mining community.[50] Though the title of chief medical officer would never be held by an African during the colonial era, Guggisberg and O'Brien did create opportunities for African doctors,

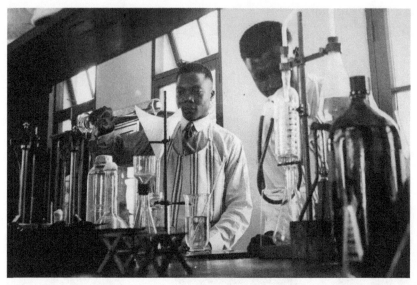

Figure 4.5. School for dispensers, circa 1945. The perspective of this photo emphasizes equipment over personnel by placing flasks in the foreground and the dispensers in their aprons and Western attire in the background. The position of dispenser offered upward mobility to young men hoping to practice medicine or conduct medical research alongside physicians at the Medical Research Institute. (Source: Basel Mission archive photo, ref #: QD-30.102.0009.)

nurses, dispensers, and technicians to advance up the ranks of the colonial medical services.

The memories of former Korle Bu employees reflect the social distinction offered by working at the Gold Coast Hospital. In particular, clothing and uniforms form a vivid part of their recollections. In the old quarters of Accra, the priests and spirit mediums announced their presence by wearing white robes, white body paint, and elaborate hairstyles and jewelry, the costume and finery associated with the traditions of worship and healing.[51] Across the lagoon at Korle Bu, nurses wore starched white accoutrements that defined cleanliness by revealing any trace of dirt.[52] Male employees were similarly uniformed in white robes or aprons and were expected to wear a Western attire of

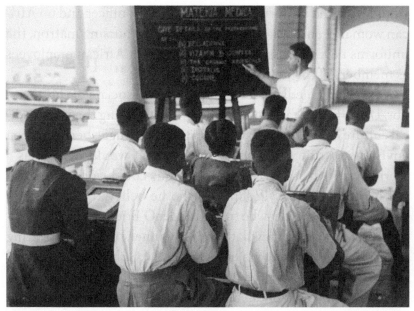

Figure 4.6. School for dispensers at Korle Bu. Mr. E. Allman lecturing to third-year students, circa early 1940s. In this photo, a White instructor points to a chalkboard listing the sorts of *materia medica* nurses and dispensers were expected to use, including belladonna (an alkaloid extracted from nightshade, used to dilate pupils for examination), vitamin B complex (used for nutritional deficiencies like pellagra), organic arsenical (a drug used to treat syphilis and trypanosomiasis, marketed under the trade name of Salvarsan), digitalis (a chemical derived from foxglove, used as a heart antiarrhythmic agent), and Cocaine (used as a topical anesthetic in eye, nose, and throat surgery). These reagents were new, imported tools of healing, and their curative properties spurred demand at the hospital. (Source: Basel Mission archive photo, ref # QD-30.102.0008.)

shirts, ties, and trousers underneath their hospital gear. Just as imported suits and ties were *de rigueur* among the gentlemanly ranks of African merchants and professionals, and just as Christians distinguished themselves from so-called heathens by adopting European dress codes, the dispensers and nurses at Korle Bu wore their medical attire as a "social skin" that marked them as participants in colonial medicine.[53] Although no African man would wear the uniform of the chief medical officer and no African woman would wear the white cap of the nursing matron, the uniforms nevertheless served to distinguish African employees as members of the new secular medical class.[54]

As the chief medical officer and a close associate of the governor, Dr. O'Brien was instrumental in establishing the new medical culture of the Gold Coast Hospital. Like Guggisberg, O'Brien envisioned Korle Bu as an institution that would operate as a meritocracy where Africans and Britons could work in unison, but his leadership style showed who he believed should be in charge.[55] As a dispenser who trained under O'Brien recalled, the hospital director was "somewhat gruff in manner, of military bearing and lame. He had been a major in the R.A.M.C., had been wounded in the First World War and won the military cross. He was a strict disciplinarian and worked like a beaver. . . . Because Dr. O'Brien was lame his footsteps had a characteristic rhythm which made it possible to identify his approach by sound at a distance and thereby give everybody a chance 'to put his house in order!'"[56]

Indeed, O'Brien had been injured during the war in British East Africa, so severely that he almost did not survive.[57] When he recovered, he trained as a physician and joined the colonial medical service, happy to return to a post in Africa. To the Gold Coast Hospital, he brought a sense of fair play and respect, evidenced by the way he knew everyone at Korle Bu by name and followed their careers closely. However, he also brought a severity to the institution that was forever seared into the memories of those who worked with him. Former employees recalled that O'Brien became furious if he saw anyone sleeping on duty and sometimes sacked them on the spot.[58] Though the staff at Korle Bu appreciated his egalitarian ethic, they did not lionize him in their memories. Unlike Guggisberg, who was revered as the founder of their institution, O'Brien embodied a hybrid form of colonial, military, and medical authority at Korle Bu, and as the patrimonial leader of the institution, he was feared and respected but not loved.

Though exacting in his standards of professionalism, O'Brien also promoted a lively social life at the institution. Sports activities were prominent in the memories of former staff members, who recalled that the hospital had football and cricket teams and that a golf course on the perimeter of the campus was open to employees.[59] Despite his war injuries, O'Brien was an avid tennis player, and he even encouraged some of the staff to join him on the lawn tennis courts on campus after work. The camaraderie on the court sometimes extended into O'Brien's domestic space, as he occasionally asked hospital staff over to his house for drinks after a match.[60] Though the African staff would have been familiar with colonial sports like cricket and football, lawn tennis and golf were novelties in Accra, and their initiation into the sports came exclusively from their White supervisors.[61] The colonial setting of the hospital still prevented Africans and Europeans from being equals, but their social relationships could be cordial and even friendly.

At Christmas, the institution came to represent a new form of Christian modernity that was emerging in the city. The staff decorated the wards and brought in trees to decorate and sing around.[62] On Christmas day, everyone joined together to cook a large feast, at which everyone, White and Black, administrators and staff, sat together, ate together, and sang Christmas carols together. Dr. O'Brien played the role of Father Christmas, handing out presents and cash to the nurses and dressers, as well as candies and toys to the patients in the children's ward.[63] Employees exchanged presents too, and nurses recalled with fondness the imported gifts they received from their White colleagues, such as perfumes.[64] The celebration of Christmas at Korle Bu signaled a transition away from *Homowo*, the annual harvest festival that for centuries had dictated the social health of the Ga people. Unlike *Homowo*, which followed strict protocols on noisemaking under the threat of fines and confiscation of property, and week after week of ritualized fishing, crop-planting, and drumming

ceremonies, Christmas at Korle Bu reinforced the British yule-
tide traditions and Christian menology propagated by churches
in the city, creating a substantial cultural space between the colonial medical institution and the African religious and healing
traditions of Accra.

Another special occasion was the annual Korle Bu Hospital
Ball, a major social event that attracted medical professionals from around the colony, White colonial officials, the Black
elites of Gold Coast Society, and any dignitaries who happened to be in the colony at the time.[65] In Accra, Ga healers
and the spirits within them danced to Kpele and Akon drumming rhythms, but at Korle Bu, people danced to a new beat
coming out of America—jazz. The 1920s and 1930s brought
an era of youthful rebellion and musical freedom, and Accra
was no exception. Pianos somehow found their way onto the
hospital grounds, and former nurses remember that songs like
Irving King's "Show Me the Way to Go Home" formed the
soundtrack of the early years of the hospital. Many of these
jazz hits would later be translated into Ga and sung in the
dance halls and drinking spots of the city, which, over time,
gave birth to a hybrid local music known as highlife, but at the
Korle Bu Hospital Ball, Whites and Blacks danced together to
an exclusively jazz beat.[66]

The degree of familiarity between British colonial officials
and African staff members at Korle Bu came to generate some
mutual respect. Ghanaian nurses mostly remembered British
matrons as gracious mentors who treated the staff with civil-
ity.[67] Similarly, some British-trained African physicians had fond
memories of their supervisors. Dr. Nanka-Bruce recalled how, on
a voyage to Liverpool, his supervisor, Dr. Le Fanu, invited him
up to the first-class section of the ship and boldly engaged the
junior colleague in a conversation in fractured Twi. In an age of
segregation and social exclusion, Dr. Le Fanu was the only White
person to speak to Nanka-Bruce during the whole two-week
voyage, while the rest of the Europeans "could hardly conceal

their resentment of having a 'native' in that part of the ship."[68] Similarly, C. E. Reindorf recalled that, on a similar voyage, Gordon Guggisberg violated race and class protocols by engaging the young graduate in a long conversation, offering him a position at the Venereal Diseases Centre (which had yet to be built) if he specialized in the treatment of syphilis during his medical training at Edinburgh.[69] These stories might be overly nostalgic, but they suggest that a professional camaraderie emerged among the builders of the institution at Korle Bu, despite the overt racism that existed in the colony and around the empire.

But while the people working at Korle Bu shared many of the same goals of the colonial medical project, and though some forms of fraternization were acceptable on the hospital campus, a strong differentiation between colonial master and colonial subject remained. At the top of the hierarchy were the resident medical officer and the hospital matron, and it was understood that these positions would never be held by Africans.[70] Not surprisingly, some of the African staff members resented this fact. As one British-trained African physician phrased it, the Black employees at the hospital were required to work under the "pressure of white supremacy" with no prospect of advancement into upper management.[71] The memories of nurses who worked at Korle Bu also contain instances of the abuse of authority.[72] One head nurse, Sister Evans, was particularly reviled as an exacting perfectionist and was described as "one of those Europeans with an imperialistic stamp about them."[73] Another head nurse, Miss Marr, was described as someone "who exuded imperial arrogance from every pore and was obsessed with the idea of 'putting the native in his place.'"[74] Guggisberg's hope of seeing "white nursing sisters and black nurses combine together to look after the sick natives of the country" had been realized, but the racial hierarchies of colonial rule remained.[75]

The depth of racism, and sexism, at Korle Bu is most poignantly evident in the story of Agnes Savage, a young woman with a

Nigerian father and a Scottish mother, who graduated from medical school at Edinburgh with first-class honors in 1929 and won the Dorothy Gilfillan Memorial Prize for the best woman graduate. Dr. Savage soon found work at Korle Bu as a junior medical officer, but despite being born in Scotland, she was paid African wages, expected to board in the quarters with African nurses, and denied the paid leave granted to her White colleagues. Savage spent years petitioning the Colonial Office to remedy the unfair situation, but she did not receive a promotion to medical officer until 1945, just two years before she retired. Eventually, Savage gave up on the Gold Coast and moved back to Scotland.[76]

Savage had the luxury of moving home to the British Isles, but the African staff had no choice but to endure the arrogant racism of their White supervisors. Talking back to a superior was simply not tolerated, and hospital employees could be summarily dismissed for any form of insolence.[77] As one dispenser recalled, African staff members were obliged to tolerate the racial slurs thrown their way. His strategy was to brush them off as motivational: "[As] much as the staff worked hard to justify a good report from superior officers, there were the usual abuses showered on them whenever there happened to be some slight fault. The abuses were in the form of 'Hurry you son of a bush man' 'You silly ape' or 'You Western Kangaroo'. Funny enough these abusive expressions rather spurred the staff on to do better than expected."[78]

These invectives may not have been remembered as grave insults, but they were never forgotten. The employees of Korle Bu resented the way in which White supervisors belittled their subordinates, but they were compelled to endure such treatment as a normal part of working at a colonial institution.

Guggisberg had envisioned Korle Bu as a hospital that would serve everyone in the colony, but the new institution never did attract large numbers of White patients. Despite being the most technically advanced hospital in British West Africa, colonial officials and employees of European firms still preferred to be treated at their homes in Accra or to travel back by steamer to their home country. And there are hints that the few White patients who did seek help at Korle Bu were treated differently from African patients. A nurse who worked at Korle Bu in the 1920s recalled that one of the hospital wards was often reserved exclusively for White patients—using a sign that said "Isolation Block"—even without the presence of any infectious disease.[79] Quite simply, the ethic of meritocracy that employees hoped the new institution would represent was not powerful enough to break the patterns of racial division that had established themselves in colonial Accra decades before.

FROM NAA EDE OYEADU, TO MOTHERCRAFT, TO THE SOCIAL MEDICINE OF CICELY WILLIAMS

Naa webii ne;
Wohe ye feeo tso
Moko na wofee.
Oshi Akwan webii ne;
Naa Ede webii ne;

This is grandmother's family;
We are very beautiful,
Someone wishes to be like us.
This is the road blocker's family;
This is Naa Ede's family.[80]

This song, recorded by anthropologist Marion Kilson in the 1970s, was sung in dedication to Naa Ede Oyeadu, the Ga goddess of birth and regrowth. For decades, perhaps centuries, the priest of Naa Ede Oyeadu had played the role of interlocutor between women and the spirits of fertility, thereby generating a public discourse of Ga motherhood.[81] One of the rules of the Naa Ede Oyeadu shrine was that Ga women who died in childbirth could not be interred in household burial grounds but had to be "left on the ground exposed to the elements" in the bush outside the city.[82] Because the death of the mother during childbirth was believed to create a social rupture that excluded her from ancestral status, the property of the deceased was forfeited to the house of Naa Ede Oyeadu until the paternal home of the woman was purified by Naa Oyeadu Ede's priest.[83] During the colonial era, the cost of purification—one sheep, several chickens, a dozen eggs, dozens of yards of cloth, and an additional cash fee in the range of £60—was so steep that it raised the ire of the colonial administration.[84] In 1905, the district officer of Accra arrested the priest of Naa Ede Oyeadu, charged him with extortion, and sent the Gold Coast Police to demolish the shrine.[85] It was the only shrine in Accra that was officially gazetted as "suppressed" under colonial rule.[86]

Naa Ede Oyeadu was a prominent deity in Accra because the Ga, like many African societies, paid great respect to women who were able to produce many healthy children.[87] Because of the high infant mortality rate in the city, women with large families were considered spiritually powerful, as they were able to defeat the invisible forces that threatened to block conception and birth. Women who entered into marriage contracts were expected to produce children in order to maintain the conjugal union, and women who produced many children and grandchildren could garner the elevated title of *amenye*.[88] Failure to produce a child could result in a loss of status for a wife within her husband's kinship group, her own kinship group, and her own household, especially if there were other wives. Women who could not produce children were thought to reside in a liminal gender state, as incomplete women suffering from a spiritual blockage of their fertility. They might even be suspected of being witches, the embodiment of an evil jealousy that devours life rather than creating it.[89] Naa Ede Oyeadu was not a paramount deity in the city, and her shrine was located in a small compound, but Ga women both revered and feared her because she was the one goddess who specialized in helping women reproduce.

The suppression of the Naa Ede Oyeadu shrine eliminated the priest's role as a mediator in the culture of birth and mothering in the city, creating a unique opportunity for colonial medical practice.[90] In a remarkable turn of events, the Princess Marie Louise Hospital for Mothers and Infants, along with a number of well-baby clinics, quickly filled the cultural vacuum created by the absence of the fertility goddess, propagating a new culture of parenting based on scientific standards of nutrition and hygiene. Quite suddenly, the women of the Gold Coast found themselves introduced to the methods of mothercraft, a wave of child-rearing culture that was sweeping the British Empire. As a result, public motherhood, which had previously been embedded in Ga social and religious institutions, became more highly medicalized than any other component of health and healing in Accra.[91]

The significance of maternal and infant care was first brought to the attention of the colonial administrators in 1915 by Dr. Nanka-Bruce, who, in a speech to the Gold Coast Legislative Council, announced that the infant mortality rate in Accra had reached 360 per thousand.[92] He argued that it was unconscionable for a colonial government to permit such a high death rate among children because it would result in demographic stagnation.[93] Nanka-Bruce implored the colonial government to construct a maternity hospital to train midwives and provide prenatal care for mothers, but during the war, the Medical Department was unable to initiate a maternal and infant health strategy.[94] When funding did become available during the cocoa boom, Governor Guggisberg reiterated Nanka-Bruce's fears of stagnant population growth to rally support for the construction of the Gold Coast Hospital, which was always intended to have a maternity ward.

When it opened in 1923, Korle Bu did have the necessary beds to care for mothers and babies, but it did not yet have a resident specialist in maternal or infant care. At the time, the only infant welfare clinic was on the opposite side of the city in a swish hut behind the Basel Mission in Christiansborg, operated by Scottish missionary Dr. Jessie Beveridge. Mothers in Osu thronged to Beveridge's practice, creating demand that earned the clinic a grant-in-aid from the government to pay for drugs, equipment, and the salary of an interpreter.[95] In 1924, Medical Officer G. J. Pirie, head of the health branch and a veteran of the West African medical services, conceived of a plan for government-run infant welfare clinics around the colony and convinced the Health Department to open one on Derby Avenue (north of Ussher Town) in 1925.[96] Both the Christiansborg and Ussher Town clinics charged nominal fees for the treatment of infants, and they were well patronized. The statistics are incomplete, but those that are available show that the Christiansborg clinic saw 2,700 children in the second half of 1924, and Ussher Town Clinic treated 549 children in the months of February and March alone.[97]

Just as they had at Korle Bu, injections drove demand at the well-baby clinics of Accra. Starting in the 1920s, nurses at the clinics began to offer free injections of chloroquine, a treatment that would have been tremendously helpful for children who could not swallow herbal remedies for malaria. Smallpox vaccinations were also offered for free, but it was the treatments for yaws that became emblematic of infant care in Accra.[98] Nurses and doctors recalled seeing children who were so badly mutilated by yaws that they had sores on their faces, missing noses, and legs so damaged that they were permanently disabled. Not surprisingly, mothers were happy to line their babies up for the weekly "yaws mornings" held at the clinics.[99] The injections of bismuth silicate were a drastic and painful therapy for children, but compared to the drawn-out treatments offered by African healers, they could rapidly dry out wounds and prevent disfigurement.[100] Yaws treatments were so popular that one doctor recalled giving 150 shots in a single morning.[101]

The overall demand for vaccinations left doctors wondering whether they were subjecting some children to the needle more than once, as indicated in a statement made by Dr. May at the Christiansborg clinic in the 1920s: "In a way we're becoming too popular. Take vaccination, for instance. I think it's important that all the children should be vaccinated, so I buy huge tins of sweets. Every child gets a sweet with the injection, and now they seem to come just for the sweet. I suspect that I am vaccinating a large proportion of the child population of Christiansborg at weekly intervals."[102]

When mothers brought their children to be vaccinated, they might not have fully understood the science of the procedure, but they were nonetheless eager to participate in the urban culture of mothering, which included treating their children to imported candies.

In the face of the rapid growth of medicalized childbirth and childcare, the authority of traditional African midwives began to diminish. Until the 1920s, midwifery was an esteemed part-time vocation, learned by apprenticeship with elderly women. The census of 1921 lists the occupation as an "age-long practice" that combined knowledge of herbal remedies for enhancing fertility and solving pregnancy complications with the practical experience of delivering babies and feeding infants.[103] Midwives had passed on their knowledge orally in a gendered sphere of women's knowledge for generations, beyond the purview of the Ga or the British colonial state. However, without the spiritual framework that Naa Ede Oyeadu had provided, and without any coordinated professional association, African midwives had difficulty maintaining control over practices of childbirth and infant care in Accra, and their numbers began to dwindle. This transition from traditional midwifery to mothercraft did not happen by accident; it was the stated goal of the Gold Coast Medical Department. In its 1924 report, the officials at the Medical Department proclaimed that clinical maternal care could offer the mothers of the city a "break from tradition" as they publicly declared themselves to be followers of colonial medicine.[104]

Perhaps the finest expression of the Medical Department's quest to bring colonial medical praxis deeper into the life cycles of the subjects of the Gold Coast was Health Week, a festival inaugurated in 1922 that included public health lectures and a general cleanup of the city, led by schoolchildren and civic groups.[105] A key partner in promoting Health Week was the Gold Coast League for Maternal and Child Welfare, a charity group made up of White women medical officers, nurses, and the wives of colonial officers, who worked together with some of the matrons of elite African families. The league organized a variety of activities to increase awareness of sanitation during the festival, including household visits encouraging mothers to follow colonial methods of child rearing,[106] but the crowning achievement of the league was the baby show.[107] Held in the heart of Ga territory, at Bukom Square, the baby show offered women a chance to show their dedication to public motherhood by presenting their babies to the ladies of the league for assessment. Hundreds of onlookers thronged the baby show as the governor's wife presented trophies to the healthiest babies in different age categories and handed out consolation prizes for all the contestants.[108] In 1925, over 150 mothers presented their babies for judging with the hope of winning a silver porringer sent by Mary, the queen consort herself.[109] As Jennifer Beinart, a historian who has studied photographic images of the African child in the twentieth century, has argued, this was an era when children were brought out of the background of visual representations of empire and put on display as evidence of the benefits of a new era of maternal colonialism. At the same time, the baby show offered a venue for Ga and other African women in Accra to aspire to the title of *amenye*, "woman with many children."

The circulation of printed material also enabled the rise of colonial maternal and infant care in Accra. During the 1920s and 1930s, the *Mothercraft Manual*, a pamphlet on the science of infant care based on the work of New Zealand health reformer

Dr. Truby King, was widely read around the British Empire.[110] In Accra, some young women treated it as an authority on rearing children according to colonial medical principles.

In an essay competition held by the Methodist Book Depot in December 1935, a young woman recommended the book to girls who planned to be mothers: "Each time or at any time I read [it] I feel still much interested as if I have not read it before. I hope to become in future a careful and healthy mother to mind my children according to the methods and instructions given in my most favourite book. For fear of forgetting some good parts in it I am treating it as my bosom friend."[111]

Even for nonliterate mothers, the book was influential because it included before-and-after graphics—images of sickly infants transformed into healthy babies though techniques of nutrition and hygiene.[112] In 1926, the Medical Department printed a short book authored by Dr. Beveridge for distribution as an instructional manual for feeding and caring for babies in the tropics. Entitled *Healthy Babies: Advice to Mothers*, the book was translated into Ga and Twi and circulated around the city of Accra with the hope that the women of Accra would start to raise their babies according to British colonial standards.[113] There are no extant copies of the translated versions, so the precise terminology used to translate concepts of maternal and infant care into Ga or Twi terminology is lost, but the simple fact that they were translated speaks to both demand from African mothers and the desire of nurses and doctors to introduce the women of the city to the practices of mothercraft.

The success of the infant welfare clinics spurred the government to put aside money for a full-fledged maternity hospital at Korle Bu. Construction began in 1925 with much fanfare, when philanthropist and traveler Princess Marie Louise (one of Queen Victoria's granddaughters) laid the cornerstone for the building.[114] In the princess's own words, "Accra in its entirety was present" at the groundbreaking, as Governor Guggisberg reiterated the evils

of infant mortality in a stirring speech, and Marie Louise bowed
to touch the stone as it was lowered into the ground at Korle Bu.
The Princess Marie Louise Hospital for Mothers and Infants took
three more years to complete, but when it did open in 1928, it offered two wards for expecting and nursing mothers, a dispensary,
a pathology laboratory, and lodging for nurses and doctors.[115]
Prominent Presbyterian women in Accra, such as Mrs. Wilkie
(the wife of a Scottish missionary) and Miss Wulff (a member of
a prominent African family in Osu), worked together to encourage women to patronize the new hospital, making it headquarters
for mothercraft in the city.[116] By the early 1930s, the number of
children treated at the maternity hospital rose to over one hundred thousand per year, and it quickly became overcrowded.[117]
So pervasive was the impact of the hospital on women's culture in
Accra that the term *kolebu* took on yet another significance—as a
word for the maternity aprons that pregnant women wore when
they were admitted to the hospital to give birth.[118]

The maternity department was administered separately from
the main Gold Coast Hospital by the first woman medical officer
in Accra, Dr. Grace Summerhayes. After training as an orderly at
a women's hospital in France during the First World War,[119] Summerhayes went home to pursue a medical degree at Edinburgh
and graduated with a specialization in obstetrics and gynecology.
With prodding from missionaries in the Student Christian Movement, she started looking for a way to combine her profession
with her faith. When the Gold Coast Maternity Hospital position was posted at Edinburgh, she applied, and during an interview conducted by a group of male doctors, she asserted that she
felt perfectly qualified for the position. She got the job and, after
two weeks of seasickness, she found herself in an empty hospital,
scrambling to fill it with furniture and equipment. By 1928, Summerhayes had established a prenatal clinic, a birthing room, and
a midwife training center and had employed six nurses.[120] All she
needed were pregnant women.

Summerhayes recalled sitting in the newly furnished hospital, waiting for patients:

> We wondered whether we would ever get any because both the witch doctors and the people were against us. I think they didn't really want us. So I sent a summons to all the witch doctors to come and have tea with me at the hospital. The Africans like having tea parties and afterwards I got up onto the platform and addressed them. I said that I hadn't come to take away their patients, but if they got into any trouble they were welcome to bring me their messes. And then the next day, we looked up and there was one of these old women bent double, with a row of eighteen little pregnant girls following behind her! We were in business. I did the first Caesarean birth out there, and this was a tremendous thing for them to see. The next day they all came saying, "We want our babies the easy way", and I had to explain to them that it wasn't necessarily the easy way and I'm afraid I couldn't oblige.[121]

The tone of this recollection is patronizing and uses the anachronistic term of "witch doctor" to refer to African midwives, an odd turn of phrase considering that Margaret Field was living in Accra and could have easily introduced the new doctor to the specificities of Ga healing culture. However, the passage also demonstrates how quickly the British physicians in charge of maternal care in Accra were able to overcome cultural boundaries, in this instance by offering much-needed help to women who might have had difficulty giving birth. In its first year, the staff at the maternity hospital delivered a modest count of 100 babies, but by 1931, the number of annual deliveries had quadrupled to over 450, and the maternity wards were soon overcrowded.[122] At the same time that the nurses were delivering babies, the hospital was admitting hundreds of pregnant women per year as inpatients, the majority of them with cases of anemia due to malaria.[123] Additionally, Dr. Summerhayes was tasked with training midwives because of a new Midwives Act passed by the Gold Coast government in 1931, which brought the training, examination,

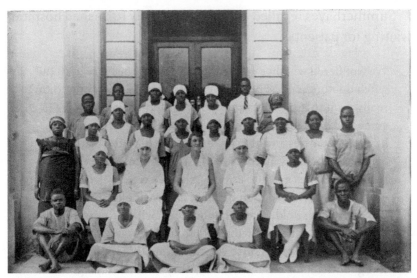

Figure 4.7. "Grace with the staff of the Maternity Hospital she started at Korle Bu, Ghana." This photo, provided with permission by the Summerhayes family, was probably taken in the late 1920s. As in other photographs taken at Korle Bu, the hierarchy of profession and duties is evident here, as the tall and lanky Dr. Summerhayes looms large at the center, flanked by her matrons, African nurses, nurses in training, male orderlies, technicians, and dispensers, as well as some pregnant women who were invited into the frame. The congenial spirit of the maternity hospital is evident in some of the smiles on the faces of staff members, uncharacteristic of photos of this era. (Source: Whitty Summerhayes MacRae Grant family.)

registration, and practice of midwifery under the purview of the Medical Department.[124] To manage increasing demand, Summerhayes continued to recruit nurses, orderlies, dispensers, and technicians until, as demonstrated by a photo of her in front of the hospital entrance (fig. 4.7), she was soon flanked by a small army of employees.

Dr. Summerhayes held the position of administrator until 1931, when she married Dr. Alexander MacRae, a British doctor working at Korle Bu. When she became pregnant, she left the Gold Coast to have her children in England. She returned a few years later, after her children had grown out of the toddler stage, but this time only as the wife of Dr. MacRae, who was now chief medical officer of the Gold Coast Hospital.[125] Her departure as head of the maternity hospital, and the distance she subsequently kept from Korle Bu, was notable—despite her previous tenure as the administrator of the most technologically sophisticated maternal-care facility in West Africa, she still did not regard the Gold Coast as a suitable place for White women to give birth or raise small children. Unlike African mothers, who built social and cultural capital via their role as mothers, Mrs. MacRae retreated to private motherhood, stepping down from her role as maternal leader of the mothers of Korle Bu. She eventually returned to her family village in England, where she raised her family and worked as a general practitioner. [126]

In 1934, the appointment of Dr. Cicely Williams as director of the maternity hospital signaled a notable change in the approach to infant and women's health on the Gold Coast.[127] Born in Jamaica as the daughter of a White British medical officer, Williams was one of the first women to earn a medical degree from Oxford, and she began her career as medical officer in a variety of clinics around the Gold Coast. She was ideologically influenced by the work of Andrija Stampar, a professor of hygiene and social medicine at Zagreb University who argued that infant care was a fundamental part of improving the health of society at large. Using Stampar's model, Williams planned to incorporate "social medicine" into the mandate of the hospital, as a way to root out the causes of childhood illness in Accra.[128] While in Accra, Williams worked diligently to learn some Ga so she could communicate effectively with her patients, and she allowed mothers to sleep beside their babies in the children's ward so that she could observe local methods of childcare—an unorthodox approach that strained her relationship with hospital administrators who believed in isolating sick patients, no matter what their age.[129] Williams's interest in local child rearing paid dividends when she found a cure for a type of malnutrition suffered by hundreds of babies in Accra.[130]

Kwashiorkor is now known to describe the symptoms found in children lacking protein in their diet, but at the time, Cicely Williams did not know how to diagnose the many sick babies that she encountered with distended bellies and brittle reddish hair.[131] Since she could not precisely determine the cause of the symptoms, she asked one of her locally trained nurses what she thought was ailing the baby. At Korle Bu, nurses normally deferred to doctors, and they were not accustomed to offering their opinions about disease causality, but in this case a Ga nurse named Christine Bryant told Williams that the baby was suffering from what was locally known as *kwashiorkor*—a word that doesn't translate well into English but refers to an illness contracted by an older child when it is weaned to make way for a new baby.[132] When Williams followed up with the parents of the sick child, she found that the baby had indeed been weaned early and given a diet of only maize porridge. The result was a severe protein deficiency that led to edema and anemia. Williams knew that if a child suffered from *kwashiorkor* for months on end, the sickness could lead to cirrhosis of the liver and possibly death.

To combat the disease, Williams encouraged mothers to add vitamins and protein to their children's diets. Her nurses suggested the easy, local solution of adding fish to their babies' maize pap to increase protein content, but Williams was convinced that mothers should supplement the porridge with staple commodities used in Britain, such as canned butter, tinned milk, bottled cod-liver oil, jars of marmite, and malt drinks.[133] Cicely Williams would later become famous for her campaign against using sweetened condensed milk as a breast milk substitute, but when she worked in Accra, she promoted tinned milk as a supplement for babies because it was produced under sanitary conditions, contained less fiber than cornmeal, and did not contain hot pepper (which she considered too strong for children).[134] Williams even wanted to help the Nestlé representative in the Gold Coast promote tinned milk by providing the company with the data of the success rates she had had at curing *kwashiorkor,* but Governor Slater disapproved because Nestlé was not a British firm. Williams's efforts to spur the consumption of imported goods is not surprising. Since the nineteenth century, when public health officials discovered that contaminated fresh milk supplies were a major factor in infant mortality, pasteurized milk became a necessity for mothers interested in perfecting mothercraft.[135] In Accra, a city without a dairy industry, Ga- and Twi-speaking mothers would not have known the historical significance of tinned milk and the anxieties about hygiene that spurred its consumption in Britain, but they would have quickly realized that, like attendance at infant welfare clinics and vaccinations, the consumption of imported foods was an integral part of the performance of mothercraft.[136]

The Princess Marie Louise Hospital for Mothers and Infants and the satellite infant-welfare clinics made colonial medicine an integral part of raising a family in Accra, but as doctors at Korle Bu quickly learned, women were still loyal to their African healing traditions. Women continued to use consecrated preparations to ritually wash their vaginas before going to the hospital to give birth, and they used herbal concoctions to dress the umbilical cord.[137] Williams carefully noted these practices and became aware that pregnant women and mothers hedged their bets by transiting between healing systems. In one particular case, Williams attempted to treat a baby who suffered from muscle spasms and an arched back, symptoms that she assumed were signs of tetanus. Williams thought that there was nothing she could do to save the baby, so she discharged the mother and child. Without complaint, the mother left and took her baby to Ata Ofori, a highly regarded local healer who specialized in treating convulsions in children with malaria. Ofori was well known to patients at Korle Bu as an herbalist who offered drumming and dancing sessions at his home as part of his healing services for spiritual problems and curses.[138] To Williams's amazement, the mother brought her baby back to the hospital a few days later, showing no signs of illness.[139] Intrigued by the dramatic recovery, Williams visited Ata Ofori at his home in James Town, and her biographer, Sally Craddock, offered this account of their meeting:

> Cicely called on one dignified, rather bald African witch doctor called Ata to "learn our medicine", hoping that in return he might teach her his. For three years Cicely sent patients on to him if she thought there was nothing she could do. For three years he maintained his proud secrecy, keeping up an amicable relationship with her but always more than arm's length. Suddenly one day two very small boys arrived carrying a vast bundle wrapped in handwoven cloth. Behind them was Ata, in ceremonial robes. This was obviously a visit of great importance. He told the boys to open the wrapping and onto the floor tipped a smelly pile of curious, almost unrecognizable things. Dried-up roots, leaves, the droppings of unidentifiable birds, lizard legs, desiccated bits of chicken wing, insects, twigs, all crazily jumbled together and all deeply significant. As he explained their uses, Cicely took notes. She was not a botanist and one piece of desiccated meat looks much like another, but she managed to list eighty items before the witch doctor and his retinue had gone, leaving her excited and flattered by his unprecedented display of confidence in a white fellow practitioner.[140]

Williams regarded this as a cultural breakthrough, believing that she had developed a relationship with an African healer to the point where he revealed his tools of healing. Over the next year, she spent much of her spare time with Ofori, taking walks with him to gather herbs and discuss their healing properties. Under Ofori's instruction, Williams collected hundreds of specimens, which she brought back to England during her furlough for further analysis. According to Williams's biographers, when she took the samples to the London School of Hygiene and Tropical Medicine, she encountered such a degree of male chauvinism, medical intransigence, and outright racism that no one would help her investigate their worth as medicines.[141] The whereabouts of the specimens today are unknown.

Williams's recollections of her time spent in Accra demonstrate that women in the city were very much in charge of their own reproductive health. She noted that, irrespective of the Ga cultural emphasis on fertility and the colonial drive to produce more and healthier babies, women privately attempted to retain as much control over their reproductive capacity and marital status as possible.[142] Williams learned early on that women in Accra felt immense pressure to produce children, so much so that they sometimes offered bribes to hospital nurses for a certificate to show they were pregnant.[143] This troubled Williams, as she realized that women were being threatened with divorce if they could not contribute children to a marital union. Conversely, she recalled that women came to her clinics with "their vaginas stuffed with all sorts of curious things, from grated ginger to ornaments, as treatments, cosmetics or contraceptives" and that they often asked her for advice about how to space their births and avoid unwanted pregnancies. Initially, Williams suggested inserting "a sponge soaked in cocoanut oil" into the vagina as a short-term solution, but she knew that this was not the most effective method, so she began to order Dutch cap diaphragms from England.[144] Williams had always been convinced that women would choose a few healthy children over many malnourished offspring, and her convictions just happened to suit the demands of the women who sought her help at Korle Bu.[145]

Cicely Williams was a nonconformist who tried to refresh the rules of mothercraft with the goal of aligning scientific mothercraft with the tender aspects of African mothering, and the recollections of her work in Accra offers a window on patient behavior in the city. Unfortunately, her innovative approaches were not always welcome because they challenged patriarchal orthodoxies about control over infant care. In 1934, a feud between

Dr. Selwyn-Clarke and Williams began over whether the hospital should focus on infant or toddler care. Selwyn-Clark stepped boldly into Williams's domain, demanding that she focus on reducing the infant mortality rate by focusing on newborns. Williams retorted that more attention should be paid to toddlers with *kwashiorkor*. Their dispute came to a climax in 1935 when Williams allowed a child with tuberculosis to remain with her mother in the children's ward, violating the hospital protocol on infectious diseases. Williams feared the child would die without its mother nearby, but Selwyn-Clarke used this as an opportunity to transfer her out of the Gold Coast.[146] In disgrace, she was relocated to Malaya. After her departure from Korle Bu, the hospital staff continued to promote mothercraft as part of women's lives in Accra, but the progressive spirit of social medicine and cultural interchange faded away.

Interlude: *Naa Korle Onamereko*—Interwar Attempts to Engineer the Korle Lagoon

For centuries, the people of Accra had set their calendars to the swelling and receding Korle Lagoon. Naa Korle is one of the founding deities of Accra. It is said that the female water spirit was discovered when a group of hunters found two large pots containing beads at the edge of the lagoon. When the hunters took the beads home to their encampment, a woman named Dede saw them and became filled with the spirit of the lagoon goddess.[147] Afterward, Korle became the guardian of the waters of the lagoon, and the Ga state placed the entire watershed under the stewardship of the priest of the Korle *wulomo*.[148] In the family of deities in Accra, Korle became the daughter of Nae, the goddess of the sea, and the wife of Sakumo, the god of war. According to oral tradition, she is a moral force in the city, a spirit that distances herself from petty rivalry, as suggested by her slogan: *Naa Korle onamereko*—"Elder woman Korle, you will see me passing by" (as a spiritual force that is present yet aloof and beyond reproach).[149]

The Korle Lagoon, as a geographical site, is also significant as a palimpsest of memories for the people of Accra, a place where stories about the goddess are stored and retold. Oral traditions at the shrine of Korle are not as robust as they once were, but the priest still uses the water of the lagoon to bless, purify, and cure supplicants, and the stories of the goddess survive in the minds of the elders. The biography of Korle is best revealed peripatetically, by visiting the small nodes of rock piles and concrete mounds (known as *otutui*) that are tucked in and around the neighborhoods surrounding the lagoon and dotting the seashore. These are the "children" of Korle, touchstones of memory that release historical information held within the minds of the goddess's followers.[150] For example, a rocky outcrop near the lagoon's shore reminds the priest of Korle of how the goddess allowed the destruction of the city by the armies of the Akwamu in revenge against the Portuguese merchants who built salt pits on her shores.[151] Another site triggers memories of a time when Naa Korle defended Accra by taking the form of a woman who fed the armies of the Ashanti with unclean food, sickening the soldiers enough to allow the Ga to vanquish them.[152]

Like many of the lagoons along the coast of West Africa, Korle recedes during the dry season, forming mudflats and stagnant pools of water. During the months of June and July, it swells with rainfall and floods the low-lying parts of Accra. In centuries past, the lagoon burst its sandy banks every rainy season, rushing into the sea. The breaking of the bar signaled adequate rainfall for the staple crop of corn and prompted the Korle priest to perform a ceremony to inaugurate the planting season.[153] The lagoon was also a source of seafood, and the residents of Accra cast nets from the shore to catch mud fish or waded along its banks to collect crabs. The priest of Korle allowed fishing in the lagoon with the exception of two weeks in late July and August, during the *Homowo* harvest festival, when a ban on fishing was instituted as a way of asking the goddess to continue to refresh the supply of water and fish for another year. To lift the ban on fishing, the priest walked to the shore with an entourage from the shrine and symbolically threw a net into the lagoon three times, collecting the fish and sharing them with the royal and priestly houses of the city.[154] The lagoon is no longer a major source of food for the people of the city today, but it remains an annual site of pilgrimage for the followers of Korle, a source of spiritual nourishment for those who worship the pantheon of Ga deities.[155] Moreover, Korle is a marker of the Ga linguistic identity. By telling someone *ekoole ya nshoŋ* (which literally means that his/her Korle goes to the sea), a Ga speaker can validate the ethnic identity of another Ga speaker, and when phrased in the negative, the words can be used as a warning that someone is a linguistic outsider.[156] In a city that changed dramatically over the course of the twentieth century, Naa Korle was a constant that regulated Ga menology and culture.

The spiritual significance of the lagoon was threatened during the cocoa boom of the 1920s. As traffic at the port of Accra grew exponentially, the Gold Coast government hoped to eliminate the costly use of surfboats by dredging the Korle Lagoon and transforming it into a deepwater harbor, with James Town on one side and Korle Bu on the other.[157] In 1919, the Public Works Department tendered the contract to a British engineer, who made a modest down payment of £50 to the house of Korle for permission to survey the lagoon, with a promise of a much greater sum of £15,000 as payment for the lease of the waterway in perpetuity. However, the project quickly ran into difficulties when the chiefs of Accra contested rights to the lands surrounding the lagoon. When the city had expanded across the lagoon during the anti-plague campaign, it had reached into territory claimed by the chiefs of Ussher Town, and since 1908 they had conducted vigorous political and legal campaigns to assert their title to the area. In the colonial courts of the Gold Coast, subchiefs from various quarters of Ussher Town argued about who had settled the lands around the lagoon first, and contested the rights of the Korle priest to collect the harbor fees. The case was tied up for so many years that the contractor decided to abandon the project.[158]

The failure to convert Korle into a harbor was a blow to British aspirations to sanitize the city. Principal Medical Officer Selwyn-Clarke believed the stagnant waters of the lagoon were bringing forth a "plague of mosquitoes," and he continued to press the government to reengineer the waterway.[159] In the mid-1920s, the Public Works Department filled some marshy areas with refuse, but they awaited funding from the Colonial Office to completely dredge the lagoon.[160] In 1929, after two years of lobbying, Governor Slater received official consent from the Colonial Office in London for a six-year scheme to create a sea outfall that would flush the waters of Korle into the Atlantic Ocean. London deposited the hefty sum of £195,000 into the Gold Coast treasury, and colonial engineers immediately set to work building tidal sluice gates to regulate the flow of water.[161] They also made plans to dredge the lagoon and construct walls all the way up the watershed, but financial retrenchment during the 1930s forced the colonial government to abandon the scheme.[162] British engineers did build a causeway over the sandbar, but the sea outfall soon began to fill with sand due to seasonal flooding. The government admitted ten years later that the whole scheme "might never have been undertaken at all."[163] The 1930s was largely a period of stagnation in the Gold Coast sanitary services division, and no new projects were undertaken.[164] Again the forces of bio-power emerged, but again their power had waned. The House of Korle maintained its hold on the spiritual significance of the lagoon and continued to play a significant part of the healing traditions of the people of Accra. But with war looming on the horizon, the sanitation syndrome began to rear its head again, this time backed by a new type of colonial force—military medicine.

NOTES

1. *Korle Bu Hospital, 1923–1973,* 36, 97, 141–44; Addae, *Evolution of Modern Medicine,* 28.
2. Foucault and Ewald, *Society Must Be Defended,* 36.
3. Davin, "Imperialism and Motherhood," 38–39.
4. *Korle Bu Hospital, 1923–1973,* 141–44.
5. Statistics compiled from *Reports on the Medical Department by the Government of the Gold Coast* (Accra: Government Press). Prior to 1926, dispensary visits were only reported as a total for the colony. For example, in 1923–24, there were 77,492 dispensary visits (*Reports on the Medical Department,* 1923–24, 17); Patterson, "Health in Urban Ghana," 257.
6. Statistics compiled from *Reports on the Medical Department by the Government of the Gold Coast* (Accra: Government Press).
7. *Reports on the Medical Department,* 1927–28.
8. Hawkins, *Writing and Colonialism,* 200–201.
9. Horn, "Control of Disease in Tropical Africa: Part I," 24–25; Horn, "Control of Disease in Tropical Africa: Part III," 254.
10. Patterson, *Health in Colonial Ghana,* 26; C. E. Reindorf, "Problem of Venereal Disease," 8–9; Pellow, "Research Article," 420.
11. C. E. Reindorf, "Influence of Fifty Years," 118.
12. Hackett, "Private Medical Practice," 129–32.
13. *Reports on the Medical Department,* 1924–38.
14. Addae, *Evolution of Modern Medicine,* 365.
15. Addae, *Evolution of Modern Medicine,* 98–99n20.
16. Dr. Matthew Arnum Barnor, interview with the author, August 29, 2003.
17. Ayers, *England's First State Hospitals,* 61.
18. Selwyn-Clarke, Le Fanu, and Ingram, "Relapsing Fever," 414. Patterson noted that not all people who were diagnosed with an illness that could be treated by surgery were willing to stay at the hospital; see Patterson, *Health in Colonial Ghana,* 17.
19. Neill, *Networks in Tropical Medicine,* 27.
20. Barrie, "Diary Notes."
21. Patterson, *Health in Colonial Ghana,* 22. See also Eckstein, *Noguchi*; D'Amelio, *Taller Than Bandai Mountain.*

22. Patterson, *Health in Colonial Ghana*, 22.

23. Patterson, *Health in Colonial Ghana*, 16.

24. Senah, *Money Be Man*, 54.

25. For references to the design of hospitals in the colonies, see Harold Cook, "From the Scientific Revolution to the Germ Theory," in *Western Medicine: An Illustrated History*, ed. Irvine Loudon (Oxford: Oxford University Press, 1997), 81, 161; Thomas R. Metcalf, "Architecture and the Representation of Empire," 37–39; Kisacky, "Restructuring Isolation," 7; Thompson and Goldin, *Hospital*, 154–69; Rivett, *London Hospital System*, 79.

26. Butchart, *Anatomy of Power*, 28.

27. Cicely Williams, "Witchdoctors," 450; Faustina Arthur, interview with the author, May 11, 2004; Interview, Evelyn Rose Naa Ahima Gilbertson, interview with the author, April 16, 2004.

28. *Mending Bodies, Saving Souls*, 339–98.

29. PRAAD ADM 1/2/144, "Le Fanu and O'Brien to Principle Medical Officer," January 23, 1922.

30. *Korle Bu Hospital, 1923–1973*, 76.

31. John Parker, "The Cultural Politics of Death & Burial in Early Colonial Accra," in *Africa's Urban Past*, ed. David Anderson and Richard Rathbone (Oxford: James Currey, 2000), 208–9.

32. *Korle Bu Hospital, 1923–1973*, 55.

33. *Korle Bu Hospital, 1923–1973*, 82. The phrase *okum nipa* translates literally as "killer of human beings."

34. Perceptions of anesthesia differed in other parts of the continent. For rumors about the use of chloroform in Uganda, see Luise White, *Speaking with Vampires*, 104–20.

35. Extract from *West Africa Review* 22, no. 286 [July 1951], quoted in *Korle Bu Hospital, 1923–1973*, 88.

36. Gold Coast, *Medical and Sanitary Reports, 1924–25*.

37. *Korle Bu Hospital, 1923–1973*, 68.

38. Stanton, "Listening to the Ga," 156.

39. *Korle Bu Hospital, 1923–1973*, 69.

40. *Korle Bu Hospital, 1923–1973*, 76.

41. The foodstuff markets of Accra have been historically dominated by market women, who deal in goods such as dried fish, corn, yams, and vegetables, and processed foods, such as the staple of kenkey, were also made by women. Though salaried positions in the government service and a colonial education system that favored boys over girls did tilt the balance

of earning power in favor of men during the twentieth century, women's authority in the marketplace has endured until today. See Claire Robertson, "Ga Women and Socioeconomic Change in Accra, Ghana," in *Women in Africa: Studies in Social and Economic Change*, ed. Nancy J. Hafkin and Edna G. Bay (Stanford, CA: Stanford University Press, 1976), 111–34.

42. *Korle Bu Hospital, 1923–1973*, 79. Mary Adoley Mingle considered her salary of £3 to be "scanty" for the work that she did as a sewing maid at the hospital.

43. Marks, *Divided Sisterhood*, 6; Lady Clifford noted that the curriculum at government schools included hygiene and sanitation, which meant that graduates would have already been introduced to medical concepts before applying for work at Korle Bu. Clifford, *Our Days on the Gold Coast*, 206.

44. Addae, *Evolution of Modern Medicine*, 250–51.

45. *Korle Bu Hospital, 1923–1973*, 68.

46. *Korle Bu Hospital, 1923–1973*, 72.

47. Dakubu, *Ga–English Dictionary*, 31, 85. Nurse Evelyn Gilbertson, interview with the author, April 16, 2004.

48. Patton, *Physicians, Colonial Racism*, 142.

49. Patterson, *Health in Colonial Ghana*, 14. The doctors appointed were A. F. Renner-Dove, G. T. Hammond, and E. Tagoe.

50. Kimble, *Political History of Ghana*, 109.

51. Field, *Religion and Medicine*, 6–9.

52. For further discussion of the relationship between class and fashion, see Marissa Moorman, "Putting on a Pano and Dancing like Our Grandparents: Nation and Dress in Late Colonial Luanda," in *Fashioning Africa: Power and the Politics of Dress*, ed. Jean Allman (Bloomington: Indiana University Press, 2004), 85; see also Turino, *Nationalists, Cosmopolitans*.

53. Commentaries in the Korle Bu Jubilee retrospective consistently included references to uniforms. See *Korle Bu Hospital, 1923–1973*, 68–73; Stephanie Newell, "Entering the Territory of Elites: Literary Activity in Colonial Ghana," in Barber, *Africa's Hidden Histories*, 221. Turner argues that the surface of the body is not just covered out of utility but with clothes that indicate social status. Terence S. Turner, "The Social Skin," in *Not Work Alone: A Cross-Cultural View of Activities Superfluous to Survival*, ed. Jeremy Cherfas and Roger Lewin (London: Temple Smith, 1980), 112–40.

54. In hospitals in Europe, uniforms served a similar purpose of distinguishing the medical worker as a class distinct from the lower classes

that might attend the hospital as patients and distinct from the physicians who administered the hospital. See Andersson, "To Work in the Garden of God"; Poplin, "Nursing Uniforms."

55. Patton, *Physicians, Colonial Racism*, 156–58.

56. *Korle Bu Hospital, 1923–1973*, 94.

57. "A. J. R. O'Brien, C.M.G., M.B., M.R.C.P.," 508–9.

58. *Korle Bu Hospital, 1923–1973*, 81.

59. *Korle Bu Hospital, 1923–1973*, 92.

60. *Korle Bu Hospital, 1923–1973*, 86.

61. Mangan, *Cultural Bond*, 68; Moore and Guggisberg, *We Two in West Africa*, 69.

62. Wood and Thompson, *Nineties*, 179.

63. *Gold Coast Independent*, January 12, 1929, 47. A game of lawn tennis (with exclusively White players and spectators) is referenced in Frenkel and Western, "Pretext or Prophylaxis," 222.

64. *Korle Bu Hospital, 1923–1973*, 73.

65. *Korle Bu Hospital, 1923–1973*, 73, 85.

66. *Korle Bu Hospital, 1923–1973*, 68; Collins, *Highlife Time*.

67. Cardinall, *Gold Coast*, 258; *Korle Bu Hospital, 1923–1973*, 68.

68. *Korle Bu Hospital, 1923–1973*, 94.

69. Dr. Barnor, interview with the author, August 29, 2003; *Gold Coast Independent*, January 22, 1927, 111.

70. *Korle Bu Hospital, 1923–1973*, 77.

71. *Korle Bu Hospital, 1923–1973*, 77.

72. *Korle Bu Hospital, 1923–1973*, 78.

73. *Korle Bu Hospital, 1923–1973*, 68; for a parallel example from South Africa, see Marks, *Divided Sisterhood*, 103.

74. *Korle Bu Hospital, 1923–1973*, 94.

75. This is a quote from the back of a postcard entitled "A Ward in the Hospital for Africans, Accra, Gold Coast," in the Smyly Gold Coast [i.e., Ghana] Collection, 1911–1929, Cambridge University Library: Royal Commonwealth Society Library, GBR/0115/Y30448L, selected postcards of the Gold Coast [i.e., Ghana], West Africa 1924: series II, PC Gold Coast/7-11, 1924.

76. Henry Mitchell, "CAS Students."

77. *Korle Bu Hospital, 1923–1973*, 77.

78. *Korle Bu Hospital, 1923–1973*, 77.

79. *Korle Bu Hospital, 1923–1973*, 76.

80. Kilson, *Kpele Lala*, 156.

81. Grace Naa Amartefio, interview with the author, August 23, 2010.

82. Kilson, *Kpele Lala*, 156. See also Quartey-Papafio, "Ga Homowo Festival," 231.

83. Kilson, *Kpele Lala*, 156. See also Quartey-Papafio, "Ga Homowo Festival," 231–32.

84. PRAAD ADM 11/1/1437, "Suppression of Objectionable Customs," 21–22.

85. Kilson, *Kpele Lala*, 156; Kilson, *Diary of Kwaku Niri*, 30, 44. See also Parker, *Making the Town*, 101–2, 173; PRAAD ADM 11/1/1437, "Suppression of Objectionable Customs."

86. Field, *Religion and Medicine*, 6, 10–11, 18–25.

87. Field, *Social Organization of the Gã people*, 216; Samuel S. Quarcoopome, "Impact of Urbanization," 151. For details on public aspects of motherhood in other parts of Africa, see Stephens, *African Motherhood*.

88. *Amenye* also can refer to a female priestess, who has responsibility beyond her own family for the spirituality of many other children. This idea of public motherhood is common to other West African cultures; see Semley, "Public Motherhood," 601.

89. Field, *Religion and Medicine*, 93.

90. PRAAD ADM 11/1/1437, "Suppression of Objectionable Customs," 22.

91. Stephens, *African Motherhood*, 2

92. Ashitey, *Epidemiology of Disease Control*, 27.

93. Davin, "Imperialism and Motherhood," 10.

94. Addae, *Evolution of Modern Medicine*, 227; Eluwa, "Emergence of the National Congress of British West Africa," 206.

95. Addae, *Evolution of Modern Medicine*, 228. Noel Smith records this as opening in 1922. Smith, *Presbyterian Church of Ghana*, 186.

96. *Gold Coast Independent*, July 24, 1926, 802. See also Addae, *Evolution of Modern Medicine*, 230.

97. Gold Coast Colony, *Report on the Medical Department by the Government of the Gold Coast* (Accra: Government Press, 1924–25), 23.

98. Gold Coast Colony, *Report on the Medical Department by the Government of the Gold Coast* (Accra: Government Press, 1924–25), 10.

99. Dally, *Cicely: Story of a Doctor*, 28.

100. Margaret Field mentions the ubiquity of yaws among children in her novel *The Stormy Dawn*, published under the pen name Mark Freshfield (London: Faber & Faber, 1946), 79.

101. *Korle Bu Hospital, 1923–1973*, 86; Gold Coast Colony, *Report on the Medical Department by the Government of the Gold Coast* (Accra:

Government Press, 1924–25), 6; Addae, *Evolution of Modern Medicine*, 261–68.

102. Dally, *Cicely: Story of a Doctor*, 30.

103. *Gold Coast Census*, 1921, 163; Acquah, *Accra Survey*, 125–27.

104. Gold Coast Colony, *Report on the Medical Department by the Government of the Gold Coast* (Accra: Government Press, 1924–25), 10.

105. *Gold Coast Independent*, December 16, 1922, 604.

106. Addae, *Evolution of Modern Medicine*, 231.

107. *Gold Coast Independent*, November 6, 1926, 1357; *Korle Bu Hospital, 1923–1973*, 42. "Baby weeks" were also held in Nigeria and the Gambia; see Horn, "Control of Disease in Tropical Africa: Part I," 25.

108. *Gold Coast Independent*, November 6, 1926, 1357. For more information on "baby weeks" held in Britain, see Davin, "Imperialism and Motherhood," 43.

109. Marie Louise, *Letters from the Gold Coast*, 225.

110. Liddiard, *Mothercraft Manual*; Cathy Urwin and Elain Sharland, "From Bodies to Minds in Childcare Literature: Advice to Parents in Inter-war Britain," in *In the Name of the Child: Health and Welfare, 1880–1940*, ed. Roger Cooter (New York: Routledge, 1992), 177; Philippa Mein Smith, "King, Sir (Frederic) Truby."

111. PRAAD CSO 18/1/144, *Methodist Book Depot—Gold Coast*, "Report on an Essay Competition Held in the Gold Coast in December/January, 1935/1936," IG-IH; PRAAD CSO 18/1/144, IC.

112. PRAAD CSO 18/1/144, *Methodist Book Depot*, IG-IH.

113. Brackett and Wrong, "Notes on Hygiene Books," 514.

114. Collett, *Accra Diocese*, 32.

115. Marie Louise, *Letters from the Gold Coast*, 226.

116. Ahmed, *Perception of Clients*, 4.

117. Addae, *Evolution of Modern Medicine*, 231–34; Patterson, *Health in Colonial Ghana*, table 8.

118. Dakubu, *Ga–English Dictionary*, 85. Style also figures prominently in the memories of former nurses; see *Korle Bu Hospital, 1923–1973*, 68–73.

119. Crofton and Raemaekers, *Painful Inch to Gain*, 46.

120. *Gold Coast Independent*, February 22, 1941, 61.

121. Wood and Thompson, *Nineties*, 179.

122. Gold Coast Colony, *Report on the Medical Department by the Government of the Gold Coast* (Accra: Government Press, 1930–31), 165.

123. Gold Coast Colony, *Report on the Medical Department by the Government of the Gold Coast* (Accra: Government Press, 1929), 211.

124. Ahmed, *Perception of Clients*, 4.

125. *Korle Bu Hospital, 1923–1973*, 85–86; Addae, *Evolution of Modern Medicine*, 236.

126. Wood and Thompson, *Nineties*, 179.

127. Dally, *Cicely*, 46.

128. Craddock, *Retired except on Demand*, 55. For more detail on the ideas of Andrija Stampar, see Grmek, *Serving the Cause of Public Health*, 12.

129. Cicely Williams, "Witchdoctors," 450; Craddock, *Retired except on Demand*, 55.

130. Cicely Williams, "Witchdoctors," 450.

131. Dally, *Cicely*, 28.

132. Dally, *Cicely*, 48, 59. See also Craddock, *Retired except on Demand*, 62. For more detail about *kwashiorkor*, see Fuchs, "Antioxidants," 1095. Field's work also mentions the term as a form of jealousy between the first-born and the child in the womb that causes illness and wasting in the first-born. Field, *Religion and Medicine*, 165–66. Field's work on the Ga may have influenced Williams's conceptions of Ga childhood, but there is no record of them knowing each other.

133. Cicely Williams, "Nutritional Disease of Childhood," 423–33.

134. Williams, "Nutritional Disease of Childhood," 425; Craddock, *Retired except on Demand*, 67.

135. Davin, "Imperialism and Motherhood," 11, 29, 34, 37.

136. Stanton, "Listening to the Ga," 160. For similar attempts to encourage the consumption of commodities related to child rearing, see Nancy Rose Hunt, "'Le Bebe en Brousse,'" 424.

137. Ahmed, *Perception of Clients*, 4–5; Cicely Williams, "Child Health in the Gold Coast," 98–99.

138. Dr. Barnor, interview with the author, August 29, 2003.

139. Dally, *Cicely*, 76–77.

140. Craddock, *Retired except on Demand*, 71; Cicely Williams, "Witchdoctors," 452; Dally, *Cicely*, 78–79. The name of the healer has been changed to Ofori, according to Williams's spelling, rather than Oforli, as printed in Craddock.

141. Craddock, *Retired except on Demand*, 71.

142. Craddock, *Retired except on Demand*, 57–58; Nurse Evelyn Rose Naa Ahima Gilbertson, interview with the author, April 16, 2004.

143. Craddock, *Retired except on Demand*, 57.

144. Craddock, *Retired except on Demand*, 57–58.

145. Craddock, *Retired except on Demand*, 57–58.

146. Craddock, *Retired except on Demand*, 72. Williams subsequently treated the child at the mother's home but was furious because she knew the child would die if not treated.

147. Dede is a common Ga house name for the firstborn girl child.

148. Privy Council Appeal no. 31 of 1958, "H.E. Golightly and Another v. E.J. Ashrifi and Others," Judgment of the Lords of the Judicial Committee of the Privy Council, delivered on December 19, 1960, by Lord Denning, West African Court of Appeal (Accra: Guinea, 1961). This citation comes from documents in the possession of the priest of Korle We.

149. Korle Wulomo, interview with the author, December 30, 2005.

150. Korle Wulomo, interview with the author, Accra, February 16, 2005; Kilson, *Kpele Lala*, 127.

151. Carl Christian Reindorf, *History of the Gold Coast and Asante*, 22.

152. Kilson, *Kpele Lala*, 127.

153. Field, *Religion and Medicine*, 57n2; Korle Wontse, interview with the author, Accra, March 30, 2005.

154. Korle Wulomo, interview with the author, Accra, February 16, 2005.

155. Dakubu, *Korle Meets the Sea*, 12.

156. Dakubu, *Korle Meets the Sea*, 12.

157. Dickson, "Evolution of Seaports," 109; Tudhope, "Development of the Cocoa Industry."

158. PRAAD ADM 11/1/1756, C. W. Welman, *Ga State Stools: Report on Enquiry into the Alleged Destoolment of Tackie Yaoboi, Ga Mantse*, 1921, 9–11, 14–16.

159. PRAAD CSO 3/1/157, *Accra (Korle) Lagoon*, August 22, 1927, 3.

160. PRAAD CSO 3/1/164, *Korle Lagoon Measures to Prevent Spreading of Mosquitoes*, "Notes by J.P. Ross, President of Accra Town Council," August 11, 1927.

161. PRAAD CSO 3/1/157, *Accra (Korle) Lagoon*; *Gold Coast Colony Blue Books* (Accra, Ghana, 1927–28). There are no extant records showing that the project was approved by the priest of Korle, but colonial correspondence indicates that the colonial secretary of the Gold Coast recommended that the committee consult with the house of Korle and the Ga chiefs. See PRAAD CSO 3/1/167 *Korle Lagoon—Application of a Committee to*, "Notes by the Secretary of Native Affairs," October 6, 1927.

162. PRAAD ADM 5/3/46, *Malaria Control*, 2.

163. PRAAD CSO 3/1/162, *Korle Lagoon*; PRAAD CSO 11/10, 3271, *Memorandum of the Director of Medical Services*, February 2, 1943.

164. Addae, *Evolution of Modern Medicine*, 74.

THE CREATION OF AN AFRICAN "BLOODSTREAM"

Malaria Control during the Hitler War, 1942–1945

IN 1942, LIEUTENANT C. R. RIBBANDS arrived in Accra to collect data about the biting habits of mosquitoes. Ribbands was an entomologist by training sent by the British West Africa Division of the army to fight malaria in Accra. He was given command of a team of army engineers, whom he ordered to build nineteen mosquito traps, each about the size of a small shed, and install them at regular intervals along the sacred Korle Lagoon. He filled the traps with human bait, army laborers from the Northern Territories of the Gold Coast Colony who were told to sleep in sheds overnight. Each morning, army crews drove their jeeps from shed to shed, ordering the human bait out and dousing the traps with pesticides. They then collected the dead mosquitoes and brought them back to Ribbands's laboratory, where he tracked the biting and flight patterns of *Anopheles gambiae*.[1] The end result was the "anopheline index," a database of mosquito behavior that Ribbands used to craft a strategy to control, and hopefully eliminate, malaria in Accra.

The work of Lt. Ribbands was part of a new era of medical colonization wherein colonial officials began to see colonized people as a "living laboratory"—an aggregation of medical subjects within which diseases could be isolated, mapped, and controlled.[2] With the help of funding made available through the Colonial Development and Welfare Act, new medical projects began to pop up in British colonies, such as the Gambia malnutrition experiment, which sought to eliminate the root causes of illness and food scarcity, and the East African Medical Survey, which sought to map and control endemic diseases like malaria, trypanosomiasis, and onchocerciasis in Uganda, Kenya, and Tanganyika.[3] In the Gold Coast, projects to control trypanosomiasis and onchocerciasis in the Ashanti and Northern Regions received dramatically increased funding starting in the 1940s, and in Accra, the new spirit of medical colonization was best represented in the wartime effort to control malaria.[4]

Lt. Ribbands was part of a new generation of entomologists who sought to eradicate human ailments by eliminating insect vectors of disease.[5] He did not anticipate any resistance to his scientific endeavors from the local population, but he soon heard grumbling from the human bait that he had hired to sleep in the traps. At the start of the project, the British Army equipped the mosquito traps only with simple raffia mats, expecting the men to sleep on the ground. But during the rainy season, the test subjects complained that the ground was too wet, so Lt. Ribbands was compelled to place US Army cots inside each test shed.[6] Then the men complained about the stringent rules of the project, which required them to blow mosquitoes off their skin rather than slap them. In response, a frustrated Ribbands agreed to provide mosquito netting for their beds but later removed the nets when they made it difficult to collect the dead mosquitoes.[7] Another problem arose when the data showed that some of the test subjects attracted more mosquitoes than others. Ribbands's answer was to rotate the men through the traps, one week at a time, until they had done a complete circuit of the lagoon.[8] Despite these challenges, Lt. Ribbands persevered, collected several months of data, compiled his anopheline index, and mapped out a "malaria control area" along the perimeter of the Korle Lagoon. He then ordered a targeted spraying of the waterway with pesticides and larvicides, and when DDT became available, he fogged the entire city of Accra.[9] By 1945, Ribbands had declared victory, claiming that all of the mosquito larvae in the control area had been destroyed. His final report stated that only one mosquito had been found alive in the entire city by mid-1945.[10]

The residents of Accra had seen their share of sanitary technocrats, such as Drs. Quartey-Papafio, Simpson, and Selwyn-Clarke, but prior to the Second World War, any colonial official who attempted to introduce a new regime of public health in Accra encountered vigorous resistance. Lt. Ribbands, however, was able to take advantage of the unique historical circumstances of the Second World War. Emboldened by the wartime emergency and Allied paranoia about the spread of malaria, Ribbands and his crew of malariologists mobilized hundreds of personnel and requisitioned millions of dollars in material to conduct the largest sanitation scheme yet seen in the colonial capital. They were also able to sidestep Ga authorities to unceremoniously douse the sacred Korle Lagoon with chemicals, temporarily nullifying the spiritual significance of the goddess. In the process, a new type of medical and racial discourse emerged about the African population—one that aggregated Africans together as a race that harbored disease in their "bloodstream."[11]

The official history of the antimalaria campaign is detailed in a report compiled by the Inter-Allied Malaria Control Group, an ad hoc body of British and American scientists who were brought together to fight malaria in Accra from 1942 to 1945. When compared to other archival material about colonial health initiatives in Accra, the Malaria Control Group report stands out because it so boldly silences any other traditions of healing in the city. Prior to the Second World War, efforts to impose European-derived understandings of health and illness had always been half-hearted because colonial medical officials knew what a herculean task it would be to change the pluralistic healing culture of Accra. But

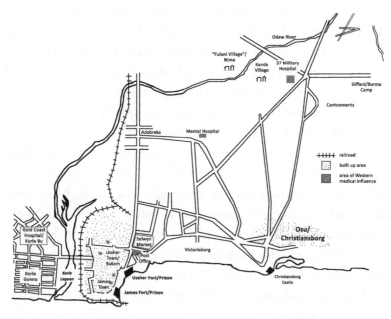

Accra 1940

Map 5.1. Map of Accra, 1940. This map shows the interior of the malaria control area, depicting the Korle Lagoon and its major tributary, the Odaw River. Allied efforts to control the mosquito population also targeted the smaller Klote Lagoon at Osu and the larger Sakumo Lagoon several kilometers to the west. The villages of Nima and Kanda are also depicted (*top*). In the 1940s, these villages were populated by Muslim migrants from Northern Ghana, Nigeria, and French West Africa. According to military records, the Allies evacuated Nima and Kanda during the war, but oral histories do not confirm that claim. Nima and Kanda are now suburbs within Greater Accra. (Source: map by author.)

according to the Malaria Control Group, local resistance during their campaign was insignificant, and the reconstruction of the urban hydrology of Accra advanced without significant delays. In fact, if we believe the military technocrats, the project was a watershed in the history of sanitation on the Gold Coast, one that should have been the beginning of the end for therapeutic pluralism in the capital city.

But though the Malaria Control Group made great strides toward a sanitized urban future, the project was almost entirely abandoned after the war. When American funding dried up, Lt. Ribbands and his colleagues packed up their equipment and left. The project to reengineer the lagoon languished, and the control over discourses surrounding the spiritual meaning of the lagoon reverted to the priest of Korle. The residents of Accra today barely remember the campaign; veterans and elders who do bear memories of the Hitler War (as it is colloquially known in Ghana) have trouble remembering the fight against malaria, and the religious elites who worship the goddess Korle do not even recollect that it happened. Within the long duration of therapeutic pluralism in Accra, a place that has witnessed the accumulation of Ga, Muslim, Christian, medical, and commercialized understandings of health and healing, the antimalarial campaign was a dramatic, but ultimately forgettable, expression of bio-power.[12] The Second World War did provide a brief opportunity to use Accra as a laboratory for the study of race, environment, and disease, but when White soldiers departed for Europe, Naa Korle reasserted her role as the goddess of the lagoon, and the shrine priest of Korle continued to guard the waterway.

CLEANSING KORLE: THE ALLIED
ANTIMALARIA CAMPAIGN OF 1942–45

As the war in Europe began, the small garrison at Accra scrambled to secure the colony from an incursion from Cote D'Ivoire, Togo, or amphibious assault by sea. A curfew was imposed in the colony, with lights off at night and car headlights shuttered. As the Allied armies suffered defeat after defeat in Europe and Asia, fear of an aerial or naval bombardment of Accra grew. Rumors flew of German submarines shooting at fishermen. In the early months of the war, it became obvious that no new troops were coming to protect the Gold Coast, and only a small number of

Royal Air Force planes were available to patrol the skies. Admitting that the home islands could do little to help the colonies, the British secretary of state called on their subjects abroad to create their own Home Guards and to retreat according to a scorched-earth policy in case of invasion. Fear was in the air.[13]

Fortunately for the residents of Accra, the Gold Coast never became a battleground during the war. However, Accra did become a hub of wartime activity when the British War Office choose the city as the headquarters of the British West African Command. General Giffard was placed in command of the West African forces and turned Accra into a marshaling yard for goods and personnel departing for India. The arrival of thousands of soldiers from Nigeria, Sierra Leone, and the Gambia should have created a major health concern for the city, in terms of clean housing, a healthy food supply, and adequate medicines, but since the soldiers were shipped out to India so quickly, the city required no sanitary changes to accommodate their numbers.

In addition to housing the West Africa Command, the city also became an aerial transshipment point for North Africa. In 1941, the German Army had cut off British troops in North Africa from their Mediterranean supply routes, forcing the Allies to send supplies across the Sahara Desert by air. Accra suddenly became home to a major Allied airbase. During the peak years of 1942–43, between two and three hundred aircraft landed daily at the airport for refueling and maintenance, and thousands of airmen and airport crews were stationed in the city.[14] To treat sick personnel, the British built the first military hospital, known officially as the 37th General Hospital of the British Empire, a segregated facility with two hundred European beds and eight hundred African beds. The hospital was badly needed because by 1942 malaria rates among soldiers and airmen in Accra were startlingly high. British, American, and African soldiers all suffered, but the illness was particularly bad among White soldiers who had never been exposed to the disease. In 1942, morbidity rates exceeded 50 percent per year, and an epidemic flare-up during that rainy season sent 62 percent of Allied soldiers to the hospital for treatment.[15] Worse still, Allied commanders feared the disease would spread from West Africa to the rest of the world. In the 1930s, sixteen thousand people in Brazil had died as a result of the introduction of *Anopheles gambiae* and its malaria parasites by ship from Dakar. Fearing another outbreak, the Brazilian government pressured the Americans to ensure that transport planes on the Atlantic routes did not harbor any mosquitoes.[16] The British and American armed forces, who had not anticipated being so heavily invested in operations in West Africa, felt obliged to take steps to control malaria in Accra.

Part of the Allied concern about illness among personnel was a fear of losing valuable war matériel. By 1942, 25 percent of the pilots flying from Accra to Egypt were landing in Cairo with malarial symptoms.[17] Trained pilots were in short supply, and to ensure the safety of both the airmen and airplanes, it was crucial that the British keep them healthy during their short stay in Accra.[18]

The Royal Air Force argued strongly for the case of a mosquito vector control scheme around the airport, claiming that "malaria control of an airfield (especially in the case of an essential airfield) shows a large credit, for the loss of only two or more heavy bombers, resulting from a poor landing by a pilot attacked with malaria during the flight (a thing very liable to happen in high altitudes of flying when the pilot has parasites in his blood), more than pays for the cost of the scheme. The cost of a Superfortress is in the region of $600,000."[19] When stated in such plain logistical and financial terms, the need to stop the spread of malaria in Accra became obvious to the Allies.

Not surprisingly, American medical officials added a racial component to the discourse about malaria, expressing concern that Africans might infect White soldiers.[20] For the US Army, segregation between the so-called races was a well-established protocol, so it was not surprising that they used the fear of disease to justify the separation of their soldiers from the African population of the Gold Coast. The British were less convinced that segregation was an appropriate strategy to fight malaria. They had already attempted to dismantle institutional segregation in the colony, and since quinine was widely available in pill form at colonial post offices or by injection at Korle Bu, they did not see the need to further divide the races.[21] However, the rapid influx of troops and a dramatic increase in construction near the airport led to rates of malaria that the British had never seen before in Accra. The fear of epidemic malaria was further amplified when the Japanese invaded Java in the Dutch East Indies, cutting off the world's largest source of natural quinine. By 1942, Allied malariologists were in agreement that they desperately needed a new strategy for controlling malaria in Accra, even if it required segregation.[22]

To coordinate antimalaria efforts, the British Army brought Major O. J. S. Macdonald of the Indian Medical Services to Accra to serve as an official area malariologist. Macdonald was a specialist in wastewater treatment, and when he arrived in Accra he echoed Selwyn-Clarke's belief that the Korle Lagoon was "swarming with Anopheline larvae" and he proposed that the two armies fund an antimalaria initiative along the Korle watershed. The Americans were receptive to the idea, but before they would sign on to a joint drainage program, they brought their own specialist to the city to investigate the situation.[23] Captain Lowell T. Coggeshall, a specialist in tropical medicine at the University of Michigan, joined forces with Macdonald in 1942, and the pair drew up a comprehensive plan that included changes to soldiers' housing, alterations to their attire, and the excavation of forty-five kilometers of viaducts and ditches around the city. Coggeshall and Macdonald brought together several other British and American physicians and scientists to create the Inter-Allied Malaria

Control Group, and both the US Army and the British Colonial Office agreed to pay for the scheme.[24] For the first time in the history of Accra, the personnel, equipment, and funding were in place to eliminate mosquito-borne illnesses from the city.

The Allies' first step was to restructure the living quarters of their troops. Following a pattern of segregation that had led to the development of suburbs like Victoriaborg and the Ridge, the Malaria Control Group set to work building an army residential area to the northeast of the city, next to the airport. The camp that housed the White soldiers was specifically located a mosquito flight away, judged to be one-quarter of a mile, from the nearby villages of Nima and Kanda. A change in attire soon followed the change in location, as the Allies adapted military apparel to better suit the disease climate. White British and American soldiers had arrived in Accra wearing their cold-weather uniforms, including greatcoats that had to be aired weekly to prevent mold.[25] They were also issued wool pajamas, which were unbearably hot, especially under a mosquito net. The soldiers soon abandoned these for cotton pajamas or for nothing at all. The Malaria Control Group remedied the problem by distributing warm-weather clothing, but they still required soldiers to wear long sleeves, trousers, and boots to prevent mosquito bites. Any leftover bare skin was to be covered with mosquito repellent.[26] The Allies also changed the soldiers' dormitories, installing screened windows and requiring soldiers to sleep under bed nets.[27] To emphasize the need for vigilance, Allied film crews projected slides of cartoons onto screens at the barracks to exhibit the dangers of mosquito exposure. These images depicted the mosquito vector as a "fifth column" that, in collusion with the lazy soldier who neglected to mend his netting, would attack the troops in their sleep. In Accra, where there were no Axis soldiers to fight, the mosquito was the enemy.

Until 1942, Allied medics had distributed a daily dosage of five grains of quinine to all army personnel, but when supplies ran low, they experimented with synthesized versions of the drug.[28] They tested two prototypes: quinacrine (reverse-engineered by Sterling Winthrop Co. from a captured German I. G. Farben product in 1941) and mepacrine (synthesized by Imperial Chemical Industries in 1939).[29] British Army experiments showed that quinacrine was a superior antimalarial because it had few side effects, but mepacrine was in greater supply, so the Allied doctors in Accra settled on a daily dose of the latter by mid-1943.[30] The White soldiers disliked mepacrine because it caused a yellowish pigmentation on their skin, but they were forced to take it every morning with their breakfast.[31] African soldiers were required to take the drug too, but use of chemical prophylaxes stopped there. Despite the belief that the residents of Accra formed a reservoir for the disease, the Allies never considered offering malaria prophylaxes to their civilian employees or to the broader African community.

At the start of the campaign, the Allies hoped that chemical insecticides might help them avoid the expense of reengineering the Korle watershed. The Americans were especially interested in using a silver-bullet approach to control the local mosquito population because they did not want to fund infrastructure projects that they would have to abandon after the war. In April 1942, the US Army began spraying the larvicide Paris green on open water surrounding the barracks, and trucked pyrethrum aerosol bombs into British camps to clear the buildings of mosquitoes.[32] They proceeded to spray all houses within a one-mile radius of the airport, three times a week. In 1944, when adequate supplies became available, they switched to spraying with dichlorodiphenyltrichloroethane (DDT), and by the end of the year, they were spraying all villages within an eight-mile radius of their camps, including the Accra city center.[33] Because DDT was not considered toxic to humans, the Malaria Control Group believed it was safe to disperse the chemical into water supplies. By 1944, the Allies commissioned a Piper J-3 cub to aerial spray the Korle,

Kpeshi, and Klotey Lagoons, and partially spray the Sakumo Lagoon, several kilometers to the west of the city.[34]

The spraying campaigns of 1942–45 were conducted at great expense in labor and material. For instance, during a three-month surge to eliminate the presence of mosquitoes and mosquito larvae at the airport in 1944, the Americans sprayed more than one thousand pounds of Paris green, two thousand pounds of pyrethrum, and five hundred pounds of DDT, and they still found larvae in some of the streams leading into the lagoon.[35] Major Macdonald had always believed that it would be cost effective to take the time to build drainage systems that would confine water to ditches and ponds, where smaller amounts of insecticides could be used, and as the war dragged on, the Americans too began to see the necessity of longer-term planning.[36] In 1944, Allied engineers mapped out a pesticide spraying zone, re-dredged the sea outfall, and employed African crews to clear ditches and streams all the way up the Korle watershed.[37] The Royal Army Medical Services followed up by spraying and oiling the waterways on a regular basis, a method that reduced the amount of pesticides used.[38]

While the drainage scheme proceeded, Lt. Ribbands built his aforementioned Malaria Field Laboratory and began by collecting data about mosquito populations in the army camps. An expert on *Anopheles gambiae*, Lt. Ribbands had already researched the flight and biting habits of mosquitoes through a variety of experiments in India and West Africa, and his first step was to replicate a study that he had conducted in Sierra Leone, collecting mosquitoes from the Gold Coast Regiment barracks.[39] The mosquito crews spread sheets on the floors of the tents and sprayed the air with pyrethrum or DDT to kill any insects inside. Afterward, Lt. Ribbands hired local men to pick up the mosquitoes and take them to a central laboratory at the airport for identification.

Lt. Ribbands and the malariologists expected to eliminate the mosquitoes around the Allied army barracks, but when he analyzed the early results, he realized that the health of soldiers was still compromised by the in-flight of mosquitoes from nearby villages. According to the Allied records, the fear of contagion spurred the Malaria Control Group to relocate the villagers outside the airport to a newly conceived one-mile sanitary cordon.[40] If this is true, then the Allies had extended the supposed flight range of a mosquito from one-quarter of a mile to a full mile and relocated the people of nearby Nima and Kanda because they had become "reservoirs of disease."[41] But though there are brief references to the planned evacuation of these nearby villages, no particular records demonstrate that a forced removal took place. If the evacuations did occur, they would have entailed the movement of hundreds of people (mostly Muslim newcomers to the city) by truck, as well as extensive documentation of claims for property. The lack of a paper trail raises the question of whether the residents of the villages were in fact relocated, but whether they were moved or not, a new spatial reckoning of Accra had been created because of the threat posed by infected mosquitoes.

Once he had established a cordon around the periphery of Korle Lagoon, Lt. Ribbands began to track the movements of *Anopheles gambiae* using his network of mosquito sheds.[42] Built by African laborers in the employ of the British Army, the traps were single-room, timber-frame structures covered with screens and tar paper and fitted with baffles to let mosquitoes in at night. Ribbands modeled his traps on a prototype developed by American entomologist E. H. Magoon, but with a substantial difference: during his research in Jamaica, Magoon used only horses and mules to attract mosquitoes. Lt. Ribbands preferred human bait.[43] Since he was largely concerned with studying the attraction of mosquitoes to White soldiers, it would have been logical to assign an American or British soldier to live in the traps, but the Allies were shorthanded, and Lt. Ribbands did not want to risk Allied airmen catching malaria. As a compromise, he hired African workers to sleep in the traps:[44] "Africans selected as bait were

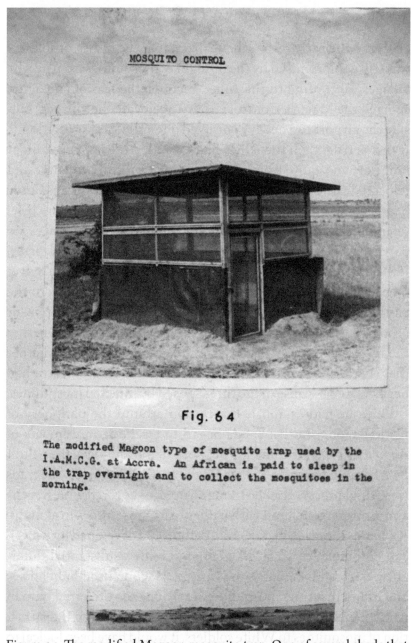

Fig. 64

The modified Magoon type of mosquito trap used by the
I.A.M.C.G. at Accra. An African is paid to sleep in
the trap overnight and to collect the mosquitoes in the
morning.

Figure 5.1. The modified Magoon mosquito trap. One of several sheds that
the Inter-Allied Malaria Control Group (IAMCG) placed around Accra to
monitor the flight of mosquitoes. The trap was a modified version of a model
designed in 1935 in Jamaica by entomologist by E. H. Magoon. Magoon used
horses, donkeys, and pigs to attract mosquitoes, but Lt. Ribbands employed
migrant workers to sleep in the traps so he could calculate the bite rate of
Anopheles gambiae on human hosts. (Source: PRAAD, Report on Service
Malaria Control, Accra and Takoradi, Gold Coast.)

chiefly men from the Northern Territories of the Gold Coast. They were chosen because most of them were homeless and it was felt that they would welcome the fine shelters provided by the mosquito traps, however only those who could speak a few words of English were hired because they had to be able to understand the simple instructions. That the traps were home to these men was soon obvious when it was seen that they preferred to remain in the vicinity even during the daytime when they were not working."[45]

The choice of migrant workers as human bait is not surprising. These men go unnamed in the military records, but they were likely drawn from the same pool of immigrants recruited by the Gold Coast Medical Department as so-called volunteers in experiments at the Accra Laboratory during outbreaks of yellow fever and relapsing fever. But if they were homeless, as Ribbands suggested, it probably did not mean that they had nowhere to sleep. Newcomers to Accra usually were able to find a bed, even if that meant crowding in with their fellow migrants.[46] And even if they did lack permanent residences, it is difficult to believe that they considered the traps desirable places to sleep. The sheds were small, filled with bugs, and lacking the benefit of any breeze to cool the skin. It is also implausible that they thought of the traps as homes, considering that they were located in wooded areas and did not have locks to secure the doors. Moreover, the sheds were spread around a perimeter of several kilometers, and Lt. Ribbands rotated the men through the network of sheds at weekly intervals.[47]

The military records also show that the hired bait did not always follow the rules. The men were required to stay in their sheds from sunset to sunrise. When they awoke, they were to leave the traps, carefully closing the baffles to catch the mosquitoes inside as they left, so that the spraying crews could lay down a tarpaulin, spray the sheds, and collect the insects. To monitor the sleeping patterns, Lt. Ribbands sent soldiers around the perimeter to ensure that the men serving as bait were actually sleeping in the traps and to prevent a reported "tendency to sit outside the trap at night"—an indication that the Africans who took part in the Malaria Control Group studies were not always willing and forthright participants.[48] Though there is no record of outright resistance, the migrants did take measures to avoid mosquito bites and preserve their dignity.

Though Lt. Ribbands and his fellow malariologists were tasked with fighting the spread of malaria, they were not particularly interested in whether the men used as human bait contracted the disease. None of the men who slept in the mosquito traps were named, nor is there any mention of whether they fell ill. The express purpose of the anopheline index was to collect entomological data to determine which parts of the Korle watershed to target with pesticides and larvicides. Nor was Ribbands particularly interested in spraying campaigns' effects on the local population. The Malaria Control Group sprayed DDT on African houses and into wells and ponds without asking because it was the only way to break the fourteen-day larvae-mosquito-human cycle of malaria transmission, thereby clearing incubated plasmodia from what Ribbands called the African "bloodstream."[49] At the same time as they mapped out the habitat of the mosquito, Lt. Ribbands and the Allied malariologists began to think of the inhabitants of Accra as a reservoir of malaria—one that could be cleansed with the liberal application of chemicals.

The residents of the old quarters of Accra did not share Lt. Ribbands's enthusiasm for malaria control. Having endured the indignity of sanitary inspections, they were reluctant to let the spraying crews into their compounds.

Details about local resistance are limited because there are no memories of the event at the Korle shrine house, but a brief, revealing passage does appear in an American report on the antimalaria campaign: "The application of larvicide to [lagoon] areas was strongly resented by the local native population who

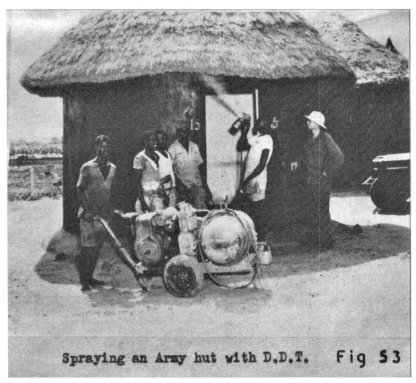

Spraying an Army hut with D.D.T. Fig 53

Figure 5.2. "Spraying an army hut with DDT." This photo places the disinfecting machine in the foreground, emphasizing the primacy of technology in the fight against malaria. The unnamed technocratic White expert supervises the spraying while the unnamed African employees pose for the camera. No personal precautions were taken to protect people from the insecticides because the long-term effects of chemicals like DDT were not known at the time. (Source: PRAAD ADM, Report on Service Malaria Control, Accra and Takoradi, Gold Coast.)

associated a high religious significance to these lagoons . . . [but the] natives [were] placated through negotiation by British authorities with the African chiefs."[50]

This passage offers evidence that the residents of Accra were quite aware of the impact of a citywide spraying campaign and were concerned about encroachment on their sacred spaces, but it also shows how colonial indirect rule allowed the British to

curry favor with local chiefs as a way of disenfranchising the religious authorities of the city. How exactly the British appeased
the chiefs is unknown, but it probably involved sums of money
to pay for the temporary rights to spray the lagoon, distributed
in a manner that would allay resistance to the campaign.[51] It
so happened that the antimalaria campaign occurred during
a period of fierce stool disputes among the Ga subchiefs in the
city, a time when the priestly stool of Korle stood vacant. The
Ga indigenous understanding of health and healing remained
firmly in place, but the figureheads who championed the social
health of the Ga, and the environmental health of the paramount gods, were temporarily absent. Without traditional
leadership, and under conditions of martial law, the residents
of the city must have struggled to voice their concerns about
the spraying campaign.[52]

MEMORIES OF THE ANTIMALARIA
CAMPAIGN DURING THE HITLER WAR

The ascent of bio-power during the antimalaria campaign barely
registers within the collective memories of the residents of Accra. The oral history of the event is difficult to collect because so
few veterans of the "Hitler War" remain. Nonetheless, several
ex-soldiers did remember basic elements of the Malaria Control
Group operations, such as being locked in their barracks while
the Americans sprayed their buildings, forced to take yellow
mosquito tablets, and ordered to dig through riverbeds with iron
bars and rakes.[53] However, only a few of them recalled anything
about the war on mosquitoes conducted by Ribbands and his
colleagues, a surprising gap the collective memory considering
the extent of the campaign.

Those who did recall the mosquito traps expressed resentment
about how inhumanely the human bait was treated. Otia Badu, a
Ga veteran who fought in Burma, remembered that soldiers were

forced to sleep in the traps as punishment if they disobeyed orders. Badu himself never slept in the tent, managing to get guard duty in the camp when he faced disciplinary measures. Choosing to sleep in the tents was a death sentence, he claimed, because everyone who slept there is now dead. Badu also recalled that British officers forced African soldiers to test "mosquito capes," overcoats with holes in the cloth that were covered with sticky glue to trap insects.[54] According to Badu, the soldiers were ordered to wear the capes when they went out at night as a way of attracting and collecting mosquitoes, but there is no evidence of such attire in the military records.[55] Another former member of the Gold Coast Regiment, Oblitey Commey, stated that all of the "northerners" who slept in the traps must have died shortly afterward because they had "challenged their spirits" by giving in to their colonial masters.[56] At the end of his interview, Commey declared that if the British had wanted to catch mosquitoes, they should have slept in the traps themselves.[57] Yet another veteran indicated that the residents of Accra were not happy to see their homes doused in chemicals and that during the campaign rumors circulated that the British were trying to poison the local population.[58] But all of the veterans emphasized that, despite the inhumane treatment the Gold Coast subjects faced during the Hitler War, no one dared to challenge the authority of their officers.[59] As retired soldier John Borketey bluntly asserted, resistance was never an option: "Whatever they tell you, you do it. Colonial days. You have no choice."[60]

Apart from the recollections of a handful of elderly veterans, memories of the antimalaria campaign within the general population of Accra are sparse. No one at the Korle shrine has any recollection of Allied airplanes dousing the lagoon with DDT, and people living in the older quarters of Accra have forgotten the story of the antimalaria campaign. Even in Nima, the suburb that likely provided the migrant workers used as human bait, religious leaders and elders have no recollection of the spraying campaign, the mosquito traps, or even the evacuation of their suburb. As a way point for migrants from points north of Accra, Nima has always had a transient population, but it is still surprising that no one remembers the campaign. Considering that the residents of Accra rioted against British attempts to fill the reservoir in Bukom in 1889 and stoned the plague-fighting crews that tried to demolish houses in Ussher Town during Simpson's anti-plague program, it is difficult to believe that the residents of Nima simply walked away from their settlement to accommodate the one-mile cordon sanitaire.

The reason that the antimalaria campaign failed to embed itself within the collective memory of the people of Accra remains a puzzle. One explanation is that the feverish activity of the 1940s fragmented and damaged memories of the wartime experience. Soldiers training in Accra can hardly be expected to have become knowledgeable about the campaign considering they were so young and so busy preparing to fight in Burma, and the migrant workers who suffered the most by participating in the campaign were probably newcomers to the city who moved on after the war, taking their memories with them. And the absence of memories among the Ga-speaking population can be attributed to the lack of a priest at the House of Korle due to succession disputes. During the 1930s, the chiefly houses of the city had contested legal rights to lands surrounding the Korle watershed, and the ownership of the property remained unresolved until 1946, when the Korle elders installed Priest Nummo Ayiteh Cobblah II. In the interim, the annual customs of the shrine that sedimented traumatic occurrences into ritual commemorations were put on hold, and the antimalarial campaign was mnemonically orphaned within the collective consciousness of the residents of Accra.

Another reason the antimalaria campaign has been forgotten is because it was censored or buried under propaganda. In 1939, the Gold Coast government created a Department of Information to disseminate news about the war in Europe, and they produced propaganda in African languages to be broadcast on radio.[61] The colony also produced a weekly newspaper entitled the *Empire at War*, which celebrated the achievements of troops from the colonies but did not once mention the antimalarial campaign.[62] Nor was the campaign mentioned in the *Gold Coast Independent*, edited by Ghanaian physician Dr. Nanka-Bruce. It may be that Nanka-Bruce objected to the antimalaria campaign, but since Nanka-Bruce had always advocated vigorous sanitation efforts (and often railed against the activities of African healers), it is more likely he supported it. We are left guessing whether resistance to the event was censored or simply ignored by the Accra press.

Memories of the antimalaria campaign also may have faded because they occurred at a time when chemical therapies for diseases and chemical treatments for insect infestations were widely regarded as beneficial to humankind. In 1945, the *Gold Coast Independent* ran advertisements that portrayed mepacrine as a weapon of war that was "more deadly than a dive bomber."[63] And in a radio broadcast during the same year, British epidemiologist G. M. Findlay exhorted residents to destroy the breeding places of mosquitoes as part of the war effort and encouraged them to take a daily dosage of mepacrine, which he claimed had no "poisonous effects" on the human body.[64] It is quite possible that the inhabitants of the city, who were already accustomed to vaccination campaigns and quinine pills and injections, actually welcomed the decline of the mosquito population.[65] If their fears of poisoning were allayed, the residents of Accra might have seen the spraying campaign as nothing more than a nuisance, making it, ultimately, a forgettable event.

KORLE AFTER THE SECOND WORLD WAR

But the major reason that the antimalarial campaign of the Second World War was forgettable is because it was never completed.

By 1945, just as Lt. Ribbands and Major Macdonald declared victory over the mosquito, the Allies had opened up the Mediterranean, and transshipment across the Sahara was no longer necessary. The number of troops stationed in Accra dwindled, and the Americans hastily terminated their involvement in the antimalaria campaign.[66] From 1942–45, the Gold Coast government had been responsible for funding only 8 percent of the work done by the Malaria Control Group, while the rest had been covered through the Lend Lease program (65%) and by the British armed forces (25%).[67] In 1945, the Allied forces left the Gold Coast Public Works Department with the entire cost of maintaining the massive drainage works built on the Korle watershed as well as the responsibility of spraying DDT around the city.[68] A year later, it was evident that the Gold Coast government would never muster enough funding to keep a perpetual campaign against malaria going—the Public Works Department did not even have a budget to screen the windows of bungalows in the city, let alone reinforce miles of concrete embankments along the Odaw River.[69] Major Macdonald's attempt to squeeze infrastructure funding out of the Americans had worked temporarily, but the war was simply too short to complete the project.

In 1946, crews working for the Gold Coast Public Works Department were further disheartened when aerial photos revealed dozens of quarries, salt pans, and borrow pits around Accra, too numerous to monitor and too expansive to spray regularly.[70] The effects of human habitation had created a niche for mosquitoes to flourish, and any dream of eradication was untenable. The British returned to a policy of malaria management—by relying on quinine prophylaxis and the occasional spraying of waterways to prevent mosquito infestations. In the short term, the effects of DDT made the city notably healthier, and use of the chemical became commonplace. For the price of only four pence a tin, DDT even found its way into homes, where people used it to control lice and bedbugs.[71] Kingsway, the largest department store in Accra, dispensed the drug at their chemist department and advertised it as a product created for the "eternal benefit of mankind."[72] Unfortunately, the mosquitos in the area quickly developed a resistance to the chemical, as they did in many other parts of the world.[73] By the 1950s, the Korle Lagoon and its tributaries became mired in silt, and malaria was once again endemic in Accra.[74]

When the soldiers were demobilized and the spraying crews departed, the identity of the lagoon as a goddess among the Ga was easily revitalized. In 1946, after several years of bitter disputes over the stool, Nummo Ayiteh Cobblah II was installed as the priest of Korle. Cobblah became a prominent religious leader in Accra, as a moderate during anticolonial riots in 1948 and as a friend to Ghana's first president, Kwame Nkrumah.[75] When Cobblah was enstooled, he resuscitated the rituals of the annual harvest festival of *Homowo*, establishing his rights to communicate with the spiritual forces that inhabit the lagoon. As she had for centuries, Naa Korle asserted herself as a moral force within Ga culture, a goddess with the ability to define states of collective well-being in the city.

Interlude: Healing the Sickness of Colonialism

In the early 1950s, when the colony of the Gold Coast was on the verge of independence, a unique type of healing culture developed among a group of Zarma-speaking migrants from western Niger, known in Accra as the Zabarima. At the time, the Zabarima were the fastest-growing segment of the Muslim population in Accra, reaching four thousand by 1954.[76] Working in the most menial of jobs, such as carrying loads around the market, recycling used flour bags, or scavenging for used tins and bottles, the Zabarima survived on the margins, and their religious and healing practices reflected their social station.[77] The Zabarima had immigrated from a part of Africa that had been Islamized for hundreds of years, but many of them were also worshippers of a pantheon of deities known as the *Hauka* (a Hausa word meaning "crazy").[78] Jean Rouch, a French filmmaker who followed the activities of migrants around West Africa, claimed that at the peak of the Hauka movement, there were approximately one hundred Hauka gods in West Africa and that approximately 30 percent of Zabarima migrants to the Gold Coast were possessed. Unlike Ga priests and spirit mediums, who worshipped and practiced in public, the followers of the Hauka operated in secret. Indeed, their ceremonies would have remained largely unknown if not captured on film by Rouch, who was invited to one of their gatherings in a village suburb of Accra.

Jean Rouch's footage of a Hauka spirit possession ceremony is striking. It includes several men and one woman gathered around a Hauka shrine in a courtyard decorated with fluttering Union Jacks. Rouch, the narrator, tells the viewer that those gathered are suffering from illnesses caused by sorcery and witchcraft and that they have come to seek the help of the Hauka deities. On the cue of a single note from a violin, the participants are slowly filled with spirits representing different colonial characters, perambulating chaotically before the camera, making grotesque faces, and foaming at the mouth. The most powerful god was *Gomno*, the "governor," a deity represented by a colorful mound with a pith helmet—an image that Rouch paralleled by interposing a scene of the Gold Coast governor Arden-Clarke wearing full regalia at an official ceremony in Accra. Other prominent characters represented the network of colonial officials, including the train engineer (who marches relentlessly back and forth), the sergeant at arms (who berates the participants), and a doctor's wife (who mediates disputes). The film climaxes with a series of heated arguments between the spirits, and a frenzied meal of dog-meat soup.[79] After they eat, the spirits slowly leave the bodies of the possessed, and the exhausted migrant workers load themselves onto a truck, bound for their regular lives in Accra.

When Rouch screened the film in Paris in 1954, it created a scandal. Some critics thought the film, entitled *Les Maitres Fous* (The mad masters), was a fake made with paid actors. Others thought it was a racist portrayal of colonial subjects as ethnographic specimens.[80] Anthropologist Marcel Griaule called the film a "travesty" because it stereotyped Africans as savages; he urged Rouch to destroy it.[81] More recently, *Les Maitres Fous* has been celebrated because it depicts a form of mimicry that expresses the colonial mentalities of African subjects.[82] As Rouch had always argued, the Hauka cult made a bold statement about the psychological effects of colonialism, representing a kind of social healing that allowed immigrants to cope with their subordinate status under White colonial rule.[83] The "mad masters," he maintained, were not Africans but the colonial ruling classes, who, within the context of the cult, represented the authoritarian structure of colonialism. The antithesis of benevolent colonialism, these spirits revealed a menacing crowd of military and technocratic elites fumbling about, fighting, arguing, and screaming. Even the character of the doctor's wife, who plays the role of the mediator among the gods, becomes complicit in Hauka imaginings of colonialism, adding strength to the argument that the colonial subjects of the Gold Coast always regarded medical workers as agents of colonial power.

After decades of conscription into corvée labor, military service, and medical experiments, it is not surprising that a cult like the Hauka emerged within the Zabarima community in Accra. After all, their experience with colonial life was different from that of the established city residents. The Ga people were also suspicious of the motives of "*Gov'ment*," but they never elaborated such apprehensions in the form of a ritual complex, perhaps because they had a sense of belonging that had allowed them to fight back against colonial incursions into their urban home. Unlike the Ga, the Zabarima survived on the margins, using the Hauka spirits to negotiate their way into colonial modernity. In a city where religions and their associated therapeutic systems accumulated rather than displaced one another, the Hauka cult fitted in nicely as a type of spiritual healing that served the most vulnerable newcomers.

When Jean Rouch returned to Accra in 1955, he showed the edited film to the followers of the cult who had been filled with the Hauka spirits. He claimed that when they saw the film, they were so impressed that they intended to expand their performances of worship, integrating film into their ceremonies as a celebration of the power of their mad masters.[84] But they never had the chance—Les Maitres Fous was banned in the Gold Coast Colony in 1955 because it contained "cruelty to an animal and insult to the Queen."[85] The worshippers of the Hauka continued to practice in the city, garnering followers from people of Songhay, Zerma, Peul, Hausa, and Kanuri ethnic origins, but the nature of their procession changed after Ghanaian independence. Rouch continued to follow the Hauka and noted a striking fact: the colonial spirits disappeared from their processions after 1957. He also noted that they were never replaced by African figures of power—no god representing Kwame Nkrumah, or any other African leader, for that matter, ever took spiritual form among the Hauka.[86] Like an epidemic disease that suddenly lost its virulence, the illness of the colony had disappeared, and the spirits of the colonial mad masters disappeared with it.

NOTES

1. PRAAD ADM 5/3/46, Report on Service Malaria Control (Accra and Takoradi, May 1945), 25.

2. Graboyes, Experiment Must Continue, 4–5.

3. A. H. Kelly, "The Territory of Medical Research: Experimentation in Africa's Smallest State," in Para-states and Medical Science: Making African Global Health, ed. P. W. Geissler (Durham, NC: Duke University Press, 2015), 303–32; Graboyes, Experiment Must Continue, 2.

4. Grischow, "K. R. S. Morris and Tsetse Eradication," 381–401; Hughes and Daly, "Onchocerciasis in the Southern Gold Coast," 243–52.

5. Stepan, *Eradication*. Stepan traces the zeal for eradication among entomologists and epidemiologists with "arch-eradicationist" Fred L. Soper as her key character. Ribbands was a contemporary of Soper.

6. PRAAD ADM 5/3/46, Malaria Control, Appendix "A," 7.

7. PRAAD ADM 5/3/46, Malaria Control, Appendix "A," 7–8.

8. PRAAD ADM 5/3/46, Malaria Control, Appendix "A," 8.

9. PRAAD ADM 5/3/46, Malaria Control, Fig. 15 and Appendix "A," 14–15.

10. PRAAD ADM 5/3/46, Malaria Control, 31.

11. National Archives and Records Administration, USA (NARA), R. 705, Major Eugene L. Vickery, "History of the Medical Section Africa-Middle East Theatre, Sept. 1941, to Sept. 1945, Prepared under the Direction of the Chief Surgeon, Eugene W. Billick, Colonel, Medical Corps, Cairo, Egypt, 1945," December 11, 1945, 213.

12. Meghan Vaughan, "Health and Hegemony: Representation of Disease and the Creation of the Colonial Subject in Nyasaland," in *Contesting Colonial Hegemony*, ed. Dagmar Engels and Shula Marks (London, 1994); Butchart, *Anatomy of Power*.

13. Addae, *Gold Coast and Achimota*, 94–100.

14. Bourret, *Gold Coast*, 154–56; David P. McBride, *Missions for Science: U.S. Technology and Medicine in America's Africa World* (New Brunswick, NJ: Rutgers University Press 2002), 168; F. M. Bourret, *Ghana: The Road to Independence, 1919–1957* (Stanford, CA: Stanford University Press, 1960), 147.

15. PRAAD ADM 5/3/46, Malaria Control, 28.

16. PRAAD ADM 5/3/46, Malaria Control, 11; Packard, *Making of a Tropical Disease*, 91.

17. PRAAD ADM 5/3/46, Malaria Control, 10.

18. PRAAD ADM 5/3/46, Malaria Control, 10.

19. PRAAD ADM 5/3/46, Malaria Control, 15.

20. PRAAD ADM 5/3/46, Malaria Control, 5, Appendix B, 1–2.

21. Harrison, *Mosquitoes, Malaria and Man*, 127; Curtin, "Medical Knowledge and Urban Planning," 595; Georg, *Pouvoir Colonial, Municipalites et Espaces Urbains*, 124.

22. Poser and Bruyn, *Illustrated History of Malaria*, 93.

23. *Gazette* (London), March 20, 1942, 1276; Macdonald, *Small Sewage Disposal Systems*; PRAAD ADM 5/3/46, Malaria Control, 5.

24. PRAAD ADM 5/3/46, Malaria Control, 5.

25. Addae, *Evolution of Modern Medicine*, 158.

26. Busvine, *Disease Transmission*, 143–44.

27. PRAAD ADM 5/3/46, Malaria Control, 21.

28. PRAAD ADM 5/3/46, Malaria Control, 22. See also NARA, R. 705, Major Eugene L. Vickery, "History of the Medical Section Africa-Middle East Theater, September, 1941, to September, 1945, Prepared under the Direction of the Chief Surgeon, Eugene W. Billick, Colonel, Medical Corps, Cairo, Egypt, 1945," December 11, 1945, 219.

29. Williams and Lemke, *Foye's Principles of Medicinal Chemistry*, 9; Arrow, Panosian, and Gelband, *Saving Lives, Buying Time*, 130–32.

30. PRAAD ADM 5/3/46, Malaria Control, 22; Sneader, *Drug Discovery*, 381–82.

31. Addae, *Evolution of Modern Medicine*, 159.

32. PRAAD ADM 5/3/46, Malaria Control, 12. See also Timothy Mitchell, *Rule of Experts*, 46–47; Busvine, *Disease Transmission*, 132; Packard, *Making of a Tropical Disease*, 124–25.

33. Packard, *Making of a Tropical Disease*, 141.

34. PRAAD ADM 5/3/46, Malaria Control, 20–21.

35. PRAAD ADM 5/3/46, Malaria Control, 12.

36. PRAAD ADM 5/3/46, Malaria Control, 13.

37. PRAAD ADM 5/3/46, Malaria Control, 31.

38. NARA, R. 705, Vickery, "Medical Section," 209; PRAAD ADM 5/3/46, Malaria Control, 17.

39. PRAAD ADM 5/3/46, Malaria Control, Appendix A, 5; Ribbands, "Moonlight and House-Haunting Habits."

40. NARA, R. 705, Vickery, "History of the Medical Section Africa-Middle East," 217.

41. Addae, *Gold Coast and Achimota*, 157–58.

42. PRAAD ADM 5/3/46, Malaria Control, 25, Appendix A, 7. Ribbands duplicated this experiment on a smaller scale in Sekondi. See Ribbands, "Effects of Bush Clearance."

43. Magoon, "Portable Stable Trap," 363; Busvine, *Disease Transmission*, 169, 175.

44. NARA, R. 705, Vickery, "History of the Medical Section Africa-Middle East," 215.

45. PRAAD ADM 5/3/46, Malaria Control, Appendix A, 8.

46. For information on labor migration in the Gold Coast Colony, see Crisp, *African Working Class*.

47. PRAAD ADM 5/3/46, Malaria Control, Appendix A, 8.

48. PRAAD ADM 5/3/46, Malaria Control, Appendix A, 8.

49. NARA, R. 705, Vickery, "Medical Section," 213, 219; PRAAD CSO 11/11/124, *Accra Anti-Malaria Scheme—Financial Implications of*, "Telegram to the Resident Minister from the Colonial Office," September 22, 1944.

50. NARA, R. 705, Vickery, "Medical Section," 218.

51. PRAAD CSO 3/1/162, *Korle Lagoon*. For example, in 1937 the colonial government paid £35 to acting Korle Priest Nee Tettey Quaye Molai for the rights to fill in some marshy areas of the lagoon.

52. *Gold Coast Independent*, June 17, 1944, 150; *Gold Coast Independent*, September 30, 1945, 239.

53. Fuseni Bomba, interview with the author, December 19, 2005; Mama Moshie, interview with the author, December 20, 2005; Saidu Mossi, interview with the author, December 18, 2005; John Borketey, interview with the author, December 28, 2005; Andrew Nikoi Dsane, interview with the author, December 23, 2005.

54. Busvine records one example of the use of birdlime on clothing to collect tsetse flies in Principe in 1907, but there is no record of adhesive clothing used to collect mosquitoes in Accra. Busvine, *Disease Transmission*, 169.

55. Otia Badu, interview with the author, December 20, 2006.

56. Oblitey Commey, interview with the author, February 25, 2005.

57. Oblitey Commey, interview with the author, February 25, 2005.

58. Old Soldier Lamptey, interview with the author, February 25, 2005.

59. Old Soldier Lamptey, interview with the author, February 25, 2005.

60. John Borketey, interview with the author, December 28, 2005.

61. Bourret, *Gold Coast*, 153–54.

62. Bourret, *Gold Coast*, 155–56.

63. *Gold Coast Independent*, January 20, 1945, 13.

64. Bourret, *Gold Coast*, 237.

65. Professor Stephen Addae, interview with the author, Accra, August 19, 2010.

66. PRAAD CSO 11/11/128, *Control and Maintenance of Accra and Takoradi Anti-Malarial Drainage Scheme—European staff for*, "Letter from Resident Minister's Office, Achimota, Accra to General Headquarters, West Africa, O.C., No. 114 Wing, Accra," May 24, 1945.

67. PRAAD CSO 11/11/124, *Accra Anti-Malaria Scheme—Financial Implications of*, "Telegram to the Resident Minister from the Colonial Office," September 22, 1944.

68. *Gold Coast Medical Reports,* 1944, 6; PRAAD ADM 5/3/46, Malaria Control, 35.

69. PRAAD CSO 10/1/65, *Bungalow no. 11, Second Road, Accra, Mosquito Proofing At,* April 5, 1945, director of public works, memo to colonial secretary.

70. PRAAD ADM 5/3/46, Malaria Control, 37.

71. *Gold Coast Observer,* August 16, 1946, 162.

72. *Gold Coast Observer,* June 7, 1946, 45.

73. Stepan, *Eradication,* 162–63. Additionally, Rachel Carson's popular work *Silent Spring* raised public concerns about the effects of DDT on wildlife and led to a ban on the chemical in the United States in 1975; see Gunter, "News Media and Technological Risks."

74. Nate Plageman, "'Accra Is Changing,'" 156.

75. The ongoing disputes over the office of priest of Korle were not resolved until Nummo Ayiteh Cobblah II was installed in 1946 (Funeral Program, Nummo Ayiteh Cobblah II, 2002).

76. Acquah, *Accra Survey,* 68.

77. Acquah, *Accra Survey,* 69.

78. Rouch, *Ciné-ethnography,* 189–90.

79. The consumption of dog meat as a ritual feast was also associated with Tigare at the time. Nii Addokwei Moffatt, "Dog Meat, A New Craze In Accra," from an article written for the *Daily Graphic,* republished on modernghana.com, July 8, 2004, https://www.modernghana.com/news/58408/dog-meat-a-new-craze-in-accra.html.

80. Lim, "Of Mimicry and White Man," 40–41.

81. Lim, "Of Mimicry and White Man," 40.

82. Stoller, *Cinematic Griot,* 159–60.

83. Michael M. J. Fischer, "Raising Questions about Rouch," 140–43.

84. "Jean Rouch Talks about His Films," 1009.

85. "Jean Rouch Talks about His Films," 1009.

86. Rouch, *Ciné-ethnography,* 193.

THE RESILIENCE OF THERAPEUTIC PLURALISM ON THE EVE OF GHANAIAN INDEPENDENCE

AT THE END OF THE Second World War, the Beveridge Report guided Britain toward the goals of the welfare state, and the Public Health Act of 1947 established the groundwork for universal, socialized medicine in the metropole. By the 1950s, the colony of the Gold Coast had already benefited from the health spending during the cocoa boom and had already reached many of the goals that the National Health Service set out for Britain, such as clinical and hospital care for free or minimal charges and urban sanitation paid for by the colonial public purse. As the officials of the Gold Coast Medical Department planned their retreat from the colony in the 1950s, they began drafting their final reports, hoping to prove that their decades of travail had produced a sort of colonial medical modernity. Key to this assertion was that a paradigmatic shift had occurred in the provision of health care in the city. According to Gold Coast Medical Department reports, patients in Accra attended clinics and hospitals as their *first therapeutic choice* whenever they became ill. Moreover, the departing colonial government asserted, African medical professionals, physicians and scientists, were ready to take over the colonial medical system and transform it into a Ghanaian national health care scheme as part of a global community of Western medical practitioners.[1]

Through the lens of this colonial archive, it seemed that Western medicine was triumphant on the eve of independence, but
the appearance of hegemony was a mirage. A first caveat is that
much of the demand for colonial medicine was, as it always had
been, driven by drugs that offered quick cures for endemic illnesses. In a city where patients were always searching for new curatives, it was not surprising that arsenic compounds, sulfa drugs,
and penicillin were soon widely sought after by patients from all
walks of life. Another major qualification is that, even during the
late colonial period when Gold Coasters were looking forward
to independence, the forces of colonial bio-power, and the corresponding forces of cultural appropriation, were still in place. The
channels that had guided patients toward colonial health care
(police, courts, ambulances, etc.) in the early twentieth century
were even more robust on the eve of independence, and employees in the colonial workforce and in European firms were guided
toward colonial medicine as an occupational identity. Concurrently, elite African residents of Accra sought out medical care
as a means of identifying with national progress, encouraging
their sons and daughters to enter medical professions, hoping
that they might appropriate the forces of bio-power that exerted
control over colonial subjects. The culture of mothercraft also
remained firmly in place, diminishing the authority of African
midwives and augmenting the power of women in the national
medical fold. If colonial medicine had succeeded, it was not because of its perceived universal qualities. Rather, it was the force
of colonial power and matériel behind it that drove it forward as
a therapeutic option.

Additionally, it must be stressed that despite the advances that
were made in the immediate postwar period, Korle Bu was both
underfunded and understaffed. The equipment at Korle Bu dated
back to the 1920s, and its dispensaries struggled to keep up the
supply of new drugs. The centralizing power of Korle Bu that
had once dominated medical culture in the colony dissipated in

the face of competition from other colonial hospitals, and from clinics run by African physicians, leading to a stratification of class and race medical privilege. When a new generation of White officials arrived in the colony after the war, Korle Bu was no longer the "great African hospital" that represented an egalitarian space for the neutral provision of medicine. Instead, it was left to struggle to provide adequate services for a growing urban population. The pre-independence decline of Korle Bu contradicts the assertion that Britain had bestowed a legacy of modernity to Ghana on the eve of independence, and that Western medicine had vanquished other healing traditions. Rather, Korle Bu, despite its rapid ascent as a healing space over the past few decades, and despite its continued popularity, remained only one of many places where people in Accra could seek aid when they were ill.

By the early 1950s, Accra was a colonial metropolis with a population of almost two hundred thousand people. Migrants were flocking to the city to work at the Port of Accra, the cocoa warehouses of James Town, and the retail businesses around Makola Market. So great was the influx of newcomers that the Ga ethnic group had lost its majority status by 1957, and it continued to shrink in significance when compared to the growing Ewe, Fante, Yoruba, and Hausa communities.[2] With such a mixture of ethnicities, African therapeutic practices diversified, expanding to include diviners from Dahomey and Nigeria, shrine keepers from the Northern Territories, and *Hauka* worshippers from Niger. Ga healers continued to make up a plurality of healers in the city, but they understood that they were losing market share. In response, they created a Ga Medical Association, but this attempt to rationalize their practices was ill-fated because of the secretive and competitive nature of their trade.

Faith healing also thrived during this era, as Christians abandoned the liturgy of Western-style churches in a search for spiritual and physical health beyond the colonial Christian order. And though they continued to find themselves marginalized under colonial rule, three types of Muslim healers, the *mallam*, the *al-haji* and the *alufa*, offered a wide range of therapies, from herbal cures to Quranic apotropaics. The number of medicines available in shops and marketplaces also expanded, as Africa became increasingly important to European pharmaceutical companies, some of which began directly targeting African consumers in their print advertisements. In sum, despite the declarations of colonial medical technocrats, the multiethnic arena of Accra continued to offer a variety of healing options from which patients and their therapy management groups could pick and choose.

COLONIAL MEDICAL INFRASTRUCTURE
AND URBAN SANITATION IN THE 1950S

On the eve of Ghanaian independence, the majority of Accra residents sought "western scientific methods of healing" as an option of first choice when they were ill.[3] This was the stunning conclusion made by Ione Acquah, an English sociologist in the employ of the Gold Coast government who published a comprehensive survey of healing in the city as part of the 1958 *Accra Survey*.[4] According to her statistics, the total number of colonial medical personnel in the city had risen so sharply that they had caught up to, or even surpassed, the total ranks of African healers. The change in numbers is impressive. By the 1950s, more than three hundred medical professionals were working on the Korle Bu campus alone, while hundreds more worked in the smaller hospitals at Achimota and Ridge, as well as in numerous private clinics around the city. The majority of physicians were European, but many were African, and the vast majority of nurses, dispensers, and technicians were Africans trained in the colony. By comparison, there were only 274 "Traditional Healers," which included all of the Ga-speaking shrine priests, spirit mediums, herbalists, and other practitioners from around West Africa.[5] By sheer numbers, it appeared that colonial medicine was becoming something

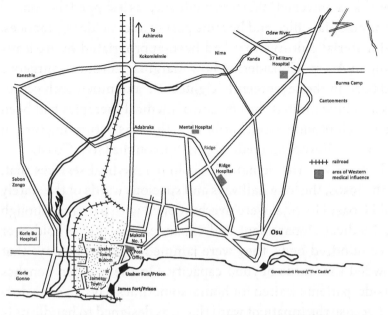

Accra 1957

Map 6.1. Map of Accra, 1957. On the eve of Ghanaian independence, hospitals were located in the suburbs of the city, and several smaller clinics, operated by African physicians, were sprinkled around the city center. Korle Bu provided the majority of colonial medical care in the city, but the Ridge Hospital in the former "European Reservation" had become the hospital of choice for Europeans. The 37th Military Hospital continued to serve the armed forces, while James and Ussher Forts, outposts of medicine during the Atlantic slave trade centuries before, had been transformed into prisons. Meanwhile, Christiansborg Castle had become the seat of the Nkrumah government. Adabraka, Nima, Kanda, and small suburbs to the north of the map housed the new Muslim immigrants arriving in the postwar period, while the new faith-healing churches sprang up in and around James Town and Ussher Town. Just to the north of Ussher Town, the Medical Department still offered quinine pills at the central post office, while Makola Market had become home to Kingsway Chemists and dozens of other merchants of over-the-counter patent medicines and pharmaceuticals. (Source: author.)

more like a universal "Western medicine," as it slipped the control of the colonial office and became part of a set of ideas, practices, and material cultures that had been appropriated by Africans living in Accra. Considering how marginal European surgeons had been in the seventeenth, eighteenth, and nineteenth centuries and how limited the efficacy of medical therapies had been prior to chloroquine and antibiotics, this was a stunning turn in fortune for European medical tradition on the Gold Coast.

So great was the demand for colonial medical services that, by the 1950s, the long hallways and spacious wards of the stately Gold Coast Hospital were overburdened with patients. Though the Medical Department had expanded the site to hold over three hundred beds, they were jammed together in ways that crowded the wards beyond capacity. On the wooden benches outside, patients waited for hours, sometimes days, to see a doctor because the inpatient ward that was designed to handle only two hundred patients a day was serving an average of eight hundred.[6] By Acquah's count, the total number of visits to Korle Bu and other hospitals and clinics in 1954 alone was 256,580, a number that exceeded the total population of the city by at least 50,000.[7] Obviously, many of these visits were by the same patients and many were by people coming to the city from other parts of the colony, but the rise in attendance showed that the exponential population growth was putting a strain on the colonial medical system.

Why were Korle Bu and the smaller hospitals and clinics so popular? The simple answer is the same as it was in the 1920s—the efficacy of new drugs. The demand for outpatient care was likely driven by four particular diseases that could be cured quickly with pharmaceuticals. The first was malaria, which was still the most significant contributor to morbidity and mortality in the city. Chloroquine or Mepacrine were available in pill form, but in severe cases when it was not possible to swallow, or in the case of babies and infants with malaria, patients would have been taken to Korle Bu for free injections of chloroquine solutions. The second disease was yaws, which could now be treated with penicillin, a miracle antibiotic that cleared up skin lesions in a matter of days.[8] The third and fourth diseases, gonorrhea and syphilis, could be remedied with injections of sulfa drugs and penicillin.[9] The demand for these sorts of chemotherapeutic treatments should not be surprising, considering that these four illnesses made up over one-quarter of the causes of death in Accra in 1953.[10]

But while the success of Korle Bu and other hospitals and clinics at treating the major endemic diseases was remarkable, it was unsustainable. In 1953, Dr. H. B. L. Russell, an administrator at the Gold Coast Hospital, reported that the hospital suffered from poorly maintained equipment, poorly organized wards, ill-equipped operating rooms, cramped inpatient facilities, and unhygienic food services. Overcrowding meant that finding adequately trained staff for the hospital became difficult. The head nurse at Korle Bu, Miss Luscombe, lamented the shortage of nursing staff in 1953, arguing that a lack of adequate housing on the hospital campus hindered the recruitment of women of a "good class."[11] Whereas Korle Bu had once been a well-funded hospital that had become home to a medical culture of the aspirant African classes, it was never given a budget that could sustain its status as the premier medical institution in the colony. By the early 1950s, nine-tenths of the equipment was out of date, and the hospital required a capital inflow of over £750,000 to pay for new equipment.[12] The new prime minister of the Gold Coast, Kwame Nkrumah, personally reviewed Russell's report, and while he may have sympathized with the predicament of overcrowding, he allocated only a modest £16,000 for improvements to the medical infrastructure of the colony and tabled any plans to renovate Korle Bu.[13] At the time, Nkrumah's focus was on political independence and economic autonomy, and the British had little interest in improving a hospital they would soon be leaving.

In the remaining years of colonial rule, the Gold Coast Hospital was improved only by small increments, and it remained grossly overcrowded.

As funding diminished and demand increased, Guggisberg's vision for the institution began to fade. Though there was no longer any formal segregation in the colony, White patients shunned Korle Bu, preferring to attend a smaller institution in the European residential area known as Ridge Hospital, which opened in 1946. Black patients were not excluded from Ridge Hospital, but its fees were higher than those charged at Korle Bu, so it remained an establishment of distinction for elites such as British officials and the European, African, Indian, Lebanese, and Syrian merchant classes.[14] As the status of the Ridge Hospital grew, Korle Bu's reputation diminished, and it began to take on the simpler moniker of the "African Hospital," signaling an end to the brief moment of the 1920s and 1930s, when Korle Bu was regarded as the "great" institution that promised to serve both White and Black populations in the city.[15] With the relocation of elite medical services to the area formerly known as the European Reservation, the city reverted to a spatialization of health care that followed patterns established in the 1890s, with the exception that non-White elite families now could now live in the former European Reservation. On the eve of independence, the racial divisions that had previously defined the geography of Accra were beginning to blur with class divisions.

By the 1950s, the sanitary infrastructure of Accra, especially in Ussher Town and James Town, was also collapsing under the weight of population growth. After the withdrawal of the US Army, the maintenance of the sanitary infrastructure was left to the Public Health Department, which reported itself to be "grossly understaffed."[16] In his annual report for 1953, the medical officer of health declared that an improvised "camp sanitation" approach could no longer be relied on to protect the health of the population and that permanent measures had to be taken to preserve

the health of the population. In particular, the city was in desperate need of a sewer system, a wastewater system, and larger
supplies of fresh water. Toilets, in particular, were hard to come
by, and would be for some time to come. In 1954, there were
only six hundred toilets in the entire city, mostly in the newly
constructed suburbs, which meant that two-thirds of the population had to use poorly maintained latrines with barrels to collect human waste. Open areas in the city were used as garbage
dumps and cesspits, which contaminated the subsoil and the
water mains that ran through it.[17] But little new money was forthcoming. Instead, the colonial government continued to fund
their small army of sanitary inspectors to monitor the behavior of Accra residents by entering their compounds and houses
in search of mosquito larvae and other sanitary violations. In
fact, Acquah's Accra Survey would not have been possible without sanitary inspectors because they used their right to enter
homes to collect information for Acquah about bathing habits,
use of latrines, food preparation, and other quotidian details
related to public health. The Survey itself is testament to the
continued presence of a colonial medical gaze in the homes of
the residents of the city, even as the sanitation syndrome began
to wane.[18]

As it had been in past decades, Korle Lagoon continued to
play the scapegoat for poor public hygiene. Sporadic outbreaks
of typhoid fever were a problem in the city, especially during the
rainy season, when people collected contaminated water from
streams leading into the lagoon.[19] As they had in the past, the
administrators at Korle Bu argued that the lagoon remained "a
menace to the hospital as a whole." They even lobbied (naively,
in the context of prior failed attempts) the Public Works Department to drain the lagoon as soon as possible.[20] The vilification of
the lagoon as an enemy to modern notions of health was repeated
in the local press too, and journalist Henry Ofori even went so far
as to deny the significance of the deity that inhabited the lagoon,

stating he thought "very little of gods who live at the bottom of black slush and odiferous waters and occupy themselves with the reproduction of mosquitoes."[21] The discourse of health and sanitation in the city had become quite divorced from the traditional beliefs of the Ga people, at least among medical and literate circles, but despite calls for further investment in sanitary infrastructure, the colonial government refused. It soon became obvious that the British were unwilling to spend millions of pounds on sanitary infrastructure only to bequeath it gratis to the government of Ghana.

Above all other diseases, malaria continued to pose the biggest health threat to the growing population. During the rainy season, the disease caused high rates of morbidity in adults and high rates of infant mortality, but the Medical Department did little to stem outbreaks.[22] Attempts to reengineer the Korle watershed had long been abandoned, and the Department of Public Works simply could not afford to continue aerial spraying DDT. The Sanitation Department had to make do with piecemeal efforts to prevent epidemics, which included sending mosquito brigades on spraying patrol around the city and prosecuting people through the so-called larvae courts. In the vain hope that increasing residents' knowledge about the illness might halt the spread of the disease, the Medical Department initiated an education campaign that included sending vans with loudspeakers around the city to spread the word about malaria control, screening educational films about the mosquito vector via the Gold Coast Film Unit, and writing curricula for health education in the schools.[23] But the Gold Coast was not included in the World Health Organization's Global Malaria Eradication Programme, nor did the Medical Department have a plan for any comprehensive malaria-fighting campaign.[24] In a way, the residents of Accra in the 1950s were lucky. Resistance to chloroquine in the *Anopheles* mosquito (the genus that spreads malaria) had not yet developed, which meant that even though malaria was widespread, it was at least curable.

The dire state of sanitary affairs in the old quarters of Accra contrasted starkly with the situation in the European Residential area. In the 1950s, the Public Works Department refitted colonial bungalows with electric lights, fans, and stoves and supplied running water for showers, bathtubs, and washbasins.[25] Refrigerators were supplied free to Europeans in the employ of the government or major commercial firms, and the sanitary crews of the Accra Town Council were hired to clean compounds. Even the so-called boys' quarters, small dwellings for servants within the compounds, were wired for lights and provided with sinks and toilets. Though urban segregation had officially ended, a new form of sanitary segregation emerged. The disparities evident in a short trip from the leafy eastern suburbs of the colonial elites through the urban core of the city to the crowded wards of Korle Bu clearly illustrated the priorities of a colonial government intent on taking care of its own while planning an exit from the capital city.

AFRICAN PHYSICIANS AS BEARERS OF MEDICAL TRADITION

The burden of meeting the demand for medical services in Accra was mollified somewhat by African physicians in private practice. By the mid-1950s, the number of Africans with their own clinics had increased to a total of six, but this was still tiny in comparison to the total of eighty-four physicians working in the colony.[26] Most African physicians were from elite families who had the means to send their sons to the United Kingdom for training, and though they operated their clinics mostly for African patients, in the heart of James Town and Ussher Town, they could only minister to the needs of as many as thirty patients per day. Evidence suggests that their clientele was drawn from all walks of life in the city, but the fees that they charged indicate that their primary clients came from a stratum of African elites.[27]

With their own clinics and dispensaries, and a new battery of pharmaceuticals at their disposal, the African-born physicians of the 1950s became wealthy, influential members of society, setting standards for upper-class social behavior by maintaining memberships at elite organizations such as the Rodger Club and the Accra Turf Club.[28] Dr. Tamakloe, the fictional sculptor-physician depicted in the Gold Coast Film Unit feature *The Boy Kumasenu* (1952), epitomizes the postwar Accra physician because he was played by the real-life Dr. Oku Ampofo, an Edinburgh-trained doctor, sculptor, and advocate for the arts community.[29] African physicians also played middleman political roles during the decolonization process. Though not at the vanguard of the independence movement, they were active on the Legislative Council, on the Accra Town Council, and in Ga chiefly politics.[30] Dr. Nanka-Bruce continued to be the most vocal public advocate for increased educational, professional, and political opportunities for the subjects of the Gold Coast. He supported increasing local control over the medical profession, founding a Gold Coast branch of the British Medical Association in 1951. Nanka-Bruce was a vocal critic of colonial medical authorities, but he had always showed his fidelity to British overrule, receiving the Order of the British Empire as well as the honor of special delegate to witness the coronation of King George VI in 1937.[31] As a member of a cadre of professionals who assumed that they would become leaders within Ghana, Dr. Nanka-Bruce thought of himself as a citizen of an independent African nation that would remain a loyal member of the British Commonwealth.

The physicians working in Accra on the eve of independence believed themselves to be the bearers of a medical tradition passed down through generations of medical professionals in both Africa and the West, but they were also well aware of the rich traditions of African healing culture, and some of them even knew African healers personally. Many of the doctors knew of Ofori Ata, the healer who had met Cicely Williams in the 1930s, and were aware that he was "held in high esteem" as a drummer, soothsayer, and herbalist by the residents of Accra.[32] And some of the physicians also had a quiet respect for locally generated therapies that made use of well-known local herbs, so much so that they even used them as home remedies.[33] Dr. Oku Ampofo, who trained at the Basel Mission in Akwapim, would later become a sponsor for the scientific study of traditional herbal medicines in that region.[34] However, as Western trained physicians, they could not conduct any professional intercourse with African healers because it might run counter to their belief in scientific treatments for illnesses.[35] As bearers of Western medical knowledge, physicians in the 1950s could entertain the possibility that herbal remedies had scientific merit, but they regarded most African practitioners as "juju men" who used fetishes to profit from the ignorance of their patients.[36]

Though they were surrounded by practitioners of African therapeutic traditions, and though they shared their patients with those healers, the African physicians of 1950s Accra were confident about their future in Accra.[37] They understood themselves as a new generation of professionals, operating on the assumption that only scientific practices could reveal pathogens and offer hope of a cure. Moreover, their social status had finally changed. Physicians like Nanka-Bruce and Ampofo had finally reached the upper classes of late-colonial Ghanaian society, a world of private clubs, horse racing, and political activity, which they shared with African lawyers and merchants in Accra. They could even envision themselves as future elites of an independent nation, and indeed, many physicians would help lead the CPP to victory, and Ghana to independence, in 1957.

THE SURVIVAL OF GA AND OTHER AFRICAN HEALING PRACTICES IN ACCRA

One of the most dramatic findings of the *Accra Survey* is the direct correlation between levels of education and the patronage of colonial medicine. Taking samples from hundreds of people, of all professions and classes, Acquah showed that the patronage of African healers had an inverse correlation with the amount of Western education a person had achieved. A straight reading of her statistics would lead one to believe that it was only a matter of time before education in the universality of scientific knowledge would make African traditional healing obsolete. In particular, Ga healing was threatened as the Ga population began to shrink in proportion to other ethnic groups in Accra. But the outcome of several decades of colonial medical expansion evades capture by the parameters of Acquah's limited questions. So skewed are the statistics in the *Accra Survey* that they read more like a congratulatory clap on the backs of the officers of the Medical Department than an honest assessment of the state of colonial medicine at independence. Considering that so many nonmedical traditions were flourishing in the city at the time, it is obvious that, just like the assertions of medical triumph made by the colonial Medical Department, Acquah's findings deserve some major qualifications.

A key problem with the *Accra Survey* is that there was little transparency in its methodology. Although we can presume that Acquah's data came from questionnaires and Town Council records, she rarely footnoted her sources. Considering how difficult communication between colonial officials and African healers had been in the past and how high tensions were between local residents and sanitary inspectors, it is likely that Acquah's data collectors did not always receive frank responses to their questions. For instance, when the survey teams queried patients about the number of times they visited the hospital versus the number of times they visited Ga healers, they did so with the use of questionnaires. How these questionnaires were formulated, printed, and distributed is not known, so it is unclear who might have filled them out in written form or who might have been asked the questions by one of Acquah's assistants. It is possible that

Table 6.1. Educational Background of 325 Males and 176 Females in Relation to Treatment Sought When Ill. These numbers, derived from questionnaires distributed by Ione Acquah's survey team, demonstrate a trend toward colonial medicine as a healing option of first resort across all educational classes. However, the data is suspect because the method of collection was not transparent and the respondents were mostly educated male residents. The vast majority of people in Accra would have fallen into category 1. (Source: Acquah, *Accra Survey*, 122.)

| | Treatment Sought When Ill | | | | | | | |
| | Scientific only | | Traditional only | | Both scientific and traditional | | | |
	Male	Female	Male	Female	Male	Female	Total	%*
1. No schooling	32	62	9	6	3	6	118	24
2. Primary schooling	14	11	—	—	4	—	29	6
3. Middle schooling	193	71	1	1	6	—	272	54
4. Commercial and technical	5	—	—	—	—	—	5	1
5. Secondary and teacher training	50	18	—	—	1	—	69	14
6. University or equivalent professional training	7	1	—	—	—	—	8	2
TOTAL	301	163	10	7	14	6	501	100

*Percentages have been rounded and therefore may not add up to exactly 100 percent.

patients were not forthright in their responses, because healing rituals conducted in the city were often shrouded in secrecy, and patronage of so-called fetish priests may have been regarded as an embarrassment, especially for Christians or Muslims.[38] Acquah herself admitted that "secrecy is maintained by many people who avail themselves of magical methods of cure or protection, it is not possible to measure the extent to which it is practiced in Accra today."[39] Without extensive participant-observer research, she did not have the capacity to make any statistical assertions about the behavior of patients in Accra.

Second, by Acquah's own admission, class distinction informed the responses to her survey. The "attitude of the more educated class," according to Acquah, was that "outwardly at least, one should show a preference for the scientific methods of treatment."[40] Moreover, employees of the government, the Town Council, and large European private firms admitted to Acquah that they "by nature of their employment, attend the hospital when they are ill."[41] This suggests that the choice of a hospital or clinic over other healing options was not always patient directed but was strongly influenced by the expectations of the workplace. Considering that approximately twenty thousand residents of Accra were working for either the colonial government or major European corporations in the 1950s, much of the demand for colonial medical services might be explained by the simple need to bring a doctor's note back to the workplace when one returned from an illness.[42] By contrast, African or religious healers could not provide documentation suitable for functionaries of the colonial state.

A third qualification is that Acquah's data contained such a strong bias toward educated respondents that the trend toward scientific medicine was overstated.[43] According to the 1948 Gold Coast Census, fewer than 20 percent of the residents of Accra had attended colonial schools, and half of those had achieved less than primary school education.[44] With so many people falling into the category of "no schooling," one can extrapolate from Acquah's own data that the vast majority of people in the city sought help from non-Western healers. Moreover, the bias toward educated informants left a major gap in statistical knowledge about women because girls were in the minority in the colonial school system.[45] Considering the influence of women in the healing culture of the city, limiting the number of responses from female patients excluded a great deal of information about reproductive health and childhood maladies. Acquah even suggested, in an aside, that much of the knowledge about herbal remedies was perpetuated domestically by elderly women.[46]

Finally, the sheer bounty of information about Ga and other African practitioners that can be found in the *Accra Survey* undercuts the assumption that patients were abandoning African healing. In contrast to her assertion that colonial medicine became the primary choice for patients, Acquah admitted that patients frequently alternated between colonial therapies and West African therapies, especially if they could not find a quick cure at a hospital or clinic.[47] The degree to which this pluralism occurred was, according to Acquah, beyond quantitative assessment because of the secretive nature of patients and practitioners, but she asserted nonetheless that many people used charms, spells, and apotropaic objects to "ward off sickness." The *Accra Survey* even includes a breakdown of several types of traditional practitioners, some of them new to the city.[48]

In the immediate postwar period, African healing traditions not only survived but were changing according to the circumstances of the times. Several descriptive passages of African practitioners in the *Accra Survey* match the ethnographic observations of Margaret Field twenty years earlier, suggesting that Acquah either discussed her findings with Field or closely read her work on the topic of Ga medicine and religion. Most of the African healers who appear in the *Survey* were described as full-time practitioners who took in patients for long-term treatments for maladies like barrenness, impotency, leprosy, convulsions,

Table 6.2. List of Traditional Healers Classified by Type and Tribe. The *Accra Survey* showed that, even in the mid-1950s, Ga healers continued to make up the plurality of practitioners in the city. Closely behind were Akan and Ewe practitioners, who may have been descended from a long line of such healers in Accra or may have been new. What is certainly new is the large number of practitioners from Northern Ghana and Nigeria. How Acquah assigned healers to these "tribal divisions" (which are actually a variety of linguistic/ethnic/regional distinctions) is not known, but the table does indicate that there were a wide variety of therapeutic options available to patients in the city. (*Source:* Ione Acquah, *Accra Survey*, 123.)

Type of healer	Tribal Divisions							Total
	Ga and Adangme	Akan	Ewe or Dahomey	Northern Ghana and beyond	Hausa or Northern Nigeria	Southern Nigeria	Sierra Leonean	
Herbalists	83	31	28	10	2	12	1	167
Midwives	6	6	1	3	—	—	—	16
Medicine men	1	3	11	2	—	—	—	17
Muslim healers	2	1	—	3	5	3	—	14
Fetish priests	—	—	—	—	—	—	—	0
Tigare cult	3	2	—	—	—	—	—	5
Individual fetishes	7	3	1	—	—	—	—	11
Fetish priestesses	20	1	2	—	—	—	—	23
Soothsayers	1	—	19	1	—	—	—	21
TOTAL	123	47	62	19	7	15	1	274

arthritis, venereal disease, and even psychological illness.[49] Because of fierce competition, practitioners could normally expect to earn only a few shillings per treatment, and they could only earn large sums by taking patients into their shrines for extended forms of therapy.[50] Notably, competition for patients led healers to devise new remedies for new problems, including medicines to help schoolchildren pass tests, spiritual assistance to help adults achieve colonial accreditations, and talismans to protect cars and trucks from accidents.[51] African healers also complemented their locally derived remedies with patent medicines and pharmaceuticals bought in the marketplace, a key point of hybridity that was touched upon only briefly.[52] Just as Margaret Field had in the 1920s, Acquah denigrated these innovations in healing, relegating them to the category of quack medicines sold by charlatans who did not conform to ethnic dogmata.[53] Her goal, like Field's, was to demonstrate that African healing traditions were on the wane, but just as Field had done, she unwittingly demonstrated that African healers were adapting to the circumstances of a rapidly changing urban healing culture.[54]

Further evidence of the vitality of the African healing community comes from outside the official record, from a group of herbalists who attempted to professionalize their work according to a code of professional standards.[55] In 1946, under the leadership of a schoolteacher who held a master's degree in science, a group of herbalists formed the Ga Medical Association, which claimed a membership of 150 by 1955. The idea of a society to promote the aims of herbalism was not new on the Gold Coast. In the 1930s J. A. Kwesi Aaba formed the Society of Herbalists in Takoradi in an attempt to coordinate knowledge about herbal cures in the Akan-speaking regions of the Gold Coast.[56] Aaba referred to himself as an "African Scientific Herbal Doctor" and published a thirty-six-page textbook that he hoped would restore the status of what he referred to as African "medical herbalism."[57] The Ga Medical Association hoped to emulate Aaba's Society of Herbalists, as an ethnically bounded organization with the goals of isolating the medicinal properties of traditional Ga remedies. Their goal was to be certified by the Medical Department to produce local remedies as mass market products, offering therapies that would preserve the "Hygienia" of the body.[58] The allusion to the Greek goddess of health was a means of framing the purposes of the society as both scientific and holistic in a way that would be understood by educated elites but that would not abandon long-standing Ga precepts about the supernatural forces that resided within healing reagents. However, despite its hopeful beginnings, the Ga Medical Association faded away without a trace in less than a decade.[59]

The drive to organize was a logical way for African healers to assert their professional rights, in particular vis-à-vis the Native Customs Regulation Ordinance, which still technically forbade the provision of nonscientific medicines, though prosecutions were exceedingly rare and only related to the use of harmful medicines.[60] However, the healers' timing was poor. In the late colonial era, the British were backing away from the colony and felt no need to rewrite laws to recognize non-Western healing traditions. Moreover, the Ga Medical Association did not have a political figure to champion their cause—it would not be until almost ten years later, in 1963, that President Kwame Nkrumah would bring together healers under the Ghana Psychic and Traditional Healers Association.[61] Without leadership in the political realm, the Ga healers of the late 1950s refused to expose their trade secrets to one another. The long-standing professional castes of the wulomei, the woŋtsemei/woyei, and the tsofatsemei of Accra may have been united linguistically, ethnically, and geographically, but they remained an internally diverse group of competitive healers who were still fending off incursions by immigrant healers from around West Africa.

It should be noted, however, that one exception to the ongoing vibrancy of African healing traditions was in the realm of maternal and infant care. Following the suppression of the Naa Ede Oyeadu shrine in 1905, the establishment of infant welfare clinics, and the construction of a children's hospital in the early 1920s, the provision of reproductive healing had fallen almost entirely into the hands of the colonial state. By the 1950s, colonial doctors, nurses, and midwives became the primary bearers of knowledge and practice about childbirth and child rearing, and thousands of women visited the hospital for prenatal, perinatal, and post-natal care. Though statistics for births are imprecise, it is likely that, on the eve of independence, the overwhelming majority of babies in Accra were either delivered at the maternity hospital or attended to by one of twenty-eight district midwives trained at Korle Bu.[62] The maternity hospital continued to sponsor weekly infant welfare clinics in different parts of the city, offering lectures on childcare, free examinations for babies and infants, and free tinned milk and cod-liver oil to mothers.[63]

So pervasive was the colonial culture of mothercraft that the *Accra Survey* could boldly state that "all children are taken to the clinic during the first year of their lives."[64] Just as they had in the 1920s and 1930s, pregnant women and mothers with babies continued to flock to hospitals and clinics, collapsing demand for African midwives, who had for centuries apprenticed with older kinswomen to learn remedies for infertility, difficult menstruation, pregnancy complications, and infant illnesses.[65] By the 1950s, the *Accra Survey* reported that most African midwives were either middle-aged or elderly, a stark contrast with the younger nurses trained at Korle Bu. The profession of the Ga midwife was in obvious decline.[66]

In the absence of African midwives, other healers continued to provide services to pregnant women and mothers. Women spirit mediums (*woyei*), in particular, offered therapies for reproductive health, evident in this summary of interview data contained in the *Accra Survey*:

> When a pregnant woman consults a Woyoo she is first given protective treatment in order that the evil acts of witches or bad medicine men will not affect her. There is a widespread belief that these

evil spirits must be warded off to safeguard the unborn babe in the womb. This protective treatment consists in making six incisions at the back of both wrists, at the base of the neck and behind the waist. Into these cuts is rubbed a black powder, the composition of which is known only to the practitioners. The pregnant woman is then given a waistband from which are suspended charms tied up in pieces of material. This waistband must be worn continuously during pregnancy, for it is said to prevent miscarriage. In addition, the pregnant woman must acquire a new sleeping mat, chamber pot, and large enamel basin which will be used after the birth of the child, and, as they are included in the protective medicinal rites, they are said to be protected from evil forces. Certain herbs are given to the woman with which she must bath [sic] on seven successive days, for through the performance of this she is committed to the care of the god. After this has been done she must then visit the Woyoo once a week for a routine examination.[67]

The *woyei* continued to generate fertility rituals that included ritual incisions, consecrated bundles, herbal baths, nutritional advice, and the evocation of the power of deities, all of which were conducted according to practices learned through apprenticeship but also through advice garnered in the spirit world. While the vocation of midwife may have been appropriated by medical experts, and while educated Christian women may have shunned African maternity customs, the power of the *woyei* over fertility and infant health remained a vibrant part of Ga culture.

As the *Accra Survey* showed, colonial medicine was expanding, but was African healing in decline? One might argue it was, if gauged in comparison to the rise of patients seeking help from colonial medical practitioners. However, the population of Accra was growing so quickly that there were actually more African healers in the city than ever before. The Ga healing professions of the *wulomei*, *woŋtsemei*, *woyei*, and *tsofatsemei* may have been in decline in proportion to colonial medical practitioners and other African healers, but they were still ubiquitous in the city, as revealed by Acquah's survey. In that respect, it is hard to say that a group of more than one hundred professionals who made up almost half of the African healers in the city, and who were still embedded within a vibrant Ga culture, were suffering diminishing status. With the exception of the near hegemony of mothercraft, Ga healing in particular, and African healing in general, continued to play a foundational role in the healing culture of the city, and were being adapted to the circumstances through the invention of new types of practices.

IMMIGRANT GODS IN POSTWAR ACCRA

After the Second World War, Accra was flooded with young immigrant men and women looking for work, and it soon became one of the largest cities in West Africa. It was a metropolis of immigrants, many of whom formed urban niches beyond the authority of the Ga state.[68] Accompanying the waves of migrant workers were migrant healers who brought with them itinerant herbalism, Afa divination, and imported deities from the Northern Territories. The Ga still made up the core network of healers in Accra, but they were competing with African traditions from farther and farther abroad.

In the 1950s, Ga herbalists still sourced most of their herbal reagents from within a twenty-mile radius of the city, gathering the same local plants they had used for generations. But on the cusp of independence, a different class of itinerant herbalists brought in medicinal flora from around West Africa, making much grander claims about their healing powers. In the absence of any regulatory bodies, traveling herbalists could claim to be familiar with the herbaria of distant regions or to be members of international herbalist associations, without any system of verification. One of these herbalists appears in the *Accra Survey* as a wandering healer:

> One educated herbalist acquired his skill, all of which he paid
> for, from non-kinsmen. First he settled in a town in Trans-Volta
> Togoland for three years, where he studied under the local

herbalists. Then he practiced for a short while there before he
went to Half Assini in Southern Ghana, where for one year he
studied under another herbalist. From there he went to Ashanti
to the villages around Lake Bosomtwi where he acquired further
herbal knowledge. In addition, his father, who lived in Northern
Nigeria, also sent him by correspondence several Hausa remedies. He is now settled in Accra as a full-time herbalist and
corresponds with healing societies in all parts of the world. In
this country he regards himself as the representative of an organisation called the Universal Religious Alliance and Permanent
World Parliament of Religions. He states that this organisation
is "a world brotherhood of friendly co-operation through all
religious fathers, fraternities and inspired philosophies under
the fatherhood of God." He appends several letters to his name:
D.D., Ph.D., D.Sc., and M.N.I.M.H. (Lond.) The latter stands
for "Member of the National Institute of Medical Herbalists
(London)." In his room is a framed certificate showing that he
has been accepted into the Fellowship of the National Institute
of Therapeutics of Calcutta (India). There is also an American
certificate bearing testimony to some religious study. He has not,
however, qualified in medicine or theology in any university. The
title he gives himself is "Botanic-Medical Practitioner of Accra"[69]

This particular healer went unnamed, but he provided an example of the type of herbalist interlopers who were congregating in
the city. The tone of Acquah's writing suggests she did not take
the claims of such herbalists seriously, and she did not bother to
verify the overseas references of her archetypical herbalist. In
fact, the Universal Religious Alliance (United Kingdom), the
World Parliament of Religions (United States) and the National
Institute of Medical Herbalists (United Kingdom) were, at one
time, real organizations, but to Acquah they were merely a veil
for charlatanism. Nonetheless, the fact that such herbalists were
wandering the city of Accra spoke to patients' interest in rare,
imported herbs and the expertise to use them.[70]

Afa diviners also rose to prominence in the 1950s. Probably carried by soothsayers from Nigeria and Dahomey, Afa divination

brought a type of diagnostics to Accra that involved casting beads, cowrie shells, or kola nuts into earthenware pots. Afa soothsayers probably carved out a space for themselves by claiming to be able to predict the future, but like the other African healers in town, they also made a living by tending to a wide variety of bodily and social illnesses.[71] To heal specific ailments, they prescribed herbal concoctions that they claimed could cure "lunacy, impotency, sterility, paralysis, rheumatism, stiffness, epilepsy, eye troubles, [and] wounds."[72] As an example of a soothsayer therapy session, the Accra Survey includes an account of an elderly patient seeking to discover why her grandson was ill:

> The soothsayer sat on the floor before the altar. He took a two-shilling piece from the client and then took the chains and other articles from the canvas bag. After fingering the two-shilling piece he handed it back to the woman, instructing her to place it between her lips and to whisper to it all that she desired on her grandson's behalf. Meanwhile the diviner, through incantations, was in communication with Afa. He passed his fingers through the chains and other objects taken from the canvas bag, constantly picking up the chains and throwing them towards the enamel dishes and the red earthenware pot under the altar. The position in which the objects on the chain fall reveals the message which Afa has for the enquirer. Each combination of positions has a special name and significance.[73]

Unlike Ga practices, which involved the slaughter of chickens in divination ceremonies, Afa practices included nuts or shells being strung together and cast onto the dishes to provide yes or no answers to any questions asked.[74] The incantations were part of a set of verses of poetry that could be selected by the diviner according to his or her assessment of the needs of the client.[75] In this particular reading, the soothsayer concluded by divining that the grandson would soon recover his health, but only if the woman refused to take him to a colonial physician and made regular two-shilling sacrifices to the soothsayer's deities to prevent further illness.[76]

Afa soothsayers were unique because they offered their clients extended regimens of healing as well as visions of health in the future. The cost of a first reading was only two shillings, but further treatments could be very expensive, reaching over one pound per session.[77] Acquah notes that soothsayers had a clientele made up of wealthy patients and that charging fees as high as £40 for serious illnesses was not unusual.[78] The cost of their services (a sum equivalent to more than a month's salary for a senior physician at Korle Bu) may have been exaggerated to elevate their status, but it reflects the presence of clients willing to pay for divination. Unfortunately, there is no data that specifies whether their customers came from Yoruba, Fon, Ewe, Ga, or other ethnic groups or what social strata they might have been drawn from. However, the high price of hiring a soothsayer speaks to a stratification within the African healing market. It may be that, in the same way that the elite classes of Accra aligned themselves with colonial medical care, wealthy immigrants in Accra distinguished themselves by having a soothsayer in their employ.

The African healing traditions present in Accra were further diversified by the arrival of mobile deities from the Northern Territories of the Gold Coast. Immigrant gods were not unknown to the people of Accra, and the colonial government had outlawed several sects regarded as cults in the early twentieth century, but importing a god was not an easy process, and it is not entirely clear what motivations drove supplicants to travel to distant locations to the north, buy the rights to the cult of a foreign god, and trundle southward with the deity's paraphernalia to build a new shrine.[79] If one follows the logic of Margaret Field, who argued that the rise of foreign gods in the southern Gold Coast was a result of jealousies generated by prosperity in the cocoa economy, these new deities may have been sought after as foils against witchcraft, which by some accounts was an increasingly dangerous force in Accra.[80] It may have been that the new gods were considered bulwarks against a rising number of witches, but considering how competitive the healing business was in 1950s Accra, they were also just another edge that healers could gain on their rivals.

Some of the better-known newcomer gods who arrived in Accra in the 1950s were Kwaku Fri from the Ashanti Region, Kunde from the Black Volta, and Tongnaab from the White Volta. Each of these deities has a migration story to tell; however, the most famous of all was Tigare, a god from Ipare, a small village in the far western corner of the Northern Territories.[81] Tigare was expensive to acquire, but once a fee ranging from £40 to £600 was paid to his shrine, the god became a spirit that could be worshipped anywhere. Initially, Tigare was brought to the city to fight a perceived outbreak of witchcraft, but the god's powers broadened, as the priests of his shrine adapted it to local concerns about health, fertility, and good fortune.[82] Tigare was a uniquely accessible deity—one could request his help simply by eating a kola nut in front of the priest and paying the initiation fee.[83] Oral tradition holds that a man named Elder Kwabena brought Tigare to southern Ghana to increase the fertility of local farms in the wake of a series of vicious witchcraft attacks.[84] Elder Kwabena had been a spirit medium who channeled multiple deities from the Southern Gold Coast, but the power of the savanna gods drew him northward to Ipare, and he returned to establish the first shrine to Tigare in Accra in 1943.[85] By 1948, Elder Kwabena claimed that three hundred devotees were worshipping Tigare, at a shrine in a suburb of Accra.[86] Shrines later sprang up at Nsawam to the north and in Labadi to the east, and by 1955, there were five Tigare priests in and around Accra, each with an average weekly attendance of fifteen to thirty devotees.[87]

Initially, Tigare was known as a god of fertility, and his followers were largely women who believed that witches were devouring their wombs. A passage from a 1949 court case shows that a married couple joined the Tigare cult because they had suffered the deaths of several newborns and they wanted to protect their three remaining infants.[88] Other imported gods, like Tongo, had been employed as fertility spirits in the past, but Tigare was particularly well-known as a foil to witches, provided that his supplicants followed the taboos of his shrine.[89] Tigare rapidly took on the role of a prophylactic cult that allowed patients to take preventive action against future problems. The suppression of the shrine of Naa Ede Oyeadu, which had created a gap that was already being filled by colonial maternal and infant medical care, may have also offered an opening for Tigare, especially considering that popular opinion held that the malicious forces of witchcraft were on the rise in Accra.[90]

The uniqueness of its shrine culture also enhanced the authority of Tigare. The steadfast nature of the god's rules borrowed liberally from Christian doctrine and included the following six decrees:[91]

1. Thou shalt not steal
2. Thou shalt not covet thy neighbour's wife
3. Honour thy father and thy mother
4. Thou shalt not bear false witness against thy neighbour
5. Love thy neighbour as thyself
6. Thou shalt not administer medicine of noxious or poisonous nature[92]

To this mixture of biblical commandments and colonial legalese were added a number of uncodified pledges against the use of curses or witchcraft.[93] Like the oath medicines used during the Atlantic slave trade, anyone who violated the taboos of the shrine was expected to suffer misfortune, illness, or even death.[94] Tigare also added a novel subculture of music, dance, dress, and material culture to the healing traditions of Accra. The priest of Tigare danced to unique rhythms, which meant that a shrine had to employ a retinue of musicians, including someone who knew the lead role of the *odono* (a double-headed, hourglass-shaped drum strung with leather chords to alternate tones) and someone who could play a Tigare bell pattern, which differed substantially from the Ga or Fante rhythms. The dancing differed too. Tigare's movements contained elements of Muslim Sufi whirling, with accentuated twists and twirls of a heavy cotton smock emblazoned with consecrated leather bundles. While in trance, a Tigare priest knelt before elders and touched his hands to the ground, actions alien to coastal dances.[95]

The material culture of Tigare's shrines also diverged from local practices because they followed the aesthetic of the savanna, including accoutrements like black pots, swords, and carvings of lions.[96] Tigare also accepted different gifts than the Ga priests. Instead of livestock, alcohol, and cloth, his oblation of choice was kola nut, a mild stimulant used as an offering to deities north of the rain forest. Tigare, a foreigner to Accra, established himself as neither Ga nor Christian nor Muslim, an identity that allowed his followers to mix together powerful ideas, practices, and material cultures from several religious and healing traditions. He was broadly understood as coming from the northern regions, but his priests and followers made sure that the god dealt with the local problems faced by supplicants in Accra.

From the perspective of patients, migrant gods complemented the work of local deities, but the priests of the major Ga shrines were nonetheless displeased by the presence of Tigare, and they sought to persecute his worshippers. For this reason, Tigare priests tended to live outside Ussher Town and James Town, in the newer suburbs of the city. For example, a famous Tigare medium who practiced well into the twenty-first century, Okomfo Numo, chose to build his shrine in Bubuashi, north of Korle Lagoon, to avoid interference by the Ga religious elites.[97] The colonial government also saw Tigare as an interloper and sought to discredit his followers. Okomfo Numo claimed he was persecuted by the government for years, and he related a story about how he had been harassed by the police at the request of the Accra Town Council. This sort of persecution is confirmed in the postwar court records of the city, which contain examples of Tigare priests being jailed and fined for using "obnoxious medicines," for conducting trials by ordeal, and for sexually exploiting patients at their shrines.[98] No such efforts were ever taken to suppress the major shrines of Korle, Sakumo, or Nae, most likely because the British wanted to maintain cordial relations with the Gas of central Accra by upholding the medico-religious status quo in the capital city.

The new healers and deities that arrived in Accra during the postwar period may have posed a threat to the established healing culture of the Ga and to colonial control over the religious and cultural makeup of Accra, but they were welcomed by patients, who were looking for everything from herbal cures to clairvoyance to witchcraft inoculation. Though it is possible that particular immigrant groups did patronize their own healing traditions more than others, it is hard to see a deity like Tigare growing powerful simply by serving migrants from the Upper West region of Ghana. Acquah herself noted that a "high number" of patients in Accra placed "reliance on all forms of healing available." She was not able to quantify this movement among African healers, but data taken from oral interviews clearly shows lateral movement between traditions. And Okomfo Numo based his status as a powerful healer on the claim that he drew clients from near and far—from the majority Ga population as well as numerous other ethnic groups. For patients accustomed to living within a pluralistic healing culture, immigrant practitioners with new gods were not a threat. On the contrary, they offered renewed hope in the fight against illness and misfortune.

CHRISTIAN FAITH HEALING AND NEW HEALING PRACTICES IN MUSLIM COMMUNITIES

One hundred years after being codified in Ga and Twi by the Basel missionaries, the spiritual forces of God, Jesus, and the Holy

Spirit began to play a daily role in defining how people in Accra understood states of health. And about eighty years after the establishment of the first Muslim community in Accra, Islamic healing practices finally became entrenched in the city, serving both followers of Islam and other patients who sought their aid. Thousands of Accra residents flocked to the new services provided by pastors who promised both physical and spiritual health, while thousands of others took advantage of a network of dozens of Muslim priests and healers living in the city. No longer were Christians and Muslims segregated in salems and suburbs. By the 1950s, the major religious healing traditions had become an integral part of the pluralistic healing culture of Accra.

The growth of Pentecostal and charismatic church movements today has been noted as an era of the so-called megachurches, led by pastors who offered new methods of healing based on the power of Christ to wash away sins and cleanse the spirit.[99] But the Christian faith healing movement was already well underway by the 1950s. Before the Second World War, the Christian community was composed of the four major so-called mainline denominations of Roman Catholic, Methodist, Anglican, and Presbyterian.[100] Unlike in western Nigeria, which was swept by the Aladura revivalist movement in the 1930s, the new Christian churches that emerged in the 1920s and 1930s had little impact in Accra. Only one Aladura church, the Christ's Apostolic Church, won converts in the city before the war, and it had faded into a small congregation by the 1950s. Even the prophetic movements of William Wade Harris and Samson Oppong, which were so influential in other parts of the Gold Coast, made little headway in Accra.

In the 1950s, a Christian revival movement finally began to sweep through the city. Several Gold Coast subjects who traveled to Nigeria came back as founders of congregations like the Eternal Sacred Order of Cherubim and Seraphim Society (1949), the Church of the Lord (1953), and the Redeemed Church of Christ (1955). Unlike the mainline congregations, who built their churches on the periphery of Ussher Town and James Town, these new churches established branches right in the heart of these quarters, holding public, outdoor baptisms for new members.[101] There are no records of membership in these churches, but interviews with elders and ministers of mainline churches indicate that the less educated classes made up the largest proportion of followers.[102] The mainline churches, with their links to the educated strata of Accra society, maintained their role as social arenas for the elites of the city and continued the traditions of attire, music, liturgy, and theology established by European missionaries in the nineteenth century.[103] But the promise of healing at the new churches, in particular for the perennial concern of infertility, must have appealed to all classes of Accra society. Every single one of the new churches in postwar Accra was founded by a former member of a mainline congregation who developed an interest in faith healing.[104]

The two most successful congregations in postwar Accra were the Nazarite Healing Home (based on the faith-healing principles of Zionist churches in South Africa) and the Musama Disco Christi Church (established by a Fante faith healer from the Central Region).[105] During public services, the pastors of these churches did not diagnose the illnesses that would be treated. Rather, the patient/congregant made a public declaration about what was making them sick, to which the pastor and the congregation would respond with boisterous rituals that included exuberant singing, dancing, drumming, and tambourine shaking, in a combination of European hymns and African rhythms. The pastors also anointed sufferers with oil, laying hands on the congregants and using group prayer to call on the power of the Holy Trinity.[106] Many services were held in Ga, but English and Twi were also spoken, and multilingual services, with assistants translating the sermon into different languages simultaneously, were common. The 1950s began a time of improvisation, when the core elements of the Bible, such as the power of *Nyoŋmo*, the cleansing virtues of the blood of *Yesu Kristo*, and in particular the breath of the *mumo kroŋkroŋ*, could be redeployed for the purpose of healing.

Some churches emphasized the healing power of the Holy Trinity to the extent that they rejected any sort of healing not based on faith. Members of the Musama Disco Christi Church were initially forbidden to accept health care from any source, either local or colonial, unless they were required to produce a note from a doctor for an official government purpose.[107] Even local antimalarial herbal medicines were prohibited. In the place of African and European healing, congregants prayed for the health of sick church members, gathering over their sickbeds in the case of major illnesses.[108] It was only in the late 1950s that prohibitions against using medicines were relaxed, because of pressure from educated members of the congregation who demanded the right to choose local or colonial medical care.[109] The Nazarite Healing Home did not restrict its members to one type of healing, but its pastors urged their followers to pray for divine intervention to stop the progress of illness, and the congregations utilized the same methods of group prayer and performance as the Musama Disco Church.

Despite the fact that none of these new congregations had established priesthoods or permanent buildings, they expanded rapidly. As movements rather than institutions, they made their presence known by praying in public, marching through streets with brass bands, gathering on beaches for mass baptisms, or meeting in groves for silent devotionals.[110] In particular, they offered hope for patients who felt their well-being was compromised by the malicious occult forces that had troubled the residents of Accra for so long.

The revivalist energy of the faith-healing movement is well expressed by a poster for James Town–based Redeemed Church of Christ that advertised a service led by the Nigerian Prophet,

Apostle Dr. Ade Ola Ajasa: "PREACHING AND REVIVAL SERVICE. . . . Do you want life and salvation free of charge? If so, come quickly. You who are barren and sick and whom the physician has failed to heal and you who have difficulties in life. BRING ALL YOUR TROUBLES. With faith, You will be helped and healed by prayers. It is free. If you are worried by witches, come with one mind. If you are thirsty for the word of God, come and drink from the fountain without charge."[111]

A minister of this type would have been expected to improvise and preach by heart in an open-air public space—any spot that the pastor could reserve or rent in the city—and his success would have been judged by the exuberance of his oration and the perceived healing outcomes of his performance. If people were impressed, they would have shown their gratitude when the pastor called for a collection and would have spread the word about the abilities of the preacher.[112]

As historian of religion J. D. Y Peel noted about the rise of Aladura churches in Nigeria, two motivations drove the growth of locally generated Christian worship in West Africa.[113] The first was a desire to Africanize worship by purging churches of the trappings of European culture that limited the freedom to express one's spirituality. For instance, the Aladura churches removed colonial dress codes that excluded the use of African cloth and changed musical repertoires to include African rhythms during services. In this sense, the new churches were part of a burgeoning African nationalism that sought to localize Christian worship on African cultural terms. The second motivation was a desire to emphasize the role of the Holy Spirit as a tool of blessing, revelation, and healing. These churches promised total salvation—for the bodily self, the social self, and the spiritual soul—a holistic approach that merged religion with healing in a way that African healers had been doing for centuries in Accra, and in a way that African patients in Accra demanded.

The healing practices within the Muslim community also diversified during the postwar period. By 1954, the number of Muslim inhabitants had risen to an estimated forty-five thousand, almost one-quarter of the total population of Accra. These numbers included a rising number of Ga converts, amounting to two thousand by 1951. Converts sought out Islam for a variety of reasons: dissatisfaction with indigenous notions of spirituality, concerns that Christianity was a colonial imposition, or as part of a personal spiritual quest, and their numbers boosted the presence of the religion in the city.[114] However, the rapid growth of Islam was largely due to immigration, including soldiers in the Royal West African Frontier Force, migrants from parts of West Africa, and, to a lesser extent, families from Lebanon and Syria. The Muslims of Accra were still lumped together colloquially in British records as Hausas,[115] but it was evident that the Islamic community in Accra was diversifying.

With increasing ethnic variety came an increasing number of Islamic healing practices, derived from Ga, Akan, Hausa, Yoruba and other immigrant groups, some of which had undergone "years of schooling in Muslim schools."[116] This tally excludes many of the Muslim clerics already living in the city who would have dabbled in medicines, as well as the many Muslims who had lay knowledge of herbalism or some sort of specialized tradition of divination. With a city population of over forty thousand, the number of Muslim clerics and healers likely totaled in the hundreds, and according to the *Accra Survey* they divided themselves into three levels of specialization: the *mallam*, the *alhaji*, and the *alufa*.

The first two groups of Islamic healers were rough categories encompassing people from a variety of walks of life. The term *mallam* referred broadly to any sort of Muslim cleric who studied and taught the Quran as well as anyone dabbling in healing on the side.[117] The healing practice of a *mallam* might include praying for a follower or making consecrated medicines inscribed with Quranic text, but those acts were peripheral to the work they would do at the *madrassa* and the mosque. Though it is not recorded, it is there that *Al-Tibb al-nabawi*, the medicine of the Prophet, might have been in use. As Muslim clerics, *mallams* were presumably better versed in the Islamic *hadith* related to healing than less-educated Muslim practitioners. The category of *alhaji* was different from *mallam* in the sense that it referred to someone who had made the pilgrimage to Mecca. These men may not have been identifiable as clerics, but they had the financial means to travel to Mecca, and some of them returned having gained proficiency in *Unani Tibb*, such as herbal remedies (made from local and imported herbs), circumcision (for boys), inoculant scarification (with different varieties of *ti*), and animal horn cupping (according to centuries-old healing traditions based on balancing fluids in the body).[118] Holding the title of *alhaji* might have signified that one had learned healing techniques during pilgrimage, but this is unlikely—most of these practices were already known to the residents of mid-twentieth-century Accra, because of the mixing and matching of Islamic and local therapies within Hausa and Tabon communities.

The most powerful subgroup of healers within the Islamic community in Accra were the *alufa*, medicine men who specialized in preventive apotropaics and rituals of divination.[119] The term *alufa* was brought to the Gold Coast by Yoruba speakers, and in Accra it seems to have been applied specifically to people with specialized learning and experience in the Islamic healing arts. A qualitative supplement to the *Accra Survey* includes a particular *alufa* who had conducted the pilgrimage and become a highly regarded healer with many wealthy Syrian and Lebanese clients.[120] Born in the Northern Territories of the Gold Coast, the cleric took on the title of *alufa* after he had apprenticed as an herbalist, while at the same time attending a *madrassa*. While living in Accra, he had adapted his therapies to include local concoctions that resembled those of Ga healers. He was able to make a version of *ti* comprising sulfur and crocodile scales, but he was also profi-cient in the production of amulets and other Islamic therapies.[121]

The *alufa* is hailed by the *Accra Survey* as the quintessential Muslim medicine man, but in reality, all of the categories of "Muslim healer" in the *Accra Survey* blur together. The *alufa* pro-duced medicines that were identifiable as part of Islamic healing tradition, such as the production of slate wash or amulets con-taining passages, but they also practiced herbalism within a West African idiom. Moreover, the material culture of their apotropaic medicines followed local motifs. In fact, there is nothing that strictly separates the work of the *mallam*, the *alhaji*, or the *alufa*, names that may reflect distinctions of social rank and levels of education rather than divergent subgroups of healing practice. But what these titles do tell us is that particular ethnicities, such as Hausa, Yoruba, and Ga, seem to have little bearing on heal-ing authority within the Muslim community, because healers mixed and matched Islamic practices with indigenous traditions. They also reveal the tolerant nature of the Islamic culture that had developed in the city, one that was not concerned with legal distinctions between categories like *Al-Tibb al-nabawi* (Prophetic medicine as passed down through hadith), *Sunnah* (normative Islamic tradition), or *bid'ah* (practices regarded as innovations, breaking with tradition).

There is no data to indicate whether Muslim healers in Accra had non-Muslim clients. However, considering the conversion activity in the city, the dissatisfaction with Ga or Christian faiths, and a commitment to pluralistic healing among the residents of Accra, it is likely that people from all walks of life patronized Mus-lim healers.[122] Snippets from the court records support this as-sumption. In one specific case in 1948, a driver named Mr. Nell, who was not Muslim, paid a *mallam* named Alhadji Tidjani £12 for a talisman to protect his car from road accidents.[123] Additionally, interview evidence from the work of anthropologist Bruce Gindal in the 1970s demonstrated that Sisala migrants from Northern

Ghana sought help from *mallams* irrespective of their devotion to Islam.[124] And further evidence from Accra today suggests that the majority of patients who seek help from Muslim healers come from non-Muslim traditions.[125] All of this suggests that by the 1950s, Muslim practitioners were serving people both inside and outside the Islamic community.

PATENT MEDICINES AND THE AFRICAN
CONSUMER IN THE 1940S AND 1950S

After the war, the markets of Accra had become clearinghouses for medicinal products. The market for herbs and herbal remedies continued unabated at Makola and other outlets, and the demand for patent medicines continued to grow until they filled the shelves of department stores like Swanzy's and Kingsway. Pharmaceuticals were also in demand. Though normally distributed through Medical Department dispensaries, they began to leak out of the stores at Korle Bu and other infirmaries and were redistributed through the marketplace.[126] The demand for mobile medicines, on terms privately dictated by each individual patient, was now an established part of the healing culture of Accra.

So strong was demand for imported medicinal products that medicine ads made up as much as one-third of the advertising content of the newspapers of the Gold Coast Colony.[127] The *Gold Coast Independent* of January 18, 1945, for instance, contained advertisements for Vogeler's Curative Compound, Mendaco Mouthwash, Kolynos Dental Crème, Milk of Magnesia, Clark's Blood Mixture, and Zam Buk Herbal Ointment, all on a single broadsheet page.[128] The tried-and-true proprietary medicines of Atwood Bitters, Woodward's Gripe Water, and Sloan's Liniment were still on the shelves, but their advertisements had become less frequent by the 1950s, perhaps because they had already established themselves in the marketplace. While patent medicines had begun to disappear from the shelves of stores in the United Kingdom and the United States by the 1940s, they continued to sell well in Africa, and wholesalers pitched their medicines directly to the individual consumer as aids to personal health. Most of the advertisements were produced in the United Kingdom or United States and then merely replicated in Gold Coast newspapers, but starting in the 1940s, images of Africans began to appear in ads for some of the most popular brands, reflecting the importance of the West African market and the long tradition of self-medication in places like Accra.[129]

The United Africa Company's Kingsway Department Store in particular began to target Africans as its primary market for patent medicines, antibiotics, and antimalarials. To promote its large stock of medicinal products, Kingsway hired an advertising agency to draw up images of Africans consuming imported medicines as a means of staying healthy and increasing personal productivity. In 1943, a Kingsway ad (fig. 6.1) appeared in the *Gold Coast Independent,* promoting "medicines and tonics" such as Dr. Lynn's products, as well as some Kingsway-branded products such as aspirin, cough syrup, and eucalyptus oil. The ad contained two images of Black colonial workers, including a porter in the background taking core samples of a bale of cocoa and a clerk in a pith helmet counting and weighing a sample of beans. For the first time in the history of the Gold Coast, newspaper advertisements depicted African workers as significant actors in the colonial economy, but their success, according to the advertisement, depended on maintaining "vigour" in the workplace, something that imported medicines promised to provide.

The Kingsway advertisement was one of a new generation of images containing African characters that emerged during the Second World War, linking individual achievement and bodily health to the consumption of imported medicines. Vogeler's Curative Compound, a diuretic invented by Charles Vogeler in Baltimore, Maryland, in the 1880s, was sold in the United Kingdom

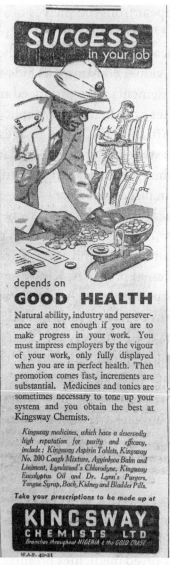

Figure 6.1. Advertisement for Kingsway Chemists, 1943. This advertisement links the healthy lifestyle provided by the consumption of pharmaceuticals to the health of the cocoa economy. A causal relationship is created between the consumption of pills and medicines (listed at *bottom*) and physical and mental vigor at work, symbolized by the laborer taking a core sample of a cocoa bale and a clerk wearing an iconic pith helmet while grading the beans. (Source: *Gold Coast Observer*, January 15, 1943, 479.)

using images of robust, scantily clad women, who extolled the virtues of the medicine as a blood purifier.[130] Vogeler's Curative Compound disappeared from British and American markets when the company folded in 1913, but when the patents were sold to the American Home Products Corporation (now known as Wyeth Pharmaceuticals), the Curative Compound found a ready market in West Africa.[131] The marketing of Vogeler's changed radically in 1945, when an image of an African medical worker appeared in an advertisement. Previous advertisements for Vogeler's in Gold Coast newspapers had featured White nurses instructing African women and children to take the medicine, but this image was the first to feature an African pointing to the label, as if explaining its medicinal virtues. The image of the Black biotechnician was intended to catch the eye of African consumers and associate the consumption of patent medicine with modern living in Accra. It was also a point of discursive hybridity, where colonial medical knowledge formed a backdrop for the consumption of mobile medicines in public.

Sarsaparilla, an American medicinal root that was sold in the city in the eighteenth century, disappeared from the historical record for over a century but reemerged in the 1940s as a purgative called Dr. Lynn's Iodised Sarsaparilla. Dr. Lynn's was just one of many advertisements for purgatives in the newspapers in Accra, but it stands out because of the imagery: a Black man transformed from a slouched position of poor health into a vigorous, striding colonial worker (fig. 6.2).[132] Drawing on iconic images of the ape-to-man progress of evolution, this advertisement portrayed the colonial subject as a rapidly evolving consumer of imported medical goods, with a final image of a man in khaki trousers and a white shirt, rolling up his sleeves to work.[133] In a marked change from its former role as an herbal simple used to cure the "clap," sarsaparilla was now part of a patent medicine that could invigorate the colonial workforce.[134]

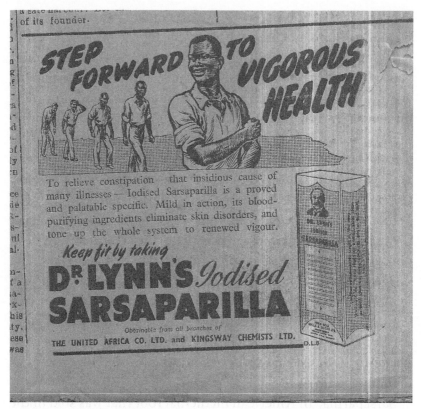

Figure 6.2. Advertisement for Dr. Lynn's Iodised Sarsaparilla. Drawing on iconic images of the progress of evolution from ape to man, this advertisement shows the progress of the colonial worker from a state of lassitude to "vigorous health." Sarsaparilla had been available as an herbal simple on the Gold Coast since the eighteenth century but was never grown locally. After the Second World War, it was marketed as a blood cleanser, iodized to make it more palatable and easier to digest. (Source: *Gold Coast Observer*, April 30, 1948, 631.)

Advertisements for Paludrine, a branded antimalarial tablet sold throughout West Africa in the 1950s, also contained localized images.[135] The active ingredient in Paludrine was a new compound called proguanil hydrochloride, which was synthesized in 1945 at the Liverpool School of Tropical Medicine.[136] When it was turned into a consumer pharmaceutical at Imperial

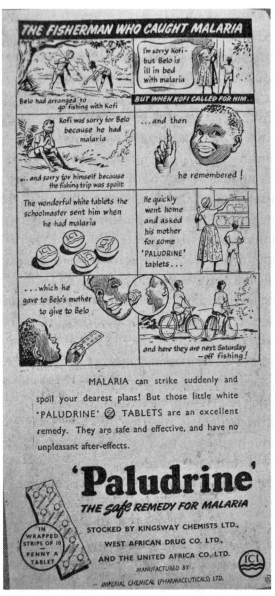

Figure 6.3. Advertisement for antimalarial Paludrine. Paludrine, produced in the United Kingdom by Imperial Chemical, was the most common brand of synthesized quinine on the Gold Coast. The advertisement branded Paludrine as a lifestyle drug and marketed it to mothers and children. (Source: *Ghana Daily Express*, September 5, 1953, 2.)

Chemical Industries in 1947, it set a new trend as an over-the-counter medicine in West Africa.[137] Chloroquine was still effective and available at a reasonable price, but Paludrine was able to carve out a market share in the city because of its low cost of one penny per pill, its unique bubble-pack strip packaging, and its advertisements that featured African characters.[138] In a cartoon for Paludrine (fig. 6.3), the advertiser used local names for its characters, including two common names for boys in Accra (Kofi, an Akan day name for a boy born on Friday, and Belo, a Muslim name commonly used in West Africa). Paludrine ads targeted mothers and children by distinguishing the modern mother and child from those who might treat malaria with herbal remedies, an extension of the medical practices of mothercraft that had been established in the 1920s. It also showed a schoolmaster recommending the pills to Kofi, linking colonial education and the consumption of imported medicines. Here was a new form of lifestyle marketing, one that offered a vision of family life linking health to both the colonial education system and the market for imported goods, using gender archetypes that followed Western norms.[139] It presented its product as distinct from its competitors by using close-up depictions of the ICI brand name on the strip of pills. Though herbal remedies were still widely available, the affordable pill form of synthesized quinine became a popular remedy for malaria, and residents of Accra bought and sold the product beyond the control of colonial medical authorities. The presence of a strongly branded quinine-derivative medicine like Paludrine may have laid the groundwork for future branding and marketing campaigns for drugs like Larium (mefloquine), Malarone (atovaquone/proguanil), and Flavoquine (amodiaquine).[140]

In the postwar period, older varieties of patent medicines, such as Atwood's Bitters, Sloan's Liniment, and Woodward's Gripe Water, no longer dominated advertising space in the newspapers of the Gold Coast. They were still around, but they were complemented by new medicines, some produced explicitly for the West

African market, complete with regional ad campaigns. Unfortunately, there are no oral memories for medicines like Vogeler's Curative Compound or Dr. Lynn's Iodised Sarsaparilla, likely because their ads disappeared from the pages of newspapers in the 1960s and seem to have disappeared from the marketplace by the 1970s. Some brands were simply unable to stand the test of time in the open markets of Accra, and the financial crises of the 1970s and 1980s led to balance-of-payments crises that diminished the number of imported goods available in general. However, in the 1950s the ad campaigns for prominent brands of mobile medicines offered a new vision of health for Gold Coast subjects, and evidence that the city's culture of self-medication continued. Despite the rise of new African deities, colonial medicine, Christian faith healing, and Islamic healing, the open exchange of medical goods in the marketplace continued to thrive, adapting to the private needs and personal dispositions of African consumers.

NOTES

1. Acquah, *Accra Survey*, 122–23.
2. Acquah, *Accra Survey*, 176.
3. Acquah, *Accra Survey*, 122–23.
4. Dowd, "Review of *Accra Survey*," 165.
5. Acquah, *Accra Survey*, 131–37.
6. Acquah, *Accra Survey*, 131, 136.
7. Acquah, *Accra Survey*, 137.
8. Patterson, *Health in Colonial Ghana*, table 24; Findlay, Hill, and MacPherson, "Penicillin in Yaws and Tropical Ulcer"; Messent "Use and Effectiveness of Anti-malaria Drugs," 629; C. E. Reindorf, "Fifty Years of Scientific Medicine," 119.
9. R. R. Willcox, "Venereal Disease in British West Africa"; Pellow, "STDs and AIDS in Ghana," 420; Addae, *Evolution of Modern Medicine*, 359.
10. Acquah, *Accra Survey*, 140.
11. PRAAD, RG 5/1/23, *Buildings of the Gold Coast Hospital Korle Bu Accra: Additions and Alterations*, 1953, "Minutes of the Meeting Held in the Prime Minister's Office. 29th July, 1953, Gold Coast Hospital," 2.

12. PRAAD, RG 5/1/23, *Buildings of the Gold Coast Hospital*, 62.

13. PRAAD, RG 5/1/23, *Buildings of the Gold Coast Hospital*, 3.

14. Acquah, *Accra Survey*, 132–33.

15. Belam, "Random Reminiscences."

16. Acquah, *Accra Survey*, 137.

17. Acquah, *Accra Survey*, 138.

18. Acquah, *Accra Survey*, 60.

19. Acquah, *Accra Survey*, 139.

20. PRAAD, RG 5/1/23, *Buildings of the Gold Coast Hospital Korle Bu Accra: Additions and Alterations*, 1953, "Notes on Visit to Gold Coast Hospital," 2.

21. *Sunday Mirror*, March 29, 1955, from Plageman, "'Accra Is Changing,'" 156.

22. Acquah, *Accra Survey*, 137.

23. UNESCO, *Visual Aids in Fundamental Education* (1952), 82–85; Acquah, *Accra Survey*, 138–39.

24. Nájera, González-Silva, and Alonso, "Some Lessons for the Future."

25. Acquah, *Accra Survey*, 62.

26. Patterson, *Health in Colonial Ghana*, table 2.

27. Acquah, *Accra Survey*, 134; Dr. Barnor, interview with the author, August 29, 2003; H. B. L. R., "F. V. Nanka-Bruce."

28. H. B. L. R., "F. V. Nanka-Bruce," 289–90.

29. Bloom and Skinner, "Modernity and Danger."

30. Edwin et al., "Development of Cardiac Surgery in West Africa."

31. H. B. L. R., "F. V. Nanka-Bruce," 290.

32. Dr. Barnor, interview with the author, August 29, 2003.

33. Dr. Barnor, interview with the author, August 29, 2003; Dr. Evans-Anfom, interview with the author, March 24, 2005; Dr. Quartey-Papafio, interview with the author, September 9, 2003.

34. Osseo-Asare, *Bitter Roots*, 133–40.

35. Dr. Barnor, interview with the author, August 29, 2003.

36. *Gold Coast Independent*, July 8, 1933, 630; Dr. Barnor, interview with the author, August 29, 2003; Dr. Evans-Anfom, interview with the author, March 24, 2005.

37. Dr. Barnor, interview with the author, August 29, 2003. According to Dr. Barnor, a special study conducted by Dr. C. O. Easmon indicated that herbalists did 70% of the work of healing in the city, while medical doctors provided only 30%. The whereabouts of this documented report are not known.

38. Acquah, *Accra Survey*, 123.

39. Acquah, *Accra Survey*, 122.

40. Acquah, *Accra Survey*, 123.

41. Acquah, *Accra Survey*, 123.

42. In 1954, Acquah's data showed that 13,578 men were working for the colonial government, 3,239 for the Municipal Council, and approximately 3,000 for the United Africa Company. It is likely that hundreds more were working for European companies in the city or were in the colonial armed forces. Acquah, *Accra Survey*, 64. Some examples from the *Gold Coast Independent* of patients directed into colonial medical care include a homicide where the body was sent to the mortuary for postmortem (March 15, 1941, 85), a woman sent to the medical department for observation and subsequently declared a lunatic (March 22, 1941, 89), and a girl who was hit by a bus and was sent to Korle Bu and then to the mortuary (June 17, 1944, 149).

43. Acquah, *Accra Survey*, 122.

44. Acquah, *Accra Survey*, 108.

45. Acquah, *Accra Survey*, 111–12.

46. Acquah, *Accra Survey*, 123.

47. Acquah, *Accra Survey*, 123.

48. Acquah, *Accra Survey*, 123, 8–9.

49. Acquah, *Accra Survey*, 125.

50. Kilson, *African Urban Kinsmen*, 89.

51. Acquah, *Accra Survey*, 123; Freshfield, *Stormy Dawn*, 23, 130.

52. Acquah, *Accra Survey*, 124; *Gold Coast Independent*, January 18, 1945, 11.

53. Acquah, *Accra Survey*, 124.

54. Acquah, *Accra Survey*, 124–25.

55. Acquah, *Accra Survey*, 125.

56. Osseo-Asare, *Bitter Roots*, 139.

57. Patterson, *Health in Colonial Ghana*, 29.

58. Acquah, *Accra Survey*, 125.

59. Weinberg, "'Mental Healing' and Social Change," 263.

60. Mensah, "Status of Traditional Medicine Development in Ghana."

61. Twumasi and Warren, "Professionalisation of Indigenous Medicine," in Last and Chavunduka, *Professionalisation of African Medicine*, 122.

62. Acquah, *Accra Survey*, 133–36.

63. Acquah, *Accra Survey*, 134–35.

64. Acquah, *Accra Survey*, 135.

65. Acquah, *Accra Survey*, 125–27.

66. Acquah, *Accra Survey*, 126.

67. Acquah, *Accra Survey*, 126–27.

68. Parker, *Making the Town*, 237.

69. Acquah, *Accra Survey*, 124.

70. All-Asia Great Modern Spiritual Revival Movement, *Spiritual Front and Moral Forces*. The National Institute of Medical Herbalism offered a correspondence course; see *Postal Domestic Course in Medical Herbalism*.

71. Mbiti, *African Religions & Philosophy*, 173.

72. Acquah, *Accra Survey*, 130.

73. Acquah, *Accra Survey*, 130.

74. Field, *Religion and Medicine*, 138.

75. Morton-Williams, Bascom, and McClelland, "Two Studies of Ifa Divination"; Peel, "Pastor and the 'Babalawo,'" 342–44.

76. Acquah, *Accra Survey*, 130.

77. Acquah, *Accra Survey*, 130.

78. Acquah, *Accra Survey*, 27.

79. For a map and a brief description of the provenance of these deities, see Allman and Parker, *Tongnaab*, 136–41.

80. Field, *Search for Security*, 87.

81. Acquah, *Accra Survey*, 164.

82. Field, "Some New Shrines," 141; James B. Christensen, "Tigari Cult," 392–93.

83. Christensen, "Tigari Cult," 392.

84. Okomfo Numo, interview with the author, February 6, 2004. Okomfo Numo passed away in 2012.

85. Okomfo Numo, interview with the author, February 6, 2004.

86. Acquah, *Accra Survey*, 143.

87. PRAAD RG 16/2/144, "D. Ako Anogywan vs Agoe Toboase," case no. 442/49, July 12, 1949, 97–98; Acquah, *Accra Survey*, 143.

88. PRAAD RG 16/2/151, "Ama Amoahba vs Owula Cobblah/Simons," case no. 103/53, February 17, 1953, 29.

89. PRAAD RG 16/2/17, 536–41; PRAAD RG 16/2/140, "Dadjamah Quarshie vs Aba Nye," case no. 587/48, December 22, 1948, 723–51.

90. Okomfo Numo, interview with the author, February 6, 2004. Okomfo Numo passed away in 2012.

91. Christensen, "Tigari Cult," 393; Acquah, *Accra Survey*, 143.

92. Acquah, *Accra Survey*, 143 (from Busia, *Sekondi-Takoradi*, 80).

93. Acquah, *Accra Survey*, 143; Busia, *Sekondi-Takoradi*, 80; Christensen, "Tigari Cult"; Okomfo Numo, interview with the author, February 6, 2004.

94. Acquah, *Accra Survey*, 128–29.

95. Christensen, "Tigari Cult," 396.

96. Parker, "Witchcraft, Anti-witchcraft," 412; Christensen, "Tigari Cult," 392–94; Interview with Okomfo Numo and apprentice Kwabena Nia, February 4, 2004.

97. Okomfo Numo, February 6, 2004.

98. PRAAD RG 16/2/167, "Tow Seyino vs Wia," case no. 551/62, November 23, 1962, 614–18; PRAAD RG 16/2/31, "Yao Adobia and Nkran Quaye vs Obosomfo Amartey," case no. a25/50, April 26, 1950, 425–88, 432–36, 440–54, 465–66; Christensen, "Tigari Cult," 395–96.

99. Gifford, Ghana's New Christianity; van Dijk, "Contesting Silence"; Meyer and Geschiere, Globalization and Identity.

100. Noel Smith, Presbyterian Church of Ghana, 140–41.

101. Baeta, Prophetism in Ghana, 119.

102. Theresa Tanor, interview with the author, June 29, 2010; Anglican Minister Quayson, interview with the author, August 1, 2003; Pastor Abednego Agoe Bortey, interview with the author, August 6, 2003.

103. Acquah, Accra Survey, 146–47.

104. Acquah, Accra Survey, 149.

105. The Musama Disco Chisti Church was founded by Joseph William Egyanka Appiah, a Fante from Abura Edumfa in the Central Region of the Gold Coast Colony. Baeta, Prophetism in Ghana, 26–62. Acquah does not state who founded the Nazarite Healing Home, but it was a very strong witch-finding and sorcery-fighting movement in South Africa. Sundkler, Bantu Prophets in South Africa, 254.

106. Acquah, Accra Survey, 149; Baeta, Prophetism in Ghana, 50–54.

107. Baeta, Prophetism in Ghana, 54.

108. Theresa Tanor, interview with the author, June 29, 2010.

109. Theresa Tanor, interview with the author, June 29, 2010.

110. Acquah, Accra Survey, 150.

111. Acquah, Accra Survey, 149.

112. Mullings, Therapy, Ideology, and Social Change, 45.

113. Peel, Making of the Yoruba, 264; Peel, "Syncretism and Religious Change," 128–29.

114. J.N.D. Anderson, Islamic Law in Africa, 282; Mumuni, "Islamic Nongovernmental Organizations," in Weiss, Social Welfare, 142.

115. Acquah sometimes lumps together the Muslim population as Hausa but at other times divides the Muslim population by ethnicity. Acquah, Accra Survey, 35, 117, 128, 144.

116. Acquah, Accra Survey, 128.

117. Acquah, *Accra Survey*, 128.

118. Acquah, *Accra Survey*, 128.

119. Acquah, *Accra Survey*, 128.

120. Acquah, *Accra Survey*, 128.

121. Acquah, *Accra Survey*, 128.

122. Acquah, *Accra Survey*, 128.

123. PRAAD, RG 16/3/10, "N.A.P. Nell versus Mallam Alhadji Tidjani," 113–16.

124. Grindal, "Islamic Affiliations and Urban Adaptation," 339.

125. Mustapha Dowuona, interview with the author, July 2, 2003; Muhammad Musah Laryea, interview with the author, June 15, 2006; Alhaji Thunder, interview with the author, July 4, 2007.

126. Acquah, *Accra Survey*, 128.

127. *Gold Coast Independent*, 1943–46.

128. *Gold Coast Independent*, January 18, 1945, 9.

129. *Gold Coast Independent*, March 1, 1941, 65.

130. United States Patent Office, *Annual Report of the Commissioner of Patents*, 1885, 360; *Meyer Brothers Druggist* 26, no. 10 (1905), 113. Ad for "Vogeler's Curative Compound," *Black and White*, 53.

131. Corley, "Patent Medicine Industries 1708–1914," 123.

132. *Gold Coast Observer*, April 30, 1948, 631.

133. The advertisement for Dr. Lynn's Sarsaparilla preceded the iconic image of the "March of Progress" by Rudolph Zallinger, from the cover of anthropologist F. Clark Howell's Time-Life book *Early Man* (1965; revised 1968), which popularized the frontispiece of Thomas Huxley's *Evidence as to Man's Place in Nature* (Williams and Norgate, 1863), which compared the skeletons of various apes to that of man.

134. De Marees, *Gold Kingdom of Guinea*, 173–74.

135. Acquah, *Accra Survey*, 136.

136. "Paludrine: A New Anti-malarial Drug," 596–597.

137. Ryley, "Proguanil and Related Antimalarial Drugs," 424.

138. *Accra Evening News*, May 6, 1952, 4.

139. Such images were also replicated in Kingsway Chemist ads that linked health with education. See *Gold Coast Independent*, March 1, 1941, 69.

140. Dart, *Medical Toxicology*, 468.

EPILOGUE

Therapeutic Pluralism in Postcolonial Accra

THE ELECTORAL VICTORY OF THE Convention People's Party in 1956 was a significant milestone in the political context of healing in Accra. The transition to home rule marked a point where Ghanaians had fully appropriated the political power behind the national medical program. The type of medical care offered at Korle Bu and the clinics around the city had not changed—doctors, nurses, dispensers, and technicians continued their duties as they had before—but Africans began taking leading roles in the provision of medical services. Thomas Hutton-Mills Jr., a Ga from James Town and a nephew of Dr. Nanka-Bruce, became the first African to fill the role of minister of health. Dr. Eustace Akwei, another Ga, became the first African to serve as chief medical officer.[1] Ghanaian doctors also proudly announced their presence among the White doctors who dominated the World Health Organization in Geneva and the International Children's Centre in Brazzaville.[2] Not since 1895, when Dr. John Farrell Easmon came close to taking charge of the progress of colonial medicine in the Gold Coast, had Africans been in a position to seize the heights of the medical establishment. This triumphant moment is captured poignantly by a 1954 photo of Kwame Nkrumah striding through

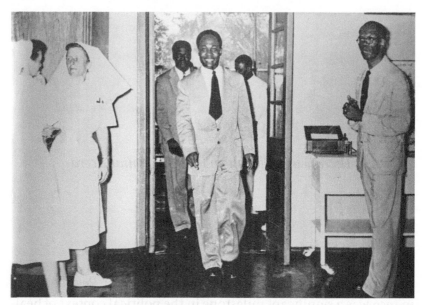

Figure E.1. Kwame Nkrumah visiting Korle Bu Hospital, circa 1954. Though the provision of medical care at Korle Bu continued regardless of whether doctors and nurses were Black or White, the transition of political power to the hands of the new citizens of Ghana meant that Africans working at the institution could advance to the highest ranks of administration, completely appropriating the levers of power at the institution. This photo is worth a thousand words because it shows the trepidation of the White nursing sisters at the arrival of the new prime minister, who is physically, and joyfully, asserting his authority over a former colonial medical outpost. (Source: *Korle Bu Hospital, 1923–1973: Golden Jubilee Souvenir* [Accra: Advent, 1973].)

the halls of Korle Bu, as White nurses look on with apprehension (fig. E.1).

But while the transition from colony to nation may have been a momentous event for medicine in Ghana, it did not necessarily signal a dramatic change in fortune for the five therapeutic traditions in Accra. Western medicine was ascendant as part of a national project of modernization, but in reality the Ghanaian government was struggling to pay for it.[3] The budget surpluses of the 1950s and early 1960s supported substantial initial investments, including a thousand more beds at Korle Bu; educational training facilities for physicians, nurses, and dispensers; and free medicines at all of its clinics and hospitals.[4] But as the price of cocoa declined throughout the 1960s and 1970s, the finances of the national government fell into disarray and funding for the national health services of Ghana became irregular. The large-scale disease-eradication projects that the British had started in parts of the country were no longer financially tenable, and hospitals around the country soon fell into disrepair. Before the Second World War, Korle Bu was a manifestation simultaneously of colonial bio-power and of colonial distinction, and its impact on the community was so profound that it became a synecdoche for all medical institutions; even in the twenty-first century, Ga speakers can be heard referring to hospitals and clinics, in general, as *korlebu*.

Kwame Nkrumah tried to keep faith with Guggisberg's dream of training doctors and nurses, but the funding to transform Korle Bu into a teaching hospital was not available until 1963, and even then the hospital struggled to provide a full set of courses.[5] To make matters worse, the departure of the last group of expatriate British medical personnel in the 1960s left Ghana with a severe lack of doctors. Nkrumah had alienated potential aid partners in the British National Health Services by reaching out to other developing countries for advice on how to build a Western medical system with a focus on tropical diseases, and as his political authority waned, he found it difficult to fund such a project.[6] It was not until 1969, while Nkrumah was in exile, that the Ghana Medical School proudly graduated its first group of students. Unfortunately their cohort would be forced to deal with the turmoil caused by coups d'etat and a retreat to a "cash and carry" fee-based system. These disruptions triggered a brain-drain of medical talent in the 1970s that became an "exodus" by the 1980s.[7] Ghanaian-trained medical professionals sought out more lucrative positions in Britain, Europe, and the United States, and despite the valiant efforts of remaining Ghanaian medical staff, the national health system declined rapidly.[8] As a side effect of this decay, the Ministry of Health's record keeping languished, making it difficult for historians to provide a robust account of Western medicine in Ghana during the second half of the twentieth century.[9]

In order to counterbalance the decline in medical services, politicians in Ghana scrambled to rejuvenate and modernize African herbal and spirit healing traditions.[10] Inspired by Maoist health reforms in China, Kwame Nkrumah sought to indigenize health provision in Ghana by hiring Mensah Dapaah to form the Ghana Psychic and Traditional Healers Association.[11] Dapaah, a scientist who had studied healing at the Akonede shrine at Larteh in the Akwapim Hills, planned to certify traditional healers with professional licenses and support the production of herbal medical products as substitutes for imported pharmaceuticals. Several physicians and scientists were sent to China in the 1960s to learn about the modernization of Chinese herbal medicine, but the association struggled after Nkrumah was deposed in 1966.[12] The only concrete outcome of the drive to Africanize health services was the Mampong Centre for Herbal Medicine, built in 1975 through the vision of Dr. Oku Ampofo and the support of the Acheampong military regime. Ampofo had already established a clinic in Mampong, but with the help of the Ghana Psychic and Traditional Healers Association, he was able to transform his practice into an innovative laboratory for plant medicine. In its early years, the Mampong Centre struggled to produce quality herbal medicines in large volumes, but it survived through lean years of funding by focusing on the production of antimalarials. In the 1980s, it partnered with the World Health Organization, and today it distributes more than thirty different herbal products to markets around Ghana. Its success provided the foundation for the proliferation of private herbal medicine producers in the country today and offers a tidy example of how therapeutic traditions can adapt and change rapidly according to shifting social and political contexts.[13]

Independence marked a change in the political context of healing in Accra, but the actions of the national government could do little to moderate the impact of a demographic explosion in the capital city. In 1954, Accra was home to 200,000 people. Ten years later, the population had swelled to 350,000. By 1984, the city held more than 1 million people, and by 2011, the population had ballooned to 4 million.[14] The most significant impact of this demographic change was a dramatic shift in city's ethnic composition. In 1948, the Gas made up only 52 percent of the population. It is safe to assume that they were a minority in the city by the time of independence a decade later.[15] Today, Ga speakers make up less than 30 percent of the total population of Accra, and proportionally, their numbers are shrinking. Immigration from Akan-speaking parts of Ghana has been the biggest contributor to the decline of Ga influence, and it is fair to say that Accra is largely an Akan city today because the descendants of Fante, Asante, and Akwapim migrants make up more than 40 percent of the urban population and because Twi is arguably the most widely spoken language. Ewe speakers are also a significant part of the Accra community, making up 18 percent of the population.[16] Smaller groups of Lebanese, Chinese, and Europeans make up the rest of the population of the city, amounting to less than 10 percent of the population, but unreported residents from other African countries probably number in the hundreds of thousands.[17] The dramatic ethnic diversification of Accra has led to countless new permutations within African healing traditions, helping therapy management groups find new treatments for their ailing patients.

Adversely, the population explosion has created a dangerously unsanitary environment. Like most cities in West Africa, Accra has no sewer system, and raw sewage is still dumped by the truckload into the Atlantic Ocean at Korle Gonno, just south of the Korle Bu Hospital. A promise by the Israeli government to build a sewer system in Accra as a gesture of friendship collapsed in the 1970s when Ghana supported the Arab nations fighting in the Yom Kippur War.[18] No effort to build a sewer has been put forward since. The water supply in the city is also a major source of concern because the water mains laid by the British one hundred years ago are leaking and the supply of piped water is irregular. In most parts of the city, water for washing is delivered inefficiently via water trucks that pump indiscriminately from the Weija Dam—a body of water that is not effectively protected from erosion and pollution. Drinking water is also delivered in a manner that offers portability but produces plastic waste, in the form of plastic sachets and bottles that have been implicated in the spread of waterborne illnesses. The environmental damage caused by discarded plastics is also a concern because they clog the local waterways, exacerbating flooding in ways that can lead to immense property damage and tragic deaths.

After a pause of several decades, the sanitary hysteria associated with the Korle Lagoon found new life in the form of the $89 million Korle Lagoon Restoration Project. Funded by the Arab Bank for Economic Development in Africa, work commenced in 2002 when a Belgian engineering firm was hired to dredge the waterway, construct a new sea outfall, and build a pumping station to try to flush contaminated water from the lagoon. The project was completed in 2008, but its pumps have struggled to handle the volume of human waste and garbage floating downstream from Kwame Nkrumah Circle.[19] The resistance to eviction by the squatters of Agbobloshie (a.k.a. Sodom and Gomorrah), an improvised village perched on the northern edge of the lagoon, has delayed and harried the project in a manner uncannily similar to Ga chiefs' and priests' resistance to the sanitary reforms of the British colonial regime. The Accra Metropolitan Assembly has made several half-hearted and incomplete attempts to evict the squatters, but they remain in the location today.[20] The horrific gas station explosion of 2016, caused by inadequate drainage into Korle, was supposed to be a wake-up call for the Accra Metropolitan Assembly, but little has been done to prevent further flooding.[21] These are just a few tangents of the larger crisis of postcolonial sanitation, which has its roots in the colonial era and the antimalaria campaign of the Second World War but which has become much more complicated as Accra has grown into a major metropolis. The Accra Metropolitan Assembly continues to look to the Ghanaian government for aid, just as the Town Council sought funding from the Gold Coast government. Meanwhile, the Ghanaian government looks to international funding bodies for financing, just as the Gold Coast governors used to appeal to the Colonial Office. By the time that major projects are realized, their capacity to change the health environment is diminished by underfunding, corruption, and local intransigence. If colonial bio-power was a force that influenced states of health during the twentieth century, the postcolonial bio-power of the twenty-first century is a mere simulacrum by comparison.

The density of the population in postcolonial Accra has also dramatically altered the disease environment of the city, making it a haven for insect-borne illness. By the early 1970s, mosquitos were resistant to DDT, and the promise of liberating Africa from mosquito-borne illnesses, a goal that had energized the past generation of entomologists and epidemiologists around the world, faded away.[22] Moreover, the growth of the urban landscape had created innumerable alleys, ditches, and rubbish piles for mosquitos to breed in, which probably led to higher rates of malaria than in any previous period in the history of the city. By the 1970s, the cost of imported antimalarial pharmaceuticals was the largest tranche of health care spending in Ghana, equivalent to the wages and salaries of all of the employees of the Ghanaian Ministry of Health. The rising resistance of parasites to chloroquine and its derivatives has been mollified by the use of a new line of artesunate drugs, but malaria still accounts for almost half of all illnesses reported at outpatient facilities in the city.[23] Worse still, the psychiatric side effects of antimalarial drugs have recently come under investigation, and a great danger looms because of the prevalence of counterfeit products. There is also a real possibility that in the near future the *Anopheles* larvae will become immune to the most common over-the-counter medicines. Though the Gates Foundation has made bold promises to eradicate malaria with the help of a vaccine (to be partially developed at the Noguchi Medical Research Institute at the University of Ghana), the cost of relying on pharmaceutical curatives for malaria remains the single most significant therapeutic burden for patients in Accra.[24] As Professor Stephen Addae, the late esteemed historian of medicine in Ghana, noted, the Gold Coast regime "passed on to the new African government a medical legacy which was largely curative- rather than preventive-oriented."[25] In other words, neglect of sanitation infrastructure and malaria prevention in favor of a reliance on "bum punching," yellow pills, and herbal bitters is a harmful legacy of the colonial era.[26]

New diseases have also arrived in the city, including HIV/AIDS in the 1980s. Accra maintained a relatively low rate of infection at only 3.1 percent during the peak of the epidemic in the 1990s—low only in comparison to Southern Africa, where rates skyrocketed into the double digits.[27] However, these statistics can be considered as estimates in a place where testing for HIV was only conducted among pregnant women and some transfusion patients. The human cost of the disease was still high, as approximately forty thousand people carried HIV in the city during the peak of the epidemic, with few of them able to pay for antiretroviral drugs. The death of thousands of people, cut down in the prime of their lives, made a significant impact on almost everyone in the city. During research for this book, it was not uncommon to hear of people dying from wasting diseases, refusing to admit that they had AIDS. I lost one of my friends to an illness that was almost certainly brought on by AIDS, though he vehemently denied it until the end, causing his friends and family much grief. Autopsies are still rare in Accra, and few people were willing to admit that their friends or loved ones were infected, even after they passed away. What may have slowed the epidemic was a widespread public awareness campaign following the "ABC" model of abstention, being faithful, and wearing a condom.[28] Though campaigns that assumed people would stay sexually inactive to prevent disease were criticized by Western donors, the ABC model was applauded in Accra, where a conservative discourse on sex talk prevails. Defeating HIV/AIDS will be a challenge in a city where imported medicines remain expensive, where taboos connected to naming an illness remain, and where women of low socioeconomic status are more vulnerable to high-risk sexual activities.[29]

Another worrying disease for the residents of Accra is cholera, which has stubbornly entrenched itself in the Korle Lagoon, causing thousands of cases of illness and scores of deaths every few years.[30] Cholera is preventable and treatable, but it continues to flare up occasionally because so many people are still making use of the soiled waters of the lagoon, which now has thousands and thousands of people living along its shoreline. The goddess Korle's relationship with the state of the lagoon continues today, and the current priest of the shrine has asserted, with some bitterness, that he cannot protect the inhabitants of the city from the ravages of disease if they do not heal the environment of the waterway. Naa Korle has been vilified by Christians as a diabolic water spirit associated with Mami Wata, but in the hearts of Ga traditionalists, she remains a spiritual force who can both harm and heal. Her followers believe her power still emanates, as seen in a small patch of greenery on a small island in the middle of the lagoon, seemingly untouched by the environmental ravages that surround it.

Looming in the epidemiological future is the threat of Ebola, which killed almost twelve thousand people in nearby Liberia, Guinea, and Sierra Leone from 2014 to 2016.[31] Though nurses and doctors in Accra are trained to handle outbreaks of such an infectious disease, they would never have the resources to contain a nationwide outbreak of such a deadly hemorrhagic fever. There are also some eerie similarities between the marginal neighborhoods within the capitals of Liberia and Ghana. The impoverished and densely populated neighborhood of Westpoint in Monrovia is home to many people who were unable to acquire land or lodging in the established parts of the Liberian city, and who live without sewers, proper toilets, or a clean water supply. The residents of this vulnerable corner of the city were targeted as vectors for the spread of Ebola and quarantined for ten days in August 2014. Though currently more prosperous than Monrovia, Accra suffers from the same inadequate sanitary infrastructure that led to the rapid spread of Ebola in parts of the Liberian capital.

The impoverished and densely populated neighborhood of Westpoint is home to many people who were unable to acquire land or lodging in the established parts of Monrovia, and who live without sewers, flush toilets, or a clean water supply. When Ebola broke out in Westpoint in August of 2014, the Liberian military quarantined the area for ten days, surrounding the neighborhood with barbed wire. One wonders what will happen in Agbobloshie, home to the most vulnerable population in Accra, should a hemorrhagic fever like Ebola take hold in the city. Almost certainly the wealthier areas of Ridge, Cantonments, and East Legon, neighborhoods now populated by African elites, will fare better during any epidemic.

Additionally, the residents of Accra now suffer from the so-called "double burden" of disease, threatened by endemic diseases like malaria as well as diseases of affluence that are typical of a developing city. Lung disease and cancer may become ongoing challenges, as air pollution takes its toll on the residents of the city. In 2010, while I was conducting my research in the city, I met a group of students from Harvard taking air samples outside the Sakumo We shrine house in Bukom. I assumed that the air quality near the ocean, with a prevailing breeze blowing off the water and to the northeast, would be fresher than in other parts of the city, but I was wrong. Their final report demonstrated that particulate matter from automobile and charcoal pollution was highest of all in James Town and Ussher Town, the oldest quarters of the city.[32] Along with the probability of increased cancer rates, statistics from the twenty-first century thus far show a rise in obesity, diabetes, hypertension, and heart disease.[33] Anyone who has spent time in long commutes across Accra, stressed out and snacking on street food, can understand why this might be happening, but there are deeper issues related to a shift away from traditional foodways toward premade foods with higher amounts of fat and salt. Even with some technological upgrades to its equipment, Korle Bu and its associated clinics are not ready to meet the new challenge of these chronic noncommunicable diseases. The proliferation of smaller private hospitals around the city may help, but a comprehensive health care system is needed in order to identify chronic illnesses and treat patients before they are incurable. And to echo Dr. Addae once again, a shift toward preventative care over primary care is long overdue in the city.

The postcolonial period has also been a time of tremendous religious revival in Accra, with a significant effect on how people understand health and healing. There are very few people in the city today who are not associated in some way with either a Christian church or the Muslim community. This represents a dramatic change from the nineteenth century, when there were fewer than a thousand Christians and Muslims combined. Accra is predominantly Christian, at 83 percent of the population. The majority of Christians now are the so-called charismatics who attend a new generation of faith-healing churches that emerged out of the revival movement of the 1940s and 1950s.[34] The Nazarite Healing Home and the Musama Disco Christi Church, two of the original faith-healing congregations, are still in existence but have dwindled to negligible significance.

Taking their place are splinter congregations, which seem to emerge regularly whenever individual pastors use their oratory and media skills to plant their own churches. In Accra, seekers of religious counsel tend to follow the same pluralist pathways as seekers of healing advice.

The influence of this new type of prosperity gospel, and its attendant structures of faith healing, has been chronicled by scholars like Birgit Meyer, Rijk van Dijk, and Paul Gifford, who have addressed the rapid growth of megachurches like Winners Chapel, Lighthouse International, and the Central Gospel Church.[35] The tale of Lighthouse International, for example, is an essential component of the postcolonial faith-healing story because it was founded by a physician, Dr. Dag Heward-Mills, who started preaching in a tiny classroom at the School of Hygiene at Korle Bu, then established his church headquarters across the street from the hospital campus. Like the other charismatic pastors, Heward-Mills claims to be able to heal the sick by laying on hands, and the church organizes massive Healing Jesus Crusades around Ghana to demonstrate his healing prowess. However, the church also coordinates practical measures for medical care around the country in the form of itinerant tent-clinics and dispensaries.[36] The megachurches continue to build larger and larger cathedrals, but they will soon be challenged by the Ghanaian government, which has planned a five-thousand-seat national cathedral for Accra, which will almost certainly be used for public faith-healing services on a scale never seen before.

Also significant are the so-called *awoyoo*, freelance Christian healers who have no attachments to major congregations. The *awoyoo* are not always highly regarded, but they are much sought after to heal bodily illness and family strife by casting out witches and other evil spirits.[37] This revolution in Christian worship speaks to changing notions of African subjectivity and global

Christian modernity, but it has its roots in the Aladura revival of the early twentieth century, which emphasized the healing power of the Holy Spirt and the deliverance offered by the blood of Jesus. Charismatic Christianity today is not by nature isolationist like the Basel Mission of the nineteenth century. Few churches forbid their followers to seek therapies outside the church, and many are building networks of clinics and dispensaries for their congregants.[38] However, the pastors of the new churches do strongly encourage their congregants to follow the tenets of faith healing and to build their therapy networks within the church community. Additionally, many of them sell consecrated healing oils, perfumes, and powders.

Muslims are still a minority compared to the Christian community, making up just over 10 percent of the urban population.[39] However, the Islamic community continues to grow as more and more migrants from northern communities and West African countries make Accra their home. Concurrently, an increasing amount of funding is being put toward the construction of mosques in the suburbs, including an enormous Ghana National Mosque Complex, funded by Turkish donors, near the old neighborhoods of Nima and Kanda. Along with the many practices of Islamic healing that arrived in the city during the twentieth century, geomancy and numerology have taken hold where immigrants from northern Ghana and the surrounding French-speaking countries tend to congregate.[40] The mixing of Hausa, Yoruba, Nigerien, Lebanese, and Syrian traditions have enabled practices such as *ruqyah* (medicines to protect against *jinn*, the evil eye, and witchcraft) and *hijama* (cupping for fevers, headaches, and other bodily maladies) to continue, and a wide variety of charms to promote general health, wealth, fertility, and wellness can now be purchased via the internet.[41] Islamic medical clinics are also springing up around the city, funded by Arab nations.[42] The abundance of these practices within the Islamic community allows Muslims to form therapy management groups within their own religious circles if they choose, but their ongoing connections to the rest of the community have not been severed. Patients from the Islamic community seek healing in much the same way that they have in the past, but a rise in militant Islam in surrounding countries may serve to label some healing practices as un-Islamic in the years to come.

The story of the research, marketing, sale, and consumption of medical products has also entered a new stage in the postcolonial period. For several decades, Ghanaian scientists have made efforts to study plant medicines with the purpose of generating an indigenous pharmaceutical industry.[43] The advances made in the study of reagents such as *Cryptolepis sanguinolenta* are significant, but endeavors to isolate the medicinal virtues of the local herbaria remain largely untold—work has continued, slowly but largely unabated, at Ghanaian universities, and a complete history of these endeavors is overdue.[44] In addition, the impact of a growing dependence on pharmaceutical imports has not been adequately gauged. According to one budgetary sample, in the 1980s, the importation of pharmaceuticals made up an estimated 75–80 percent of the operating costs of hospitals in Ghana, demonstrating that the country had become reliant on the curative values of imported drugs.[45] This dependency on imported drugs has moved into the markets and streets of Ghana, where patients continue to freely purchase patent medicines and pharmaceuticals, without the oversight of physicians. Medical anthropologist Kodjo Senah has warned that the proliferation of pharmaceuticals has turned bodily health in Ghana into a "transactionable good" by making patients beholden to market rates for medicines.[46] Other studies have shown that patients use commodified medical products to distinguish themselves as part of the upwardly mobile classes.[47] The place to investigate the growing demand for market medicines is the Okaishie section of the Makola Market, a warehousing area of several square blocks that has grown into an entrepôt for imported medicines. Every imaginable sort of pharmaceutical and patent medicine is available at Okaishie, including brand-name drugs, counterfeit derivatives, Chinese sex medicines, and smartly packaged Ghanaian herbal remedies.[48] The Ghana Standards Board attempts to regulate medicinal products, and government inspectors regularly send out alerts about counterfeit and dangerous packaged medicines, but monitoring the market for medicines in a place known for deep-seated therapeutic pluralism may prove elusive.[49] When patients enter the market for over-the-counter medicines, they follow the tenets of *caveat emptor*, just as they did in the past. Gossip about the value or dangers of portable medicines emerges rapidly as they circulate through the city, and the fear of poisoning continues to instill caution in any quests for therapy.[50]

After three hundred years of interaction and competition, the five healing traditions continue to flourish alongside one another, a testament to African patients' long-standing commitment to mix and match their options when seeking cures. The presence of therapeutic diversity over the long durée compels us to abandon the search for the singularity inherent in the logic of Occam's razor and accept that universal models of science, medicine, and the body cannot offer a parsimonious explanation of the history of disease. Rather, in Accra the waves of healing traditions arrived, took hold, and clustered together, rather than displacing one another. To be sure, the fortunes of each healing tradition have ebbed and flowed. At times, barriers to movement of patients between the traditions emerged, in the form of religious proscriptions, or the demand for paperwork, or the segregation of living spaces. Indeed, some traditions strove toward healing hegemony, threatening to end the way that therapy management groups conducted quests for therapy. But patients remained conversant in a wide variety of healing customs, maintaining what we might today describe as a cross-cultural "health literacy," a disposition that empowered them to seek aid from a wide variety of healers.[51] Correspondingly, a vast majority of healers showed tolerance toward their competitors, conceding that they might not be able to heal all of the maladies that afflicted their patients. Some points of hybridity have appeared, in the form of religious medical institutions and in the adoption of market medicines by African healers, but all of the significant attempts at syncretism have petered out, and the culture of healing in Accra has remained fractured rather than unified. Over the centuries, the Ga ethos of *hela tamo jarawoo* has held firm. It has been patients who have taken on the duty of "selling" their sickness to differing purveyors of health. In the future, it is likely they will continue shopping around until they find an appropriate cure.

NOTES

1. PRAAD, RG 5/1/23, *Buildings of the Gold Coast Hospital*, 3; Doortmont, *Pen-Pictures of Modern Africans*, 266.

2. Pearson, *Colonial Politics of Global Health*, 167.

3. Addae, *Evolution of Modern Medicine*, 97, 456–80.

4. Addae, *Evolution of Modern Medicine*, 92–93, 291–92; Mercer, "Gold Coast Development Programme."

5. Addae, *Evolution of Modern Medicine*, 289.

6. Power, *Tropical Medicine in the 20th Century*, 152.

7. Addae, *Evolution of Modern Medicine*, 457.

8. Addae, *Evolution of Modern Medicine*, 194.

9. Patterson, *Health in Colonial Ghana*, 86; Addae, *Evolution of Modern Medicine*, 89, 458.

10. *Brachott Committee Report on Professionalization of African Medicine* (Accra: Government of Ghana, Ministry of Health, 1961); *Easmon Report* (Accra: Government of Ghana, Ministry of Health, 1966); Mensah-Dapaah, "Traditional Healing"; Last and Chavunduka, *Professionalisation of African Medicine*, 132–33.

11. Twumasi and Warren, "Professionalisation of Indigenous Medicine," in Last and Chavunduka, *Professionalisation of African Medicine*, 122. Helga Fink stated in 1990 that two parallel organizations emerged in

the early 1960s with deceptively similar names—the "Ghana Psychic and Traditional *Healers* Association" and the "Ghana Psychic and Traditional *Healing* Association"—a situation that created confusion about registration and licensing among healers in Ghana. Fink, *Religion, Disease and Healing*, 38.

12. Twumasi and Warren, "Professionalisation of Indigenous Medicine," in Last and Chavunduka, *Professionalisation of African Medicine*, 121–23; Senah, *Money Be Man*, 66–67; Evans-Anfom, *Traditional Medicine in Ghana*, 42.

13. Kingsley Kumi, interview with the author, October 2002. For a more recent defense of the potential of herbal medicine in Ghana, see Akosah-Sarpong, "Herbalization of Korle Bu"; Darko, "Ghanaian Indigenous Health Practices," 50; Gyekye, *Tradition and Modernity*, 217–19.

14. Acquah, *Accra Survey*, 31; Accra Metropolitan Assembly, *MCE's Message*, accessed March 1, 2011, http://www.ama.ghanadistricts.gov.gh /?arrow=dce&_=3. The chief executive of the Accra Metropolitan Assembly estimated that approximately three million people live in Accra while about one million visit the city for business each day.

15. The population breakdown by ethnicity of a total of 129,065 was (1) Ga, 66,619 (52%); (2) Ewe, 14,343 (11%); (3) Fanti, 6,696 (5%); (4) Nigerian (south), 6,109 (5%); (5) Hausa, 4,407 (3%); (6) Adangme, 3,642 (3%); (7) Akwapim, 2,878 (2%); (8) Kwahu, 2,623 (2%); (9) Zabarima, 2,282 (2%); and (10) Asante, 2,163 (2%). See Acquah, *Accra Survey*, 176.

16. George Owusu and Samuel Agyei-Mensah, "A Comparative Study of Ethnic Residential Segregation in Ghana's Two Largest Cities, Accra and Kumasi," *Population and Environment* 32 (2011): 343.

17. Owusu and Agyei-Mensah, "A Comparative Study of Ethnic Residential Segregation," 343.

18. Addae, *Evolution of Modern Medicine*, 140.

19. Korle Wulomo, interview with the author, February 3, 2005; Korle Wulomo, interview with the author, February 16, 2005; Huchzermeyer and Karam, *Informal Settlements*, 191–94.

20. Squatters in Agbobloshie have sought legal means to stave off eviction. See Centre For Public Interest Law, "Housing Rights"; modernghana .com, "The Tale of Two evictions," accessed September 9, 2009, https:// www.modernghana.com/news/237368/the-tale-of-two-evictions.html.

21. BBC News, "Ghana Petrol Station Inferno Kills about 150 in Accra," June 5, 2015, http://www.bbc.com/news/world-africa-33003673.

22. Desowitz, "Malaria Vaccine," 175; Stepan, *Eradication*, 162.

23. Barnett, Creese, and Ayivor, "Economics of Pharmaceutical Policy in Ghana," 480; Songsore and McGranahan, "Environment, Wealth and Health," 11; Awine et al., "Towards Malaria Control."

24. Kilama, Chilengi, and Wanga, "Towards an African-Driven Malaria Vaccine"; Stepan, *Eradication*, 10.

25. Addae, *Evolution of Modern Medicine*, 36.

26. Addae, *Evolution of Modern Medicine*, 370–71.

27. Ghana, *National AIDS/STD Control Programme*, 15.

28. Afful-Mensah and Nketiah-Amponsah, "Review of HIV/AIDS"; Okware et al., "Revisiting the ABC Strategy."

29. Adanu et al., "Sexually Transmitted Infections," 157.

30. Ghana News Agency, "Greater Accra Leads Cholera Infection," March 22, 2011, http://www.ghanaweb.com/GhanaHomePage /NewsArchive/artikel.php?ID=205482.

31. CDC, *2014–2016 Ebola Outbreak in West Africa*, March 8, 2019, https://www.cdc.gov/vhf/ebola/history/2014-2016-outbreak/index.html.

32. Dionisio et al., "Air Pollution in Accra Neighborhoods."

33. Agyei-Mensah and De-Graft, "Epidemiological Transition." R. B. Duda and other scientists have found that high blood pressure is a significant health risk and cause of death in Accra for both men and women, while A. G. Amoah has found that obesity rates are rising in the city, especially for women. Duda et al., "Results of the Women's Health Study"; Amoah, "Obesity in Adult Residents."

34. Ghana Statistical Service, "2010 Population & Housing Census: Summary Report of Final Results," May 2012, 40. Accessed March 22, 2021. https://statsghana.gov.gh/gssmain/storage/img/marqueeupdater /Census2010_Summary_report_of_final_results.pdf.

35. Gifford, *Ghana's New Christianity*; Birgit Meyer, "'Make a Complete Break'"; van Dijk, "Localisation, Ghanaian Pentecostalism"; van Dijk, "From Camp to Encompassment."

36. Dag Heward-Mills Ministries, "Healing Jesus Medical Outreach," accessed March 1, 2018, http://www.daghewardmills.org/en/index.php /humanitarian/helping-the-sick.

37. Abednego Agoe Bortey, interview with the author, August 6, 2003; Rahel Roye, interview with the author, June 17, 2003.

38. Quayesi-Amakye, "Church, Medicine and Healing."

39. Ghana Statistical Service, "2010 Population & Housing Census," 40.

40. Mustapha Dowuona, interview with the author, June 12, 2003.

41. Al-Qur'an Shifaa Ruqya & Hijama/Cupping Centre, https://www.facebook.com/CeroqGhana/; Best Traditional Healer Muslim Sheikh Aazam Xulu, *Description Money Spell*, https://www.myjoymarket.com/ads/view/74192.

42. For instance, the Muhammed Al-Ayar Clinic is partially funded by the Egyptian government, while Iran has funded the Iran Clinic. "Egypt Supports Clinic in Accra," *Daily Graphic*, March 16, 2009, https://www.modernghana.com/news/206536/egypt-supports-clinic-in-accra.html; Joseph Kobla Wemakorm, "Iran Clinic Moves to Improve Healthcare Service Delivery in Ghana," *Modern Ghana*, September 9, 2015, https://www.modernghana.com/news/641785/iran-clinic-moves-to-improve-healthcare-service-delivery-in-ghana.html.

43. *World Health Organization Traditional Medicine Strategy 2002–2005* (Geneva: World Health Organization, 2002), http://whqlibdoc.who.int/hq/2002/WHO_EDM_TRM_2002.1.pdf; Osseo-Asare, *Bitter Roots*.

44. Oliver-Bever, *Medicinal Plants in Tropical West Africa*, 131; Iwu, *Handbook of African Medicinal Plants*, 163–64; Ankrah et al., "Evaluation of Efficacy and Safety"; Mshana, N.R., *Traditional Medicine and Pharmacopoeia*, 716–19. See also Osseo-Asare, *Bitter Roots*, 131–64.

45. Barnett, Creese, and Ayivor, "Economics of Pharmaceutical Policy," 481.

46. Senah, *Money Be Man*, 204.

47. Van der Geest and Whyte, "Charm of Medicines"; Whyte, *Questioning Misfortune*; Senah, *Money Be Man*.

48. Auntie Charlotte, interview with the author, June 18, 2007; Mabel Taylor, interview with the author, May 23, 2006.

49. Ghana Standards Board, *Destination Inspection Programme*, accessed March 21, 2011, http://www.gsb.gov.gh/site/pdf/Destination%20Inspection%20Programme.pdf; Ghanaweb, "Stop Buying Drugs from Peddlers—FDA warns," April 20, 2018, https://mobile.ghanaweb.com/GhanaHomePage/NewsArchive/Stop-buying-drugs-from-peddlers-FDA-warns-Ghanaians-644991.

50. Felix Dela Klutse, "Poisonous Drugs Hit Market," *Business Day Ghana*, March 7, 2017, http://businessdayghana.com/poisonous-drugs-hit-market/.

51. Centers for Disease Control and Prevention, United States, "Culture & Health Literacy," October 17, 2019, https://www.cdc.gov/healthliteracy/culture.html; Berkman, Davis, and McCormack, "Health Literacy."

BIBLIOGRAPHY

ORAL INTERVIEWS (CONDUCTED IN ACCRA, GHANA
BY AUTHOR UNLESS OTHERWISE STATED)

Amarteifio, Amarh, July 18, 2003.
Ansa, Woyoo Ankroh, June 14, 2003.
————, June 21, 2007.
Anyormisi, Ntsu, July 9, 2007.
Arthur, Faustina, May 11, 2004
Ashaley, Nii, June 16, 2003.
Badu, Otia, December 20, 2006.
Barnor, Matthew Arnum, August 29, 2003.
————, March 22, 2005.
Bentum, Nii Amartey Tagoe, June 17, 2003.
————, July 8, 2003.
————, March 5, 2004.
Bomba, Fuseni. December 19, 2005.
Borketey, John, December 28, 2005.
Bortey, Abednego Agoe, August 6, 2003.
Cedi, Nii, February 4, 2004.
————, January 26, 2005.
———— with Sakumo Wulomo, January 26, 2005.
Charlotte (Auntie), June 18, 2007.
Codjoe, Joseph, February 22, 2007.
Codjoe, Joseph, Mary Codjoe, and Richard Codjoe, February 22, 2007.

Commey, Oblitey, February 25, 2005.

Dowuona, Mustapha, June 12, 2003.

Dsane, Andrew Nikoi, December 23, 2005.

Evans-Anfom, Emmanuel, March 24, 2005.

Gilbertson, Evelyn, April 16, 2004.

Kumi, Kingsley, October 15, 2002.

Lamptey, Felicia. June 10, 2006.

Lamptey, Old Soldier, February 25, 2005.

Lamptey, Tsofatse, June 9, 2003.

Laryea, Muhammad Musah, June 15, 2006.

Moshie (Mama), December 20, 2005.

Mossi, Saidu, December 18, 2005.

Nkrumah, Ellis. December 26, 2006.

Numo, Okomfo, February 6, 2004.

Numo, Okomfo, and apprentice Kwabena Nia, February 4, 2004.

———, February 6, 2004.

Ofusu, Hannah. June 11, 2006.

———, June 20, 2006.

Otoo, Woyoo Ogbame Rebecca, July 10, 2003.

Quartey, Boi, and Lawrence Tetteh, July 17, 2003.

Quartey-Papafio, Benjamin William, September 9, 2003.

Quaye, Augustina, June 20, 2006.

Quaye, Robert Ayitey, December 30, 2005.

Quaye, Woyoo Joyce Ayile, June 18, 2003.

Roye, Rahel, June 17, 2003.

Santos, Carlos, June 9, 2006.

Sister Mary, June 13, 2006.

Taylor, Mabel, May 23, 2006.

Tanor, Theresa, June 29, 2010

Tetteh, Henry Joshua, June 16, 2003.

———, February 7, 2004.

Thunder, Alhaji, July 4, 2007.

Thunder, Tsofatse, December 22, 2006.

Wiafe, Ama, June 20, 2006.

Wontse, Korle, March 30, 2005.

Wulomo, Korle, August 10, 2003.

———, February 3, 2005.

———, February 16, 2005.

———, December 30, 2005.

Wulomo, Nae, August 5, 2002.
————, November 28, 2002.

ARCHIVAL MATERIAL

Cambridge University Library, Royal Commonwealth Society Library
Government of Ghana
NARA (National Archives and Records Administration, US)
PRAAD (Public Records and Archives Administration, Ghana)
United States Patent Office
World Health Organization

GOLD COAST COLONY PUBLICATIONS

Annual reports
Blue books
Census
Civil service lists
Government gazettes
Handbooks
Ordinances
Report of the Commission of Enquiry into the Health Needs of the Gold
    Coast, 1952
Reports on the Medical and Sanitary Departments

Government of Ghana

Brachott Committee Report on Professionalization of African Medicine. Government of Ghana. Accra: Ministry of Health, 1961.
Census Reports. Accra: Central Bureau of Statistics.
Ghana News Agency
Ghana Standards Board
Ghana Statistical Service

Newspapers

Accra Evening News
Accra Metropolitan Assembly
Accra Town Council Minutes

BBC News
Daily Graphic (print and online)
Ebifa Mu Uganda [News from Uganda]
Gold Coast Echo
Gold Coast Independent
Gold Coast Leader
Gold Coast News
Gold Coast Observer
Jamaica Gleaner
JoyOnline
Matalisi [Messenger]

Films

Amenu's Child. Accra: Gold Coast Film Unit, 1950. Film.
Rouch, Jean. *Jaguar*. Paris: Les Films de la Pléiade, (1954) 1967. Film.
———. *Les Maitres Fous*. Paris: Les Films de la Pléiade, 1953. Film.

ONLINE SOURCES

Basel Mission Archives, http://www.bmarchives.org
Ghanaweb.com
Government of Ghana Website, http://www.ghana.gov.gh
MyJoyOnline.com

DOCUMENTARY SOURCES

Abdalla, Ismail Hussein. "Islamic Medicine and Its Influence on Traditional Hausa Practitioners in Northern Nigeria." PhD diss., University of Wisconsin, 1984.
Ackernecht, Erwin H. *Medicine at the Paris Hospital, 1794–1848*. Baltimore, MD: Johns Hopkins Press, 1967.
Acquah, Ione. *Accra Survey: A Social Survey of the Capital of Ghana, Formerly Called the Gold Coast, Undertaken for the West African Institute of Social and Economic Research, 1953–1956*. London: University of London Press, 1958.
Adams, C. D. "Activities of Danish Botanists in Guinea, 1783–1850." *Transactions of the Historical Society of Ghana* 3, no. 1 (1957): 30–46.
Adamu, Mahdi. *The Hausa Factor in West African History*. Zaria, Nigeria: Ahmadu Bello University Press, 1978.

Adanson, Michel. *A Voyage to Senegal, the Island of Goree, and the River Gambia*. London: Printed for J. Nourse and W. Jonhston, 1759.

Adanu, Richard M. K., Allan G. Hill, Joseph D. Seffah, Rudolph Darko, John K. Anarfi, and Rosemary B. Duda. "Sexually Transmitted Infections and Health Seeking Behaviour among Ghanaian Women in Accra." *African Journal of Reproductive Health / La Revue Africaine De La Santé Reproductive* 12, no. 3 (2008): 151–58.

Addae, Stephen. *The Evolution of Modern Medicine in a Developing Country: Ghana 1880–1960*. Durham, UK: Durham Academic, 1996.

———. *The Gold Coast and Achimota in the Second World War*. Accra: Sedco, 2004.

Addy, Yacub. Official Website. Accessed August 18, 2009. http://www.yacubaddy.com.

Ademuwagun, Z. A. *African Therapeutic Systems*. Los Angeles: Crossroads, 1979.

Adeyemi, O. O. "Effects of Aqueous Extract of *Baphia nitida* on Isolated Cardiac Tissues." *Phytotherapy Research* 6, no. 6 (2006): 318–21.

Adjanohoun, E. V. *Contribution aux études ethnobotaniques et floristiques au Togo*. Paris: Agence de Coopération Culturelle et Technique (ACCT), 1986.

Affrifa, Kofi. *The Akyem Factor in Ghana's History 1700–1875*. Accra: Ghana Universities Press, 2000.

Afful-Mensah, Gloria, and Edward Nketiah-Amponsah. "A Review of HIV/AIDS Awareness and Knowledge of Preventive Methods in Ghana: Review Article." *African Journal of Reproductive Health* 17, no. 1 (2013): 69–82.

Agyei-Mensah, S., and Aikins A. De-Graft. "Epidemiological Transition and the Double Burden of Disease in Accra, Ghana." *Journal of Urban Health* 87, no. 5 (2010): 879–97.

Agyei-Mensah, Samuel, and John B. Casterline, eds. *Reproduction and Social Context in Sub-Saharan Africa: A Collection of Micro-Demographic Studies*. Westport, CT: Greenwood, 2003.

Agyemang, Fred. *Century with Boys: The Story of Middle Boarding Schools in Ghana, 1867–1967*. Accra: Waterville, 1967.

Ahmadiyya Movement in Ghana (Headquarters—Saltpond) West Africa 1921–1961. Saltpond: Ahmadiyya Movement Ghana, 1960.

Ahmed, Halima Opoku. "Perception of Clients and Private Midwives on Student Midwives during Clinical Sessions in Berekum District, Brong Ahafo Region, Ghana." Master's thesis, University of Cape Coast, 2011.

Ajayi, J. F. A., and Michael Crowder, eds. *History of West Africa*. New York: Columbia University Press, 1972.

"A. J. R. O'Brien, C.M.G., M.B., M.R.C.P." *British Medical Journal* 1, no. 4133 (1940): 508–9.

Akhtar, Rais. *Health and Disease in Tropical Africa: Geographical and Medical Viewpoints*. Chur, Switzerland: Harwood Academic, 1987.

Akosah-Sarpong, Kofi. "The Drugs That Kill by Default." *West Africa* (November 21–28, 1988): 2185–86.

———. "The Herbalization Of Korle Bu." *Ghanaweb.com*, January 25, 2004. http://www.ghanaweb.com/GhanaHomePage/features/artikel .php?ID=50539.

Akyeampong, Emmanuel. "Bukom and the Social History of Boxing in Accra." In "Leisure in African History," special issue, *International Journal of African Historical Studies* 35, no. 1 (2002): 39–60.

———. *Drink, Power, and Cultural Change: A Social History of Alcohol in Ghana, c. 1800 to Recent Times*. Portsmouth, NH: Heinemann, 1996.

Aladesanmi, A. J., E. O. Iwalewa, A. C. Adebajo, E. O. Akinkunmi, B. J. Taiwo, F. O. Olorunmola, and A. Lamikanra. "Antimicrobial and Antioxidant Activities of Some Nigerian Medicinal Plants." *African Journal of Traditional, Complementary and Alternative Medicines* 4, no. 2 (2007): 173–84.

Alilio, Martin S., Ib C. Bygbjerg, and Joel G. Breman. "Are Multilateral Malaria Research and Control Programs the Most Successful? Lessons from the Past 100 Years in Africa." Supplement 2, *American Journal of Tropical Medicine and Hygiene* 71 (2004): 268–78.

All-Asia Great Modern Spiritual Revival Movement. *The Spiritual Front and Moral Forces of the World: General Report of the 25th Grand Assembly of the Permanent World Parliament of Religions, Fraternities and Philosophies, under the Aegis of the Universal Religious Alliance*. Rangoon, Burma: Universal Spiritual Union, 1955.

Allman, Jean, ed. *Fashioning Africa: Power and the Politics of Dress*. Bloomington: Indiana University Press, 2004.

Allman, Jean, and John Parker. *Tongnaab: The History of a West African God*. Bloomington: Indiana University Press, 2005.

Alpern, Stanley. "What Africans Got for Their Slaves." *History in Africa* 22 (1995): 5–43.

Al-Qur'an Shifaa Ruqya & Hijama/Cupping Centre. Accessed March 10, 2018. https://www.facebook.com/CeroqGhana/.

Alubo, S. Ogoh. "Death for Sale: A Study of Drug Poisoning and Deaths in Nigeria." *Social Science and Medicine* 38, no. 1 (1994): 97–103.

American Journal of Nursing. Review of *Amenu's Child.* 56, no. 2 (February 1956): 228–29.

Amoah, A. G. "Obesity in Adult Residents of Accra, Ghana." *Ethnicity and Disease* 13, no. 2 (Summer 2003): 97–101.

Amos, Alcione M., and Ebenezer Ayesu. "'I Am Brazilian': History of the Tabon, Afro-Brazilians in Accra, Ghana." *Transactions of the Historical Society of Ghana* 6 (2002): 35–58.

Anderson, Allan. *An Introduction to Pentecostalism: Global Charismatic Christianity.* Cambridge: Cambridge University Press, 2004.

Anderson, David, and Richard Rathbone. *Africa's Urban Past.* Portsmouth, NH: Heinemann, 1999.

Anderson, Gerald H. *Biographical Dictionary of Christian Missions.* Grand Rapids, MI: W. B. Eerdmans, 1999.

Anderson, J. N. D. *Islamic Law in Africa.* London: Frank Cass, 1970.

Anderson, Stuart, and Peter Homan. "'Best for Me, Best for You': A History of Beecham's Pills 1842–1998." *Pharmaceutical Journal* 269 (2002): 921–24.

Anderson, Warwick. "Review Essay: Where Is the Postcolonial History of Medicine?" *Bulletin of the History of Medicine* 72, no. 3 (1998): 522–30.

Andersson, Asa. "To Work in the Garden of God: The Swedish Nursing Association and the Concept of the Call, 1909–1933." *Nursing History Review* 10 (2002): 4–19.

Andrews, Bridie. *The Making of Modern Chinese Medicine.* Vancouver: UBC Press, 2014.Anfom, E. E. *Traditional Medicine in Ghana. J. B. Danquah Memorial Lectures* 1, no. 17 (1986).

Ankrah, N. A., A. K. Nyarko, P. G. A. Addo, M. Ofosuhene, C. Dzokoto, E. Marley, M. Addae et al. "Evaluation of Efficacy and Safety of a Herbal Medicine Used for the Treatment of Malaria." *Phytotherapy Research* 17, no. 6 (2003): 697–701.

Anomanyo, Edward Dotseh. "Integration of Municipal Solid Waste Management in Accra (Ghana): Bioreactor Treatment Technology as an Integral Part of the Management Process." Master's thesis, Lund University, 2004.

Anquandah, James. "The Accra Plains c. AD 1400–1800: An Overview of Trade, Politics, and Culture from the Perspective of Historical Archaeology." Supplement, *Research Review* 17 (2006): 1–20.

———. "Accra Plains, Dangmeland: A Case Study in the Eclectic Approach to Archaeological and Historical Studies." *Archaeology in Ghana* 3 (1992): 1–8.

———. *Rediscovering Ghana's Past.* London: Longman, 1982.

Antwi, S., O. N. K. Martey, K. Donkor, and L.K. Nii-Ayitey. "Antidiarrhoeal Activity of *Blighia sapida* (Sapindaceae) in Rats and Mice." *Journal of Pharmacology and Toxicology* 4 (2009): 117–25.

Anyinam, Charles. "Traditional Medical Practice in Contemporary Ghana: A Dying or Growing 'Profession'?" *Canadian Journal of African Studies / Revue Canadienne des Études Africaines* 21, no. 3 (1987): 315–36.

Appadurai, Arjun. *Modernity at Large: Cultural Dimensions of Globalization.* Minneapolis: University of Minnesota, 2003.

———, ed. *The Social Life of Things.* Cambridge: Cambridge University Press, 1986.

Arn, Jack. "Third World Urbanization and the Creation of a Relative Surplus Population: A History of Accra, Ghana to 1980." *Review: Fernand Braudel Center* 19, no. 4 (Fall 1996): 413–44.

Arnold, David. *Colonizing the Body: State Medicine and Epidemic Disease in Nineteenth-Century India.* Berkeley: University of California Press, 1993.

———, ed. *Imperial Medicine and Indigenous Societies.* New York: Manchester University Press, 1988.

———, ed. *Warm Climates and Western Medicine: The Emergence of Tropical Medicine, 1500–1900.* Atlanta, GA: Rodopi, 1996.

Arrow, Kenneth Joseph, Claire Panosian, and Hellen Gelband. *Saving Lives, Buying Time: Economics of Malaria Drugs in an Age of Resistance.* Washington, DC: National Academic, 2004.

Asase, Alex, and Gloria Oppong-Mensah. "Traditional Antimalarial Phytotherapy Remedies in Herbal Markets in Southern Ghana." *Journal of Ethnopharmacology* 126, no. 3 (December 10, 2009): 492–99.

Asase, Alex, A. A. Oteng-Yeboah, G. T. Odamtten, and M. S. J. Simmonds. "Ethnobotanical Study of Some Ghanaian Anti-malarial Plants." *Journal of Ethnopharmacology* 99 (2005): 273–79.

Asenso-Okyere, W. K., A. Anum, I. Osei-Akoto, and A. Adukonu. "Cost Recovery in Ghana: Are There Any Changes in Health Care Seeking Behavior?" *Health Policy and Planning* 13, no. 2 (1998): 181–88.

Ashforth, Adam. "An Epidemic of Witchcraft? The Implications of AIDS for the Post-Apartheid State." *African Studies* 61, no. 1 (2002): 121–43.

Ashitey, Gilford A. *An Epidemiology of Disease Control in Ghana, 1901–1990.* Accra: Ghana Universities Press, 1994.

Astley, Thomas. *A New General Collection of Voyages and Travels.* Vol. 2. London, 1745.

Atobrah, Deborah. "Caring for the Seriously Ill in a Ghanaian Society: Glimpses from the Past." *Ghana Studies* 15/16 (2013/2014): 69–101.

Attewell, Guy N. A. *Refiguring Unani Tibb: Plural Healing in Late Colonial India.* Hyderabad, India: Orient Longman, 2007.

Aubrey, T. *The Sea-Surgeon, or The Guinea Man's Vade Mecum.* London, 1729.

Austin, Dennis. *Ghana Observed: Essays on the Politics of a West African Republic.* Manchester: Manchester University Press, 1976.

Awine, T., K. Malm, C. Bart-Plange, and S. P. Silal. "Towards Malaria Control and Elimination in Ghana: Challenges and Decision Making Tools to Guide Planning." *Global Health Action* 10, no. 1 (2017):1–9. https://www.ncbi.nlm.nih.gov/pmc/articles/PMC5678345/.

Ayeni, B., A. L. Mabogunje, A. Soyibo, and A. S. Gbadegesin. "Symposium on 'Mabogunje on Development and Development Policy.'" *Research Report.* Ibadan, Nigeria: Development Policy Centre, 2002.

Ayensu, Edward S. "Plant and Bat Interactions in West Africa." *Annals of the Missouri Botanical Garden* 61, no. 3 (1974): 702–27.

Ayers, Gwendoline M. *England's First State Hospitals and the Metropolitan Asylums Board, 1867–1930.* Berkeley: University of California Press, 1971.

Ayisi, N. K., and C. Nyadedzor. "Comparative In Vitro Effects of AZT and Extracts of *Ocimum gratissimum, Ficus polita, Clausena anisata, Alchornea cordifolia,* and *Elaeophorbia drupifera* against HIV-1 and HIV-2 Infections." *Antiviral Research* 5, no. 8 (March 2003): 25–33.

Azevedo, Mario J., Gerald W. Hartwig, and K. D. Patterson. *Disease in African History: An Introductory Survey and Case Studies.* Durham, NC: Duke University Press, 1978.

Azu, Diana Gladys. *The Ga Family and Social Change.* Leiden: Afrika-Studiecentrum, 1974.

Baesjou, R. "Dutch 'Irregular' Jurisdiction on the Nineteenth Century Gold Coast." *African Perspectives* 2 (1979): 21–66.

Baeta, C. G. *Prophetism in Ghana: A Study of Some 'Spiritual Churches.'* Achimota: African Christian Press, 2004.

Bagchi, Jeebesh, Monica Narula, Shuddhabrata Sengupta, Geert Lovink, and Marleen Stikker, eds. *Sarai Reader: Shaping Technologies.* Delhi: Sarai Media Lab, 2003.

Bala, Poonam. *Biomedicine as a Contested Site: Some Revelations in Imperial Contexts.* Lanham, MD: Lexington Books, 2009.

Bannerman-Richter, Gabriel. *Mmoetia: The Mysterious Little People.* Sacramento, CA: Gabari, 1987.

Barber, Karin, ed. *Africa's Hidden Histories: Everyday Literacy and the Making of the Self.* Bloomington: Indiana University Press, 2006.

———. "When People Cross Thresholds." *African Studies Review* 50, no. 2 (September 2007): 111–23.

Barbot, Jean. *Barbot on Guinea: The Writings of Jean Barbot on West Africa, 1678–1712.* Edited by P. E. H. Hair, Adam Jones, and Robin Law. London: Hakluyt Society, 1992.

———. *A Description of the Coasts of North and South Guinea.* London, 1732.

———. *A Description of the Coasts of North and South Guinea: And of Ethiopia Inferior, Vulgarly Angola . . . and a New Relation of the Province of Guiana, and of the Great Rivers of Amazons and Oronoque in South-America, with an Appendix, Being a General Account of the First Discoveries of America, in the Fourteenth Century and Some Observations Thereon, and a Geographical, Political, and Natural History of the Antilles-Islands in the North-Sea of America.* London: Henry Lintot and John Osborn, 1980.

Barnett, A., A. L. Creese, and E. C. Ayivor. "The Economics of Pharmaceutical Policy in Ghana." *International Journal of Health Services* 10, no. 3 (1980): 479–99.

Barnor, M. A. *A Socio-medical Adventure in Ghana: Autobiography of Dr. M. A. Barnor.* Accra: Vieso Universal, 2001.

Baronov, David. *The African Transformation of Western Medicine and the Dynamics of Global Cultural Exchange.* Philadelphia: Temple University Press, 2008.

Barrie, H. J. "Diary Notes on a Trip to West Africa in Relation to a Yellow Fever Expedition under the Auspices of the Rockefeller Foundation, 1926, by Oskar Klotz." *Canadian Bulletin of Medical History / Bulletin Canadien D'histoire De La Medecine* 14, no. 1 (1997): 133–63.

Barry, Jonathan, Marianne Hester, and Gareth Roberts. *Witchcraft in Early Modern Europe: Studies in Culture and Belief.* Cambridge: Cambridge University Press, 1998.

Bartels, F. L. *The Roots of Ghanaian Methodism.* Cambridge: Cambridge University Press, 1965.

Barth, Fredrik. *One Discipline, Four Ways: British, German, French, and American Anthropology.* Chicago: University of Chicago Press, 2005.

Beckerleg, Susan. "Medical Pluralism and Islam in Swahili Communities in Kenya." *Medical Anthropology Quarterly,* n.s., 8, no. 3 (September 1994): 299–313.

Behrend, Heike, and Ute Luig, eds. *Spirit Possession, Modernity & Power in Africa.* Madison: University of Wisconsin Press, 1999.

Belam, F. "Random Reminiscences of the R.A.M.C. 1909–1949." *Public Health* 64 (1951): 117–18.

Berkman, Nancy D., Terry C. Davis, and Lauren McCormack. "Health Literacy: What Is It?" *Journal of Health Communication* 15, no. 2 (2010): 9–19.

Bertrand, Monique. "Migration internationale et métropolisation en Afrique de l'Ouest: Le cas des Zabrama du Grand Accra, Ghana." *Espace, Populations, Societies* 2–3 (2010): 307–20.

Bever, Edward. "Witchcraft Prosecutions and the Decline of Magic." *Journal of Interdisciplinary History* 40, no. 2 (2009): 263–93.

Bierlich, Bernhard. *The Problem of Money: African Agency and Western Medicine in Northern Ghana.* Oxford: Berghahn Books, 2007.

———. "Sacrifice, Plants, and Western Pharmaceuticals: Money and Health Care in Northern Ghana." *Medical Anthropology Quarterly,* n.s., 13, no. 3 (September 1999): 316–37.

Bliss, Michael. *William Osler: A Life in Medicine.* New York: Oxford University Press, 1999.

Bloom, Peter J., and Kate Skinner. "Modernity and Danger: 'The Boy Kumasenu' and the Work of the Gold Coast Film Unit." *Ghana Studies* (2011): 121–53.

Blumenthal, Ivan. "The Gripe Water Story." *Journal of the Royal Society of Medicine* 93 (April 1–2, 2000): 172–74.

Boatens, E. A. *A Geography of Ghana.* Cambridge: Cambridge University Press, 1959.

Bosman, Willem. *A New and Accurate Description of the Coast of Guinea, Divided into the Gold, the Slave, and the Ivory Coasts.* London: James Knapton, 1705.

Bourdieu, Pierre. *Distinction: A Social Critique of the Judgment of Taste.* Cambridge, MA: Harvard University Press, (1979) 1984.

———. *Practical Reason.* Stanford, CA: Polity, 1998.

———. *The State Nobility: Elite Schools in the Field of Power.* Stanford, CA: Stanford University Press, (1989) 1996.

Bourret, F. M. *Ghana: The Road to Independence, 1919–1957.* Stanford, CA: Stanford University Press, 1960.

———. *The Gold Coast: A Survey of the Gold Coast and British Togoland, 1919–1946.* London, 1949.

Bowdich, T., ed. *Mission from Cape Coast to Ashantee.* London, 1819.

Boyce, Rupert. "The Distribution and Prevalence of Yellow Fever in the Gold Coast." *Transactions of the Royal Society of Tropical Medicine and Hygiene* 4, no. 2 (1910): 33–59.

Boyle, Laura. *Diary of a Colonial Officer's Wife.* London: Collins, 1970.

Brackett, D. G., and M. Wrong. "Notes on Hygiene Books Used in Africa." *Africa: Journal of the International African Institute* 5, no. 1 (January 1932): 71–74.

Brantley, Cynthia. "Kikuyu-Maasai Nutrition and Colonial Science: The Orr and Gilks Study in Late 1920s Kenya Revisited." *International Journal of African Historical Studies* 30, no. 1 (1997): 49–86.

British Dispensatory, Containing a Faithful Translation of the New London Pharmacopœia. London: Royal College of Physicians of London, 1747.

British Medical Association. *More Secret Remedies: What They Cost & What They Contain.* London: British Medical Association, 1912.

———. *Secret Remedies, What They Cost and What They Contain: Based on Analyses Made for the British Medical Association.* London: British Medical Association, 1910.

Brook, Timothy. "Rethinking Syncretism: The Unity of the Three Teachings and Their Joint Worship in Late-Imperial China." *Journal of Chinese Religions* 21 (Fall 1993): 13–44.

Brown, Candy G., ed. *Global Pentecostal and Charismatic Healing.* Oxford: Oxford University Press, 2011.

Brown, E. K., and Sarah Ogilvie. *Concise Encyclopedia of Languages of the World.* Amsterdam: Elsevier, 2009.

Brown, Spencer H. "Colonialism on the Cheap: A Tale of Two English Army Surgeons in Lagos, Samuel Rowe and Frank Simpson, 1862–1882." *International Journal of African Historical Studies* 27 (1994): 551–88.

Brummitt, R. K., and C. E. Powell, eds. *Authors of Plant Names: A List of Authors of Scientific Names of Plants, with Recommended Standard Forms of their Names, Including Abbreviations.* London: Royal Botanic Gardens, Kew, 1992.

Buel, James W. *Heroes of the Dark Continent: A Complete History of All the Great Explorations and Discoveries in Africa, from the Earliest Ages to the Present Time.* New York: Hunt & Eaton, 1890.

Burkill, H. M. *Useful Plants of West Tropical Africa.* Vol. 2. Kew, UK: Royal Botanic Gardens, 1994.

Burton, Richard. *A Mission to Gelele, King of Dahomey.* London: Tylston & Edwards, 1893.

Burton, Richard F., and Verney Lovett Cameron. *To the Gold Coast for Gold: A Personal Narrative.* Vol. 2. London: Chatto & Windus, 1883.

Busia, K. A. *Report on a Social Survey of Sekondi-Takoradi.* London: Crown Agents for the Colonies on Behalf of the Govt. of the Gold Coast, 1950.

Busvine, James R. *Disease Transmission by Insects: Its Discovery and 90 Years of Effort to Prevent It.* New York: Springer, 1994.

Butchart, Alexander. *The Anatomy of Power: European Constructions of the African Body.* New York: Zed Books, 1998.

Bynum, William. F., and Caroline Overy, eds. *The Beast in the Mosquito: The Correspondence of Ronald Ross and Patrick Manson.* Clio Medica 51, Welcome Institute Series in the History of Medicine. Amsterdam: Rodopi, 1998.

Bynum, William F., and Roy Porter. *Medicine and the Five Senses.* Cambridge: Cambridge University Press, 1993.

Callewaert, Staf. "Bourdieu, Critic of Foucault." *Theory, Culture & Society* 23, no. 6 (2006): 73–98.

Campbell, Lyle. *Historical Linguistics: An Introduction.* Edinburgh: Edinburgh University Press, 2013.

Canot, Theodore. *A Slaver's Log Book, or 20 Years' Residence in Africa: The Original Manuscript.* Englewood Cliffs, NJ: Prentice-Hall, 1976.

Capanna, Ernesto. "Grassi versus Ross: Who Solved the Riddle of Malaria?" *International Microbiology* 9, no. 1 (March 2006): 69–74.

Cardinall, A. W. *The Gold Coast, 1931.* Accra, Gold Coast: Government Printer, 1931.

Carney, Judith. "African Traditional Plant Knowledge in the Circum-Caribbean Region." *Journal of Ethnobiology* 2, no. 2 (Fall/Winter 2003): 167–85.

Carson, Rachel. *Silent Spring.* London: H. Hamilton, 1963.

Carstensen, Edward. *Governor Carstensen's Diary, 1818–1850.* Legon: University of Ghana, 1965.

Centre for Public Interest Law. "Housing Rights and Forced Eviction Cases, Issa Iddi Abass v Accra Metropolitan Authority (Ama) & Another." Accessed March 4, 2011. http://www.cepil.org.gh/files/Issah-Iddi-Vs.-AMA.pdf.

Cherfas, Jeremy, and Roger Lewin, eds. *Not Work Alone: A Cross-Cultural View of Activities Superfluous to Survival.* London: Temple Smith, 1980.

Cherry, Steven. *Medical Services and the Hospitals in Britain, 1860–1939.* Cambridge: Cambridge University Press, 1996.

Chouin, Gérard. "Seen, Said, or Deduced? Travel Accounts, Historical Criticism, and Discourse Theory: Towards an 'Archeology' of Dialogue in Seventeenth-Century Guinea." *History in Africa* 28 (2001): 53–70.

Christaller, Johannes G. *A Dictionary of the Asante and Fante Language Called Tshi (Chwee, Twi), with a Grammatical Introduction and Appendices on the Geography of the Gold Coast and other Subjects.* Basel: Evangelical Missionary Society, 1881.

Christensen, James B. "The Tigari Cult of West Africa." *Papers of the Michigan Academy of Science, Arts and Letters* 39 (1954): 389–98.

Christopher, Emma. *Slave Ship Sailors and Their Captive Cargoes, 1730–1807.* New York: Cambridge University Press, 2006.

Christophers, S. R., and J. W. W. Stephens. *Destruction of Anopheles in Lagos.* Vol. 3 of *Royal Society, Reports of the Malaria Committee of the Royal Society.* London, 1900.

Churchill, Wendy D. "Bodily Differences? Gender, Race, and Class in Hans Sloane's Jamaican Medical Practice, 1687–1688." *Journal of the History of Medicine and Allied Sciences* 60, no. 4 (2005): 391–444.

Claridge, William Walton, and William Ernest Frank Ward. *A History of the Gold Coast and Ashanti: From the Earliest Times to the Commencement of the Twentieth Century.* Vol. 2. 2nd ed. London: Frank Cass, 1964.

Clifford, Lady [Mrs. Henry de la Pasture, pseud.]. *Our Days on the Gold Coast.* London: John Murray, 1919.

Cohen, William B. "Malaria and French Imperialism." *Journal of African History* 24, no. 1 (1983): 23–36.

Collett, Dom Martin. *Accra Diocese.* London: Society for the Propagation of the Gospel in Foreign Parts, 1928.

Collins, John. *Highlife Time.* Accra: Anansasem, 1994.

Comaroff, Jean, and John Comaroff, eds. *Modernity and Its Malcontents: Ritual and Power in Postcolonial Africa.* Chicago: University of Chicago Press, 1993.

———. *Of Revelation and Revolution: Christianity, Colonialism and Consciousness in South Africa.* 2 vols. Chicago: University of Chicago Press, 1997.

Conklin, Alice L. *A Mission to Civilize: The Republican Idea of Empire in France and West Africa, 1895–1930.* Stanford, CA: Stanford University Press, 2003.

Conrad, Lawrence I., and Anne Hardy. *Women and Modern Medicine.* Amsterdam: Rodopi, 2001.

Cooper, Frederick. *Africa since 1940: The Past in the Present.* Cambridge: Cambridge University Press, 2002.

———. "Conflict and Connection: Rethinking Colonial African History." *American Historical Review* 99, no. 5 (December 1994): 1516–45.

———. *Decolonization and African Society: The Labor Question in French and British Africa.* Cambridge: Cambridge University Press, 1996.

Cooter, Roger, ed. *In the Name of the Child: Health and Welfare, 1880–1940.* New York: Routledge, 1992.

Coquery-Vidrovitch, Catherine. *The History of African Cities South of the Sahara.* Princeton, NJ: Markus Wiener, 2005.

Corley, T. A. B. "Interactions between the British and American Patent Medicine Industries 1708–1014." *Business and Economic History,* 2nd ser., 16 (1987): 13.

Craddock, Sally. *Retired except on Demand: The Life of Cicely Williams.* Oxford: Green College, 1983.

Cramp, Arthur J. *Nostrums and Quackery: Articles on the Nostrum Evil and Quackery. Journal of the American Medical Association.* Reprinted with additions and modifications. 2nd ed. Chicago: American Medical Association Press, 1921.

Crellin, J. K. *A Social History of Medicines in the Twentieth Century: To Be Taken Three Times a Day.* New York: Pharmaceutical Products, 2004.

Crisp, Jeff. *The Story of an African Working Class: Ghanaian Miners' Struggles, 1870–1980.* London: Zed, 1984.

Crofton, Eileen, and Patricia Raemaekers. *A Painful Inch to Gain: Personal Experiences of Early Women Medical Students in Britain.* N.p.: Fast-Print Publishing, 2014.

Crooks, J. J. *Records Relating to the Gold Coast Settlements from 1750 to 1874.* Dublin: Browne & Nolan, 1923.

Crozier, Anna. *Practising Colonial Medicine: The Colonial Medical Service in British East Africa.* London: I. B. Tauris, 2007.

Cunningham, Andrew, and Bridie Andrews. *Western Medicine as Contested Knowledge.* New York: Manchester University Press, 1997.

Curth, Louise H. *From Physick to Pharmacology: Five Hundred Years of British Drug Retailing.* Aldershot, Hampshire, England: Ashgate, 2006.

Curtin, Philip D. *The Atlantic Slave Trade: A Census.* Madison: University of Wisconsin Press, 1969.

———. *Disease and Empire: The Health of European Troops in the Conquest of Africa.* Cambridge: Cambridge University Press, 1998.

———. "Medical Knowledge and Urban Planning in Tropical Africa." *American Historical Review* 90, no. 3 (1985): 594–613.

———. "The White Man's Grave: Image and Reality, 1780–1850." *Journal of British Studies* 1, no. 1 (November 1961): 94–110.

Daaku, K. Y. *Trade and Politics on the Gold Coast 1600–1720.* Oxford: Oxford University Press, 1970.

Dakubu, Mary E. Kropp, ed. *Ga–English Dictionary with English–Ga Index.* Accra: Black Mask, 1999.

———. *Korle Meets the Sea: A Sociolinguistic History of Accra.* Oxford: Oxford University Press, 1997.

Dally, Ann. *Cicely: The Story of a Doctor.* London: Victor Gollancz, 1968.

D'Amelio, Dan. *Taller Than Bandai Mountain: The Story of Hideyo Noguchi.* New York: Viking, 1968.

Danfulani, Umar Habila Dadem. "Factors Contributing to the Survival of the Bori Cult in Northern Nigeria. *Numen* 46, no. 4 (1999): 412–47.

Daniell, William F. "On the Ethnography of Akkrah and Adampe, Gold Coast, Western Africa." *Journal of the Ethnological Society of London (1848–1856)* 4 (1856): 1–32.

Dansi, A., A. Adjatin, H. Adoukonou-Sagbadja, V. Faladé, H. Yedomonhan, D. Odou, and B. Dossou. "Traditional Leafy Vegetables and Their Use in the Benin Republic." *Genetic Resources and Crop Evolution* 55, no. 8 (December 2008): 1239–56.

Darko, Isaac Nortey. 2009. "Ghanaian Indigenous Health Practices: The Use of Herbs." Master's thesis, University of Toronto, 2009.

Dart, Richard C. *Medical Toxicology.* Philadelphia: Lippincott Williams & Wilkins, 2004.

Davenport, Manuel M. "The Moral Paternalism of Albert Schweitzer." *Ethics* 84, no. 2 (January 1974): 116–27.

Davidson, James Michael. "Mediating Race and Class through the Death Experience: Power Relations and Resistance Strategies of an African-American Community, Dallas, Texas (1869–1907)." PhD diss., University of Texas at Austin, 2004.

Davies, J. N. P. *Pestilence and Disease in the History of Africa.* Johannesburg: Witwatersrand University Press for the Institute for the Study of Man in Africa, 1979.

Davies, K. G. *The Royal African Company.* New York: Octagon Books, 1975.

Davin, Anna. "Imperialism and Motherhood." *History Workshop* 5 (1978): 9–65.

Debrunner, Hans W. *History of Christianity in Ghana.* Accra: Waterville, 1967.

DeCourse, Christopher. *An Archeology of Elmina: Africans and Europeans on the Gold Coast, 1400–1900.* Washington: Smithsonian Institution Press, 2001.

Delbourgo, James, and Nicholas Dew, eds. *Science and Empire in the Atlantic World.* New York: Routledge, 2008.

De Marees, Pieter. *Description and Historical Account of the Gold Kingdom of Guinea (1602).* Translated from the Dutch and edited by Albert van Dantzig and Adam Jones. Oxford: Oxford University Press, 1987.

Desai, Gaurav. *Subject to Colonialism: African Self-Fashioning and the Colonial Library.* Durham, NC: Duke University Press, 2001.

Desowitz, R. S. "The Malaria Vaccine: Seventy Years of the Great Immune Hope." *Parassitologia* 42 (2000): 173–82.

Deutsch, Jan-Georg, Peter Probst, and Heike Schmidt, eds. *African Modernities: Entangled Meanings in Current Debate.* Portsmouth, NH: Heinemann, 2002.

Dickson, K. B. "Evolution of Seaports in Ghana: 1800–1928." *Annals of the Association of American Geographers* 55, no. 1 (March 1965): 98–111.

———. *A Historical Geography of Ghana.* Cambridge: Cambridge University Press, 1969.

Digby, Anne. *Diversity and Division in Medicine: Health Care in South Africa from the 1800s.* Oxford: Lang, 2006.

Dinges, Martin, ed. *Medical Pluralism and Homeopathy in India and Germany (1810–2010): A Comparison of Practices.* Stuttgart: Verlag Stuttgart, 2014.

Dionisio, Kathie L., Raphael E. Arku, Allison F. Hughes, Jose Vallarino, Heather Carmichael, John D. Spengler, Samuel Agyei-Mensah, and Majid Ezzati. "Air Pollution in Accra Neighborhoods: Spatial, Socioeconomic, and Temporal Patterns." *Environmental Science & Technology* 44 (2010): 2270–76.

Dirks, Nicholas B., Geoff Eley, and Sherry B. Ortner, eds. *Culture/Power/ History: A Reader in Contemporary Social Theory.* Princeton, NJ: Princeton University Press, 1994.

Dobson, J. "Malaria in England: A Geographical and Historical Perspective." *Parassitologia* 36, no. 1–2 (August 1994): 35–60.

Dokosi, O. B. *Herbs of Ghana.* Accra: Ghana University Press, 1998.

———. "Some Herbs Used in the Traditional Systems of Healing Disease in Ghana—I." *Ghana Journal of Science* 9 (1969): 119–30.

Donnan, Elizabeth, ed. *Documents Illustrative of the History of the Slave Trade to America.* Vol. 2, *The Eighteenth Century.* New York: Octagon Books, 1965.

Doortmont, Michael R. *The Pen-Pictures of Modern Africans and African Celebrities by Charles Francis Hutchison: A Collective Biography of Elite Society in the Gold Coast Colony.* London: Brill, 2005.

Dowd, F. B. "Review of *Accra Survey.*" *African Affairs* 59, no. 235 (April 1960): 164–65.

Drewal, Henry John. "Performing the Other: Mami Wata Worship in Africa." *Drama Review* 32, no. 2 (Summer 1988): 160–85.

Drewal, Henry John, and Marilyn Houlberg, eds. *Mami Wata: Arts for Water Spirits in Africa and Its Diasporas.* Los Angeles: Fowler Museum at UCLA, 2008.

Drewal, Henry John, and John Mason. *Beads, Body and Soul: Art and Light in the Yoruba Universe.* Los Angeles: UCLA Fowler Museum, 1998.

Duda, R. B., M. P. Kim, R. Darko, R. M. K. Adanu, J. Seffah, J. K. Anarfi, and A. G. Hill. "Results of the Women's Health Study of Accra: Assessment of Blood Pressure in Urban Women." *International Journal of Cardiology*, April 12, 2007, 115–22.

Duffin, Jacalyn. *History of Medicine: A Scandalously Short Introduction.* Toronto: University of Toronto Press, 1999.

Dumett, Raymond E. "African Merchants of the Gold Coast, 1860–1905: Dynamics of Indigenous Entrepreneurship." *Comparative Studies in Society and History* 25, no. 4 (October 1983): 661–93.

———. "The Campaign against Malaria and the Expansion of Scientific Medical and Sanitary Services in British West Africa, 1898–1910." *African Historical Studies* 1, no. 2 (1968): 153–97.

———. "John Sarbah, the Elder, and African Mercantile Entrepreneurship in the Gold Coast in the Late Nineteenth Century." *Journal of African History* 14, no. 4 (1973): 653–79.

———. "The Rubber Trade of the Gold Coast and Asante in the Nineteenth Century: African Innovation and Market Responsiveness." *Journal of African History* 11, no. 1 (1971): 79–101.

———. "The Social Impact of the European Liquor Trade on the Akan of Ghana (Gold Coast and Asante), 1875–1910." *Journal of Interdisciplinary History* 5, no. 1 (Summer 1974): 69–101.

Dupuis, Joseph. *Journal of a Residence in Ashantee.* London: H. Colburn, 1824.

Dweck, Anthony C. "The Internal and External Use of Medicinal Plants." *Clinics in Dermatology* 27, no. 2 (March–April 2009): 148–58.

Dwight, Henry Otis, H. Allen Tupper Jr., and Edwin Munsell Bliss. *Encyclopedia of Missions: Descriptive, Historical, Biographical, Statistical.* 2nd ed. London: Funk & Wagnalls, 1904.

Dwight, Timothy, deWaal Malefyt, and Brian Moeran. *Advertising Cultures*. New York: Berg, 2003.

Eades, C. A., C. Brace, L. Osei, and K. D. LaGuardia. "Traditional Birth Attendants and Maternal Mortality in Ghana." *Social Science and Medicine* 36, no. 11 (1993): 1503–7.

Echenberg, Myron. *Black Death, White Medicine: Bubonic Plague and the Politics of Public Health in Colonial Senegal, 1914–1945*. Portsmouth, NH: Heinemann, 2002.

Echtler, Magnus, and Asonzeh F. K. Ukah. *Bourdieu in Africa: Exploring the Dynamics of Religious Fields*. Leiden: Brill, 2016.

Eckstein, Gustav. *Noguchi*. London: Harper & Brothers, 1931.

Edsman, Bjorn. *Lawyers in Gold Coast Politics, c. 1900–1945: From Mensah Sarbah to J.B. Danquah*. Stockholm: Uppsala, 1979.

Edwin F., M. Tettey, E. Aniteye, M. Tamatey, L. Sereboe, K. Entsua-Mensah, D. Kotei, and K. Baffoe-Gyan. "The Development of Cardiac Surgery in West Africa: The Case of Ghana." *Pan African Medical Journal* 9, no. 15 (2011): 15.

Ehrenreich, John. *The Cultural Crisis of Modern Medicine*. New York: Monthly Review, 1978.

Ehret, Christopher. *The Civilizations of Africa*. Charlottesville: University of Virginia Press, 2002.

Eicher, Joanne B., ed. *Dress and Ethnicity: Change across Space and Time*. Washington, DC: Berg, 1995.

Eisenberg D. M., R. B. Davis, S. L. Ettner, S. Appel, S. Wilkey, M. Van Rompay, and R. C. Kessler. "Trends in Alternative Medicine Use in the United States, 1990–1997: Results of a Follow-Up National Survey." *Journal of the American Medical Association* 280, no. 18 (November 11, 1998): 1569–75.

Elliott, W. A. *"Nyaka" the Doctor: The Story of David Livingstone, with Chronological and Distance Notes and Memoranda of Progress and Development on His Routes*. London: London Missionary Society, 1908.

Eltis, David. *Economic Growth and the Ending of the Transatlantic Slave Trade*. New York: Oxford University Press, 1987.

El-Tom, A. O. "Berti Qur'anic Amulets." *Journal of Religion in Africa* 17, no. 3 (1987): 224–44.

Eluwa, G. I. C. "Background to the Emergence of the National Congress of British West Africa." *African Studies Review* 14, no. 2 (September 1971): 205–18.

Encyclopaedia Britannica. 11th ed. Cambridge: Cambridge University Press, 1911.

Engels, Dagmar, and Shula Marks, eds. *Contesting Colonial Hegemony.* London: British Academic, 1994.

Engmann, Joyce, "Immortality and the Nature of Man in Ga Thought." In *Person and Community: Ghanaian Philosophical Studies I,* edited by Kwasi Wiredu and Kwame Gyekye, 153–90. Washington, DC: Council for Research in Values and Philosophy, 1992.

Ephson, Ben. "Herbs in Pharmacy." *West Africa,* July 11, 1983, 1605–7.

Erah, Patrick O. "Traditional or Orthodox Medicine in Africa: A New Look." *International Journal of Health Research* 1, no. 4 (September 2008): 175–76.

Eriksen, Thomas Hylland, and Finn Sivert Nielsen. *A History of Anthropology: Anthropology, Culture, and Society.* London: Pluto, 2001.

Ernst, Waltraud. *Plural Medicine, Tradition and Modernity, 1800–2000.* New York: Routledge, 2002.

Etkin N. L., P. J. Ross, and I. Muazzamu. "The Indigenization of Pharmaceuticals: Therapeutic Transition in Rural Hausa Land." *Social Science and Medicine* 30 (1990): 919–28.

Evans-Anfom, E. *Traditional Medicine in Ghana: Practice, Problems and Prospects.* Accra: Academy of Arts and Sciences, 1986.

Evans-Pritchard, E. E. Review of *Religion and Medicine of the Ga People,* by Margaret Field. *Geographical Journal* 91, no. 2 (February 1938): 177–78.

———. *Witchcraft, Oracles, and Magic among the Azande.* Oxford: Clarendon, 1980.

Extra Pharmacopoeia Martindale. Vol. 1. 24th ed. London: Pharmaceutical, 1958.

Fabian, Johannes. *Time and the Other: How Anthropology Makes Its Object.* New York: Columbia University Press, 2002.

Fage, J. D. *An Introduction to the History of West Africa.* 2nd ed. Cambridge: Cambridge University Press, 1959.

———. "Slavery and the Slave Trade in the Context of West African History." *Journal of African History* 10, no. 3 (1969): 393–404.

Falconbridge, Alexander. *An Account of the Slave Trade on the Coast of Africa.* London: J. Phillips, 1788.

Fang, Xiaoping. *Barefoot Doctors and Western Medicine in China.* Rochester, NY: University of Rochester Press, 2012.

Feierman, Steven. "Change in African Therapeutic Systems." *Social Science & Medicine, Part B: Medical Anthropology* 13, no. 4 (1979): 277–84.

———. *Peasant Intellectuals: Anthropology and History in Tanzania.* Madison: University of Wisconsin Press, 1990.

———. "Struggles for Control: The Social Roots of Health and Healing in Modern Africa." *African Studies Review* 28, no. 2/3 (June–September 1985): 73–147.

Feierman, Steven, and John M. Janzen, eds. *The Social Basis of Health and Healing in Africa*. Berkeley: University of California Press, 1992.

Feld, Steven, ed. *Ciné-ethnography*. Vol. 13, *Visible Evidence*. Minneapolis: University of Minnesota Press, 2003.

Field, Margaret Joyce. *Akim-Kotoku: An Oman of the Gold Coast*. Westport, CT: Negro Universities Press, 1970.

———. "The Otutu and the Hionte of West Africa." *Man* 43 (March–April 1943): 36–37.

———. *Religion and Medicine of the Gā People*. London: Oxford University Press, 1937.

———. *Search for Security: An Ethno-Psychiatric Study of Rural Ghana*. Evanston, IL: Northwestern University Press, 1960.

———. *Social Organization of the Gā People*. London: Crown Agents for the Colonies, 1940.

Findlay, G. M., and R. W. Brookfield. "A Fever of the Dengue Group Occurring in West Africa." *Transactions of the Royal Society of Tropical Medicine and Hygiene* 37, no. 2 (September 1943): 95–109.

Findlay, G. M., K. R. Hill, and A. MacPherson. "Penicillin in Yaws and Tropical Ulcer." *Nature* 3921 (December 23, 1944): 795–96.

Findlay, G. M., N. H. Martin, and J. B. Mitchell. "Hepatitis after Yellow Fever Inoculation Relation to Infective Hepatitis." *Lancet* 244, no. 6315 (September 9, 1944): 340–44.

Fink, Helga. *Religion, Disease, and Healing in Ghana: A Case Study of Traditional Dormaa Medicine*. München: Trickster Wissenschaft, 1990.

Firkins R., H. Eisfeld, C. Keinki, J. Buentzel, A. Hochhaus, T. Schmidt, and J. Huebner. "The Use of Complementary and Alternative Medicine by Patients in Routine Care and the Risk of Interactions." *Journal of Cancer Research and Clinical Oncology* 144, no. 3 (March 2018): 551–57.

Fischer, Michael M. J. "Raising Questions about Rouch." *American Anthropologist* 99, no. 1 (March 1997): 140–43.

Fisher, Ruth A. *Extracts from the Records of the African Companies*. New York: Association for the Study of Negro Life and History, 1930.

Flint, Karen E. *Healing Traditions: African Medicine, Cultural Exchange, and Competition in South Africa, 1820–1948*. Athens: Ohio University Press, 2007.

Forster, E. B. "A Short Psychiatric Review of Ghana." *American Journal of Psychotherapy* 16 (1962): 7–51.

Fortes, Meyer. "Book Review: Religion and Medicine of the Gã People." *Bulletin of the School of Oriental Studies, University of London* 9, no. 2 (1938): 479–81.

Fosu, Gabriel B. "Disease Classification in Rural Ghana: Framework and Implications for Health Behaviour." *Social Science and Medicine, Part B: Medical Anthropology* 15, no. 4 (Fall 1981): 471–82.

Foucault, Michel. *The Birth of the Clinic.* New York: Vintage, 1994.

———. *Discipline and Punish: The Birth of the Prison.* New York: Knopf Doubleday, 2012.

———. *The History of Sexuality.* Vol. 1, *The Will to Knowledge.* London: Penguin, 1998.

———. *The Order of Things: An Archaeology of the Human Sciences.* New York: Vintage, 1973.

Foucault, Michel, and François Ewald. *Society Must Be Defended: Lectures at the Collége De France, 1975–76.* London: Penguin, 2008.

Foucault, Michel, and Colin Gordon. *Power/Knowledge: Selected Interviews and Other Writings, 1972–1977.* New York: Pantheon Books, 1980.

Frank, Katherine. *A Voyager Out: The Life of Mary Kingsley.* Boston: Houghton Mifflin, 1986.

Frederick, J. George. *Masters of Advertising Copy.* New York: Frank Maurice, 1925.

Freeman, T. B. *Journal of Various Visits to the Kingdoms of Ashanti, Aku, and Dahomi.* London: J. Mason, 1884.

Frenkel, Stephen, and John Western. "Pretext or Prophylaxis? Racial Segregation and Malarial Mosquitos in a British Tropical Colony: Sierra Leone." *Annals of the Association of American Geographers* 78, no. 2 (June 1988): 211–28.

Freshfield, Mark. *The Stormy Dawn.* London: Faber & Faber, 1946.

Friedson, Eliot. *Professional Dominance: The Social Structure of Medical Care.* New York: Atherton, 1970.

Fuchs, George J. "Antioxidants for Children with Kwashiorkor." *British Medical Journal* 330 (2005): 1095.

Gaisie, Samuel K., and K. T. De Graft-Johnson. *The Population of Ghana.* Paris: CICRED, 1976.

Gale, Thomas S. "The Struggle against Disease in the Gold Coast: Early Attempts at Urban Sanitary Reform." *Transactions of the Historical Society of Ghana* 16, no. 2, n.s., no. 1 (January 1995): 185–203.

Gann, L. H., and Peter Duignan, eds. *Rulers of British Africa, 1870–1914.* Stanford, CA: Stanford University Press, 1978.

Gate, Daniel. *Gate's New Shepherd's Guide for Cumberland, Westmoreland, and Lancashire.* Cockermouth, Cumberland: Brash Bros, 1879.

Gatsonis, Constantine, and Sally C. Morton. *Methods in Comparative Effectiveness Research.* Boca Raton, FL: CRC Press, 2017.

Geissler, Wenzel. *Para-states and Medical Science: Making African Global Health.* Durham: North Carolina University Press, 2015.

Gelfand, Michael. *The Sick African: A Clinical Study.* Cape Town: Stewart, 1948.

———. *Tropical Victory: An Account of the Influence of Medicine on the History of Southern Rhodesia, 1890–1923.* Cape Town: Juta, 1953. Published for the Rhodes Centenary Celebration Committee Southern Rhodesia.

Gemery, Henry A., and Jan S. Hogendorn, eds. *The Uncommon Market: Essays in the Economic History of the Atlantic Slave Trade.* New York: Academic, 1979.

Gentilcore, David. "Was There a 'Popular Medicine' in Early Modern Europe?" *Folklore* 115, no. 2 (August 2004): 151–66.

Georg, Odile. *Pouvoir Colonial, Municipalites et Espaces Urbains: Conakry–Freetown des Annees 1880 a 1914.* 2 Vols. L'Harmattan: Paris, 1997.

Gesler, Wilbert M. "Illness and Health Practitioner Use in Calabar, Nigeria." *Social Science and Medicine* 13 D, no. 1 (1979): 23–30.

Gesler, Wilbert M., and Robin A. Kearns. *Culture/Place/Health.* London: Routledge, 2002.

Ghana. Ghana Districts. Accessed March 3, 2021. http://www .ghanadistricts.com.

Ghana. Greater Accra. Accessed October 21, 2014. http://www.ghana.gov .gh/index.php/about-ghana/regions/greater-accra.

Ghana. *National AIDS/STD Control Programme, HIV/AIDS in Ghana: Background, Projections, Impacts, and Interventions.* Korle-Bu, Accra: Programme, 1999.

Giddens, Anthony, and Philip W. Sutton. *Modernity and Self-Identity: Self and Society in Late Modern Age.* Cambridge, UK: Polity Press, 2014.

Gifford, Paul. *African Christianity: Its Public Role.* Bloomington: Indiana University Press, 1998.

———. "Ghana's Charismatic Churches." *Journal of Religion in Africa* 24, no. 3 (August 1994): 241–65

———. *Ghana's New Christianity: Pentecostalism in a Globalizing African Economy.* Bloomington: Indiana University Press, 2004.

Gilroy, Paul. *The Black Atlantic: Modernity and Double Consciousness.* Cambridge, MA: Harvard University Press, 1993.

Gocking, Roger. *Facing Two Ways: Ghana's Coastal Communities under Colonial Rule.* Lanham, MD: University Press of America, 1999.

———. *The History of Ghana.* Westport, CT: Greenwood, 2005.

Gold Coast, Percy Alexander McElwaine, and Patrick Francis Branigan. *The Laws of the Gold Coast: Containing the Ordinances of the Gold Coast, the Gold Coast Colony, Ashanti, the Northern Territories, and Togoland Under United Kingdom Trusteeship, Enacted on or Before the 31st Day of December 1951.* London: C.F. Roworth, Govt. printers for the purposes of this edition, 1954.

Gold Coast Colony. *Achievement in the Gold Coast: Aspects of Development in a British West African Territory.* Accra: Public Relations Department, 1951.

———. *Report on the Medical Department by the Government of the Gold Coast.* Accra: Government Press, 1924–25.

Good, Charles M. *Ethnomedical Systems in Africa: Patterns of Traditional Medicine in Rural and Urban Kenya.* New York: Guildford, 1987.

Gordon, Charles Alexander. *Life on the Gold Coast.* London: Bailliere, Tindall & Cox, 1874.

Govindaraj, Ramesh, A. A. D. Obuobi, N. K. A. Enyimayew, P. Antwi, and Ofosu-Amaah. "Hospital Autonomy in Ghana: The Experience of Korle Bu and Komfo Anokye Teaching Hospitals." *School of Public Health, University of Ghana* (August 1996). https://pdf.usaid.gov/pdf_docs /PNABZ208.pdf.

Graboyes, Melissa. *The Experiment Must Continue: Medical Research and Ethics in East Africa, 1940–2014.* Athens: Ohio University Press, 2015.

Graeber, David. "Fetishism as Social Creativity; or, Fetishes Are Gods in the Process of Construction." *Anthropological Theory* 5 (2005): 407–38.

Graham, C. K. *The History of Education in Ghana from the Earliest Times to the Declaration of Independence.* London: Routledge, 1971.

Gran, Peter. "Medical Pluralism in Arab and Egyptian History: An Overview of Class Structures and Philosophies of the Main Phases." *Social Science and Medicine* 13 B, no. 4 (December 1979): 339–41.

Grant, Richard. *Globalizing City: The Urban and Economic Transformation of Accra, Ghana.* Syracuse, NY: Syracuse University Press, 2008.

Gray, Natasha. "Witches, Oracles, and Colonial Law: Evolving Anti-witchcraft Practices in Ghana, 1927–1932." *International Journal of African Historical Studies* 34, no. 2 (2001): 339–63.

Great Britain. Secretary of State for the Colonies. *West African Pocketbook.* London: Waterlow & Sons, 1905.

Green, Edward C. *Indigenous Theories of Contagious Disease.* Walnut Creek, CA: AltaMira, 1999.

Greene, Jack P., and Philip D. Morgan, eds. *Atlantic History: A Critical Appraisal.* Oxford: Oxford University Press, 2009.

Greene, Sandra. *Sacred Sites and the Colonial Encounter: A History of Meaning and Memory in Ghana.* Bloomington: Indiana University Press, 2002.

Grell, Ole Peter, and Andrew Cunningham, eds. *Medicine and Religion in Enlightenment Europe.* Burlington, VT: Ashgate, 2007.

Griffith, William B. *Ordinances of the Settlements on the Gold Coast and of the Gold Coast Colony in Force April 7th, 1887.* London: Stevens & Sons, 1887.

Grindal, Bruce T. "Islamic Affiliations and Urban Adaptation: The Sisala Migrant in Accra, Ghana." *Africa: Journal of the International African Institute* 43, no. 4 (October 1973): 333–46.

Grischow, Jeff D. "K. R. S. Morris and Tsetse Eradication in the Gold Coast, 1928–51." *Africa: Journal of the International African Institute* 76, no. 3 (2006): 381–401.

Grmek, M. D., ed. *Serving the Cause of Public Health: Selected Papers of Andrija Stampar.* Zagreb: Andrija Stampar School of Public Health, 1966.

Grover, J. K., and S. P. Yadav. "Pharmacological Actions and Potential Uses of *Momordica charantia*: A Review." *Journal of Ethnopharmacology* 93, no. 1 (2004): 123–32.

Guggisberg, Governor Sir Gordon. *The Post War Gold Coast Report, 6th March, 1924.* Accra: Government Press, 1924.

Gumperz, John J., and Dell Hymes, eds. *Directions in Sociolinguistics: The Ethnography of Communication.* New York: Holt, Rinehart & Winston, 1972.

Gunter, Valerie J. "News Media and Technological Risks: The Case of Pesticides after 'Silent Spring.'" *Sociological Quarterly* 46, no. 4 (Autumn 2005): 671–98.

Guyer, Jane I. *Marginal Gains: Monetary Transactions in Atlantic Africa.* Chicago: University of Chicago Press, 2004.

Guyer, Jane I., and Samuel M. Eno Belinga. "Wealth in People as Wealth in Knowledge: Accumulation and Composition in Equatorial Africa." *Journal of African History* 36, no. 1 (1995): 91–120.

Gyekye, Kwame. *An Essay on African Philosophical Thought: The Akan Conceptual Scheme.* Cambridge: Cambridge University Press, 1987.

———. *Tradition and Modernity: Philosophical Reflections on the African Experience.* New York: Oxford University Press, 1997.

Hackett, C. J. "Private Medical Practice and Anti-yaws Campaigns in South Eastern Nigeria, 1925–1950." *Tropical Doctor* 10 (1980): 129–32.

Hafkin, Nancy J., and Edna G. Bay. *Women in Africa: Studies in Social and Economic Change.* Stanford, CA: Stanford University Press, 1976.

Hahn, Robert A., and Marcia C. Inhorn. *Anthropology and Public Health: Bridging Differences in Culture and Society.* Oxford: Oxford University Press, 2009.

Hale-White, William. *Materia Medica, Pharmacy, Pharmacology and Therapeutics.* Toronto: Macmillan, 1914.

Haliburton, Gordon MacKay. *The Prophet Harris: A Study of an African Prophet and His Mass-Movement in the Ivory Coast and the Gold Coast 1913–1915.* London: Longman, 1971.

Halliday, S. "Duncan of Liverpool: Britain's First Medical Officer." *Journal of Medical Biography* 11, no. 3 (August 2003): 142–49.

Hambly, Wilfrid Dyson. "Review of M. J. Field, *Religion and Medicine of the Gã People.*" *American Anthropologist,* n.s., 40, no. 2 (April–June 1938): 312–14.

Hamilton, Gary G. "Chinese Consumption of Foreign Commodities: A Comparative Perspective." *American Sociological Review* 42, no. 6 (December 1977): 877–91.

Hansen, E., and A. Ninsin. *Easmon Report.* Accra: Government of Ghana, Ministry of Health, 1966.

Hansen, Karen Tranberg. "Transnational Biographies and Local Meanings: Used Clothing Practices in Lusaka." *Journal of Southern African Studies* 21, no. 1 (March 1995): 131–45.

Harley, G. W. *Native African Medicine.* London: Cass, 1970.

Harrison, Gordon A. *Mosquitoes, Malaria and Man.* New York, 1978.

Harvey, David. *Justice, Nature, and the Geography of Difference.* Oxford: Blackwell, 2000.

Hastrup, Kirsten. "The Ethnographic Present: A Reinvention." *Cultural Anthropology* 5, no. 1 (February 1990): 45–61.

Hausman, Gary J. "Making Medicine Indigenous: Homeopathy in South India." *Social History of Medicine* 15, no. 2 (2002): 303–22.

Hawkins, Sean. *Writing and Colonialism in Northern Ghana: The Encounter between the LoDagaa and "the World on Paper."* Toronto: University of Toronto Press, 2002.

Haynes, Douglas M. *Imperial Medicine: Patrick Manson and the Conquest of Tropical Disease.* Philadelphia: University of Pennsylvania Press, 2013.

Headrick, Daniel R. *The Tools of Empire: Technology and European Imperialism in the 19th Century.* New York: Oxford University Press, 1981.

Heap, Simon. "'A Bottle of Gin Is Dangled before the Nose of the Natives': The Economic Uses of Imported Liquor in Southern Nigeria, 1860–1920." *African Economic History* 33 (2005): 69–85.

Heelas, Paul. *The New Age Movement: The Celebration of the Self and the Sacralization of Modernity.* London: Basil Blackwell, 1996.

Henige, David. "Measuring the Immeasurable: The Atlantic Slave Trade, West African Population and the Pyrrhonian Critic." *Journal of African History* 27, no. 2 (1986): 295–313.

Henley, Paul. *The Adventure of the Real: Jean Rouch and the Craft of Ethnographic Cinema.* Chicago: University of Chicago Press, 2009.

———. "Spirit Possession, Power, and the Absent Presence of Islam: Reviewing Les Maîtres Fous." *Journal of the Royal Anthropological Institute* 12, no. 4 (2006): 731–61.

Hepper, F. N. *West African Herbaria of Isert and Thonning.* Chicago: University of Chicago Press, 2000.

Hill, Poly. *The Migrant Cocoa-Farmers of Southern Ghana.* Cambridge: Cambridge University Press, 1963.

Hill, Robert A., and Marcus Garvey. *Marcus Garvey and Universal Negro Improvement Association Papers.* Berkeley: University of California Press, 1985.

Hobsbawm, Eric, and Terence Ranger, eds. *The Invention of Tradition.* New York: Cambridge University Press, 1992.

Hogerzeil, Simon J., and David Richardson. "Slave Purchasing Strategies and Shipboard Mortality: Day-to-Day Evidence from the Dutch African Trade, 1751–1797." *Journal of Economic History* 67, no. 1 (March 2007): 160–90.

Hokkanen, Markku. "Quests for Health and Contests for Meaning: African Church Leaders and Scottish Missionaries in the Early Twentieth Century Presbyterian Church in Northern Malawi." *Journal of Southern African Studies* 33, no. 4 (December 2007): 733–50.

Homan, Peter. "Medicated Cheer." *Pharmaceutical Journal* 27, no. 7280 (December 20/27, 2003): 867–68.

Hopkins, Donald R. "Dracunculiasis Eradication: The Final Inch." *American Journal of Tropical Medicine and Hygiene* 73, no. 4 (2005): 669–75.

Hörbst, V., and T. Gerrits. "Transnational Connections of Health Professionals: Medicoscapes and Assisted Reproduction in Ghana and Uganda." *Ethnicity & Health* 21, no. 4 (2016): 357–374.

Horder, Mervyn. "The Hard Boiled Saint: Selwyn-Clarke in Hong Kong."
    British Medical Journal 311 (August 19, 1995): 492–95.
Horn, Arthur E. "The Control of Disease in Tropical Africa: Part I." *Jour-
    nal of the Royal African Society* 32, no. 126 (January 1933): 21–30.
———. "The Control of Disease in Tropical Africa: Part III." *Journal of the
    Royal African Society* 32, no. 128 (July 1933): 252–60.
Horton, Robin. *Patterns of Thought in Africa and the West: Essays on Magic,
    Religion and Science*. Cambridge: Cambridge University Press, 1993.
Hostettmann, K., and A. Marston. "Countercurrent Chromatography in
    the Preparative Separation of Plant-Derived Natural Products." *Journal
    of Liquid Chromatography & Related Technologies* 24, no. 11/12 (June 15,
    2001): 1711–22.
Howard, Joel. *Technology in the Hospital: Transforming Patient Care in the
    20th Century*. Baltimore, MD: Johns Hopkins University Press, 1995.
Huber, Magnus. *Ghanaian Pidgin English in Its West African Context: A
    Sociohistorical and Structural Analysis*. Amsterdam: John Benjamins,
    1999.
Huchzermeyer, Marie, and Aly Karam. *Informal Settlements: A Perpetual
    Challenge?* Cape Town: UCT Press, 2006.
Hudson, Geoffrey L., ed. *British Military and Naval Medicine, 1600–1830*.
    New York: Rodopi, 2007.
Hughes, M. H., and P. F. Daly. "Onchocerciasis in the Southern Gold
    Coast," *Transactions of the Royal Society of Tropical Medicine and Hygiene*
    45, no. 2 (1951): 243–52.
Hunt, Nancy Rose. "'Le Bebe en Brousse': European Women, African
    Birth Spacing and Colonial Intervention in Breast Feeding in the Bel-
    gian Congo." *International Journal of African Historical Studies* 21, no. 3
    (1988): 401–32.
———. *A Colonial Lexicon: Of Birth Ritual, Medicalization, and Mobility in
    the Congo*. Durham, NC: Duke University Press, 1999.
Hunt, Nancy Rose, Tessie P. Liu, and Jean Quataert, eds. *Gendered Colo-
    nialisms in African History*. Williston, VT: Blackwell, 1997.
Hutchinson, John, and John McEwen Dalziel. *Flora of West Tropical Africa*.
    London: Crown Agents for the Colonies, 1927.
Hutchison, T. J. *Impressions of Western Africa with Remarks on the Diseases
    of the Climate*. London: Longman, Brown, Green, Longmans & Roberts,
    1858.
Hutton, William. *A Voyage to Africa: Including a Narrative of an Embassy to
    One of the Interior Kingdoms, in the Year 1820; with Remarks on the Course*

and Termination of the Niger, and Other Principal Rivers in That Country. London: Longman, Hurst, Rees, Orme & Brown, 1821.

Huxley, Thomas H. *Evidence as to Man's Place in Nature.* London: Williams & Norgate, 1863.

Iliffe, John. *East African Doctors: A History of the Modern Profession.* Cambridge: Cambridge University Press, 1998.

Illich, Ivan. *Medical Nemesis: The Expropriation of Health.* Toronto: McClelland & Stewart, 1975.

Ipsen, Pernille. "Intercultural Intimacy in Danish Guinea, 1680–1740." *Historie Netmagasinet,* December 16, 2005. Accessed April 22, 2010. https://www.historie-nu.dk.

Iqani, Mehita, and Bridget Kenny. *Consumption, Media and Culture in South Africa Perspectives on Freedom and the Public.* London: Routledge, 2016.

Irvine, F. R. *Plants of the Gold Coast.* London: Oxford University Press, 1930.

———. *Woody Plants of Ghana: With Special Reference to Their Uses.* London: Oxford University Press, 1961.

Isichei, Elizabeth. *Voices of the Poor in Africa.* Rochester, NY: University of Rochester Press, 2002.

Iwu, Maurice M. *Handbook of African Medicinal Plants.* Boca Raton, FL: CRC, 1993.

Janzen, John. *Lemba, 1650–1930: A Drum of Affliction in Africa and the New World.* New York: Garland, 1982.

———. *Ngoma: Discourses of Healing in Central and Southern Africa.* Berkeley: University of California Press, 1992.

———. *The Quest for Therapy: Medical Pluralism in Lower Zaire.* Berkeley: University of California Press, 1982.

———. "Therapy Management: Concept, Reality, Process." *Medical Anthropology Quarterly,* n.s., 1, no. 1 (March 1987): 68–84.

Jenkins, Paul, ed. *The Recovery of the West African Past: African Pastors and African History in the Nineteenth Century, C. C. Reindorf and Samuel Johnson.* Basel: Baseler Africka Bibliographien, 1998.

Jennings, Michael. "Chinese Medicine and Medical Pluralism in Dar es Salaam: Globalisation or Glocalisation?" *International Relations December* 19, no. 4 (2005): 457–73.

Johannessen, Helle, and Imre Lazar, eds. *Multiple Medical Realities: Patients and Healers in Biomedical, Alternative, and Traditional Medicine.* New York: Berghahn Books, 2006.

Johnson, John. *The Epic of Son-Jara: A West African Tradition.* Bloomington: Indiana University Press, 1986.

Johnson, Ryan. "Tabloid Brand Medicine Chests: Selling Health and Hygiene for the British Tropical Colonies." *Science as Culture* 17, no. 3 (2008): 249–68.

———. "The West African Medical Staff and the Administration of Imperial Tropical Medicine, 1902–14." *Journal of Imperial and Commonwealth History* 38, no. 3 (2010): 419–39.

Johnson, Terence. "Imperialism and the Professions: Notes on the Development of Professional Occupations in Britain's Colonies and the New States." *Sociological Review* 20 (1972): 281–309.

Johnson, Terry. *Health Professions and the State in Europe*. London: Taylor & Francis, 2005.

Jones, Adam, ed. *Brandenburg Sources for West African History, 1680–1700*. Stuttgart: Franz Steiner Verlag Wiesbaden, 1985.

———. *German Sources for West African History, 1599–1669*. Wiesbaden: Steiner, 1983.

———. *West Africa in the Mid-Seventeenth Century: An Anonymous Dutch Manuscript*. Atlanta, GA: African Studies Association Press, 1995.

Jones, Charles. *Historical Linguistics: Problems and Perspectives*. Hoboken, NJ: Taylor & Francis, 2014.

Jones-Quartey, K. A. B. "The Gold Coast Press: 1822-c 1930, and the Anglo-African Press: 1825-c 1930—The Chronologies." Archival document held at Michigan State University. Accessed June 28, 2014. http://archive.lib .msu.edu/DMC/African%20Journals/pdfs/Institue%20of%20African %20Studies%20Research%20Review/1968v4n2/asrv004002004.pdf.

Justesen, Ole, and James Manley. *Danish Sources for the History of Ghana, 1657–1754*. Copenhagen: Det Kongelige Danske Videnskabernes Selskab, 2005.

Kaba, Lansiné. "The Pen, the Sword, and the Crown: Islam and Revolution in Songhay Reconsidered, 1464–1493." *Journal of African History* 25, no. 3 (1984): 241–56.

Kalmus, H. "Obituary. C. R. Ribbands, M.A. (Cantab.), Sc.D. (Cantab.)." *Animal Behaviour* 15, no. 4 (October 1967): 402.

Karp, Ivan. "Deconstructing Culture-Bound Syndromes." *Social Science and Medicine* 21, no. 2 (1985): 221–28.

Kassim, Olakunle O., Mark Loyevsky, Biaffra Elliott, Andrew Geall, Henrietta Amonoo, and Victor R Gordeuk. "Effects of Root Extracts of *Fagara zanthoxyloides* on the In Vitro Growth and Stage Distribution of *Plasmodium falciparum*." *Antimicrobial Agents and Chemotherapy* 49, no. 1 (2005): 264–68.

Kawachi, Ichirō, and Sarah P. Wamala, eds. *Globalization and Health*. New York: Oxford University Press, 2007.

Kea, Ray. "GSGC Notes and Queries: On the Eve of the Battle of Katamanso: Translated Extracts from a Danish Document (1826)," *Ghana Studies Journal*, online. http://www.ghanastudies.com/gsa/gsc97kea2 .html.

———. *Settlements, Trade, and Polities in the Seventeenth-Century Gold Coast*. Baltimore, MD: Johns Hopkins University Press, 1982.

Keita, Maghan. *A Political Economy of Health Care in Senegal*. Leiden: Brill, 2007.

Kemp, Reverend Dennis. *Nine Years at the Gold Coast*. London: Macmillan, 1898.

Kilama, Wen L., Roma Chilengi, and Charles L. Wanga. "Towards an African-Driven Malaria Vaccine Development Program: History and Activities of the African Malaria Network Trust (AMANET)." In "Defining and Defeating the Intolerable Burden of Malaria III: Progress and Perspectives," edited by J. G. Breman, M. S. Alilio, and N. J. White. Supplement, *American Society of Tropical Medicine and Hygiene* 77, no. 6 (December 2007): 282–88.

Killingray, David. "Military and Labour Recruitment in the Gold Coast during the Second World War." *Journal of African History* 23, no. 1 (1982): 83–95.

Kilson, Marion. *African Urban Kinsmen: The Ga of Central Accra*. London: Hurst, 1974.

———, ed. *Excerpts from the Diary of Kwaku Niri (alias J. Q. Hammond) 1884–1918*. Accra: Institute of African Studies, University of Ghana, Legon, 1967.

———. *Kpele Lala: Ga Religious Songs and Symbols*. Cambridge, MA: Harvard University Press, 1971.

Kimble, David. *A Political History of Ghana: The Rise of Gold Coast Nationalism, 1850–1928*. Oxford: Clarendon, 1963.

Kingsley, Mary. *Travels in West Africa*. London: MacMillan, 1897.

Kiple, Kenneth. *Cambridge World History of Human Disease*. New York: Cambridge University Press, 1993.

Kisacky, Jeanne. "Restructuring Isolation: Hospital Architecture, Medicine, and Disease Prevention." *Bulletin of the History of Medicine* 79, no. 1 (2005): 1–49.

Kleinman, Arthur. *Culture and Healing in Asian Societies: Anthropological, Psychiatric, and Public Health Studies*. Boston: G. K. Hall, 1978.

———. *Illness Narratives: Suffering, Healing and the Human Condition.* New York: Basic Books, 1988.

———. *Patients and Healers in the Context of Culture.* Berkeley: University of California Press, 1980.

Klieman, Kairn A. *"The Pygmies Were Our Compass": Bantu and Batwa in the History of West Central Africa, Early Times to c. 1900 C.E.* Portsmouth, NH: Heinemann, 2003.

Klooster, Peter M., Johanna C. M. Oostveen, Linda C Zandbelt, Erik Taal, Constance H. C. Drossaert, Etelka J. Harmsen, and Mart A. F. J van de Laar. "Further Validation of the 5-Item Perceived Efficacy in Patient-Physician Interactions (peppi-5) Scale in Patients with Osteoarthritis." *Patient Education and Counseling* 87, no. 1 (2012): 125–30.

Köhler, Werner. "Killed in Action: Microbiologists and Clinicians as Victims of Their Occupation. Part 2: Yellow Fever and Bartonellosis." *International Journal of Medical Microbiology* 295, no. 4 (2005): 193–200.

Kopytoff, Igor, ed. *The African Frontier.* Bloomington: Indiana University Press, 1987.

Korle Bu Hospital, 1923–1973: Golden Jubilee Souvenir. Accra: Advent, 1973.

Kotey, Paul A. *Twi-English, English-Twi.* New York: Hippocrene Books, 2005.

Krause, Kristine, David Parkin, and Gabi Alex. "Turning Therapies: Placing Medical Diversity." *Medical Anthropology* 33, no. 1 (2014): 1–5.

Kuczynski, Robert R. *Demographic Survey of the British Colonial Empire.* New York: Kelley, 1977.

Kuklick, Henrika, ed. *A New History of Anthropology.* Oxford: Blackwell, 2008.

Laidler, Percy Ward, and Michael Gelfand, eds. *South Africa: Its Medical History 1652–1898.* Cape Town: C. Struik, 1971.

Lalu, Premesh. "Medical Anthropology, Subaltern Traces, and the Making and Meaning of Western Medicine in South Africa: 1895–1899." *History in Africa* 25 (1998): 133–59.

Lambek, Michael. *Knowledge and Practice in Mayotte: Local Discourses of Islam, Sorcery and Spirit Possession.* Toronto: University of Toronto Press, 1993.

———. *The Weight of the Past: Living with History in Mahajanga, Madagascar.* New York: Palgrave Macmillan, 2002.

Landau, Paul Stuart. "Explaining Surgical Evangelism in Colonial Southern Africa: Teeth, Pain and Faith." *Journal of African History* 37, no. 2 (1996): 261–81.

———. *The Realm of the Word: Language, Gender, and Christianity in a Southern African Kingdom.* Portsmouth, NH: Heinemann, 1995.

Langwick, Stacey A. "Devils, Parasites, and Fierce Needles: Healing and the Politics of Translation in Southern Tanzania." *Science, Technology, & Human Values* 32, no. 1 (January 2007): 88–117.

Last, Murray, and G. L. Chavunduka. *The Professionalisation of African Medicine.* International African seminars, n.s., no. 1. Manchester: Manchester University Press in association with the International African Institute, 1986.

Law, Robin. *From Slave Trade to 'Legitimate' Commerce: The Commercial Transition in Nineteenth-Century West Africa.* London: Cambridge University Press, 2002.

———. *Ouidah: The Social History of a West African Slaving 'Port', 1727–1892.* 2nd ed. Athens: Ohio University Press, 2004.

Law, Robin, and Kristen Mann. "West Africa in the Atlantic Community: The Case of the Slave Coast." *William and Mary Quarterly*, 3rd ser., 56, no. 2 (April 1999): 307–34.

League of Nations, Health Organization. *Malaria Commission, Principles and Measures of Antimalarial Measures in Europe.* Geneva: Publication Department of the League of Nations, 1927.

Lentz, Carola, and Paul Nugent, eds. *Ethnicity in Ghana: The Limits of Invention.* London: Palgrave Macmillan, 2000.

Leslie, Charles, ed. *Asian Medical Systems: A Comparative Study.* Berkeley: University of California Press, 1976.

———. "Medical Pluralism in World Perspective [1]." *Social Science & Medicine, Part B: Medical Anthropology* 14, no. 4 (1980): 191–95.

Levtzion, Nehemia, and Pouwels, Randall L. *The History of Islam in Africa.* Athens: Ohio University Press, 2000.

Liddiard, Mabel. *The Mothercraft Manual, Etc.* London, 1924.

Lighthouse Chapel International. "Healing Jesus Crusade." Accessed October 1, 2012. http://www.daghewardmills.org/healingjesuscrusade/.

Lim, Kien Ket. "Of Mimicry and White Man: A Psychoanalysis of Jean Rouch's *Les Maitres Fous.*" *Cultural Critique* 51 (Spring 2002): 40–73.

Lind, James. *An Essay on Diseases Incidental to Europeans in Hot Climates: With the Method of Preventing Their Fatal Consequences [. . .].* London, 1792.

Lindemann, Mary. *Medicine and Society in Early Modern Europe.* Cambridge: Cambridge University Press, 2010.

Lindenbaum, Shirley, and Margaret Lock, eds. *Knowledge, Power, and Practice: The Anthropology of Medicine and Everyday Life.* Berkeley: University of California Press, 1997.

Lindley, John. *Flora Medica: A Botanical Account of All the More Important Plants Used in Medicine, in Different Parts of the World.* London: Longman, et al., 1838.

Linnaeus, Carolus. *Systema Naturae.* Stockholm: Salvius, 1758.

Lissowska, Jolanta. "The Demographic, Social and Professional Structure of the Population of Accra between 1960 and 1970." *Africana Bulletin* 32 (1984): 113–29.

Livingston, Julie. "Productive Misunderstandings and the Dynamism of Plural Medicine in Mid-Century Bechuanaland." *Journal of Southern African Studies* 33, no. 4 (December 2007): 801–10.

Loeb, Lori. "Doctors and Patent Medicines in Modern Britain: Professionalism and Consumerism." *Albion: A Quarterly Journal Concerned with British Studies* 33, no. 3 (Autumn 2001): 404–25.

Lötter, H. P. P. *Injustice, Violence and Peace: The Case of South Africa.* Amsterdam: Rodopi, 1997.

Loudon, Irvine, ed. *Western Medicine: An Illustrated History.* Oxford: Oxford University Press, 1997.

Lovejoy, Paul E. *Transformations in Slavery: A History of Slavery in Africa.* 2nd ed. Cambridge: Cambridge University Press, 2000.

———. "The Volume of the Atlantic Slave Trade: A Synthesis." *Journal of African History* 23, no. 4 (1982): 473–501.

Lucas, Charles. *The Gold Coast and the War.* London: Oxford University Press, 1920.

Luedke, Tracy. "Spirit and Matter: The Materiality of Mozambican Prophet Healing." *Journal of Southern African Studies* 33, no. 4 (December 2007): 715–731.

Lugard, F. D. *The Dual Mandate in British Tropical Africa.* London: Frank Cass, 1965.

Lyons, Maryinez. *The Colonial Disease: A Social History of Sleeping Sickness in Northern Zaire, 1900–1940.* Cambridge: Cambridge University Press, 1992.

MacConnaughey, David Robert. *Medical Landscapes: The Perceived Links between Environment, Health, and Disease in Pre-Twentieth-Century North America.* Chapel Hill, NC: University of North Carolina Press, 1986.

Macdonald, Ogilvy James Scott. *Small Sewage Disposal Systems, with Special Reference to the Tropics.* London: H. K. Lewis, 1951.

Macfie, J. W. S. "Intravenous Injection of Tartar Emetic in Guinea-Worm Infections." *Lancet* 195, no. 5038 (March 20, 1920): 654–55.

MacLeod, Roy M., and Milton J. Lewis. *Disease, Medicine, and Empire: Perspectives on Western Medicine and the Experience of European Expansion.* London: Routledge, 1988.

Macmillan, Allister, ed. *The Red Book of West Africa: Historical and Descriptive Commercial and Industrial Facts, Figures, & Resources*. London: Frank Cass, 1968.

Magoon, E. H. "A Portable Stable Trap for Capturing Mosquitoes." *Bulletin of Entomological Research* 26 (1935): 363–69.

Maier, Diane. "Nineteenth-Century Asante Medical Practices." *Comparative Studies in Society and History* 21, no. 1 (January 1979): 63–81.

Makepeace, Margaret, ed. *Trade on the Guinea Coast, 1657–1666: The Correspondence of the English East India Company*. Madison: African Studies Program, University of Wisconsin, 1991.

Malefyt, Timothy Dwight deWaal, and Brian Moeran. *Advertising Cultures*. Oxford: Berg, 2003.

Maly, R. C., J. C. Frank, G. N. Marshall, M. R. DiMatteo, and D. B. Reuben. "Perceived Efficacy in Patient-Physician Interactions (peppi): Validation of an Instrument in Older Persons." *Journal of the American Geriatrics Society* 46, no. 7 (1998): 889–94.

Mangan, J. A. *The Cultural Bond: Sport, Empire, Society*. London: Routledge, 1992.

Manning, Patrick, and William S. Griffiths. "Divining the Unprovable: Simulating the Demography of African Slavery." *Journal of Interdisciplinary History* 19, no. 2 (Autumn 1988): 117–201.

Manson, Patrick. "An Introductory Address on the Necessity for Special Education in Tropical Medicine. Delivered at St George's Hospital [London] at the Opening of the Winter Session, October 1, 1897." *Lancet*, October 2, 1897, 843.

Marie Louise, H. H. Princess. *Letters from the Gold Coast*. London: Methuen, 1926.

Marks, Shula. *Divided Sisterhood: Race, Class, and Gender in the South African Nursing Profession*. New York: St. Martin's, 1994.

Marshall, George N., and David Poling. *Schweitzer: A Biography*. Baltimore, MD: Johns Hopkins University Press, 2000.

Martin, Marie-Louise. *Kimbangu: An African Prophet and His Church*. Grand Rapids, MI: Eerdmans, 1976.

Maynard, Kent. *Making Kedjom Medicine: A History of Public Health and Well-Being in Cameroon*. Westport, CT: Praeger, 2004.

Mazrui, Ali A. "Dr. Schweitzer's Racism." Review of *Out of My Life and Thought: An Autobiography*, by Albert Schweitzer, edited by Antje Bultmann Lemke. *Transition* 53 (1991): 96–102.

Mbiti, John S. *African Religions & Philosophy*. London: Heinemann, 1990.

M'Boloko, Elikia. "Peste et Société urbaine à Dakar: l'épidèmie de 1914." *Cahiers d'études africaines* 22, no. 85–86 (1982): 13–46.

McBride, David P. *Missions for Science: U.S. Technology and Medicine in America's Africa World*. New Brunswick, NJ: Rutgers University Press, 2002.

McCaskie, Thomas. "Denkyira in the Making of Asante." *Journal of African History* 48, no. 1 (2007): 1–25.

———. "Innovational Eclecticism: The Asante Empire and Europe in the Nineteenth Century." *Comparative Studies in Society and History* 14, no. 1 (January 1972): 30–45.

———. *State and Society in Pre-colonial Asante*. Cambridge: Cambridge University Press, 1995.

McKeown, Thomas. *The Role of Medicine: Dream, Mirage, or Nemesis?* London: Nuffield Provincial Hospitals Trust, 1976.

McKeown, Thomas, and R. G. Brown. "Medical Evidence Related to English Population Changes in the Eighteenth Century." *Population Studies* 9 (1955): 119–41.

McKeown, Thomas, R. G. Brown, and R. G. Record. "An Interpretation of the Modern Rise of Population in Europe." *Population Studies* 26 (1972): 345–82.

McKeown, Thomas, and R. G. Record. "Reasons for the Decline of Mortality in England and Wales during the Nineteenth Century." *Population Studies* 16 (1962): 94–122.

Mensah, E. N. "Status of Traditional Medicine Development in Ghana." Lecture presented in Accra, April 27, 2011. http://expressfsgroup.com/tm.co.uk/5.doc.

Mensah-Dapaah, K. "Traditional Healing." *Ghana Journal of Science* 21 (1968): 16–21.

Mercer, T. M. Kodwo. "The Gold Coast Development Programme." *African Affairs* 55, no. 218 (January 1956): 27–32.

Meredith, Henry. *An Account of the Gold Coast of Africa, with a Brief History of the African Company*. London: Cass, 1967.

Messent, J. J. "Use and Effectiveness of Anti-malaria Drugs: Correspondence." *British Medical Journal* 2 (September 12, 1953): 629.

Metcalf, Thomas R. "Architecture and the Representation of Empire: India, 1860–1910." *Representations*, no. 6 (Spring 1984): 37–65.

Metcalfe, G. E., ed. *Great Britain and Ghana: Documents of Ghana History 1807–1957*. London: Thomas Nelson and Sons, 1964.

Meyer, Birgit. "Christianity in Africa: From African Independent to Pentecostal-Charismatic Churches." *Annual Review of Anthropology* 33 (2004): 447–74.

———. "'Make a Complete Break with the Past': Memory and Post-colonial Modernity in Ghanaian Pentecostalist Discourse." *Journal of Religion in Africa* 28, fasc. 3 (August 1998): 316–49.

———. *Translating the Devil: Religion and Modernity among the Ewe in Ghana*. Cambridge: Edinburgh University Press, 1999.

Miller, Jon. *Missionary Zeal and Institutional Control: Organizational Contradictions in the Basel Mission on the Gold Coast 1828–1917*. Cambridge: Routledge, 2003.

Minocha, A. "Medical Pluralism and Health Services in India." *Social Science & Medicine, Part B: Medical Anthropology* 14, no. 4 (1980): 217–23.

Mitchell, Henry. "CAS Students to Lead Seminar on University's African Alumni, Pt. IV: Agnes Yewande Savage." *CAS from the Edge* (blog). Centre of African Studies, University of Edinburgh, November 16, 2016. Accessed March 3, 2021. https://centreofafricanstudies.wordpress.com/2016/11/16/cas-students-to-lead-seminar-on-universitys-african-alumni-pt-iv-agnes-yewande-savage/.

Mitchell, Timothy. *Rule of Experts: Egypt, Techno-Politics, Modernity*. Berkeley: University of California Press, 2002.

Moffatt, Nii Addokwei. "Dog Meat, a New Craze in Accra." *Daily Graphic*. Republished on GhanaWeb.com, July 8, 2004. Accessed August 18, 2009. http://www.ghanaweb.com/GhanaHomePage/NewsArchive/artikel.php?ID=61222.

Mohr, Adam. "Capitalism, Chaos, and Christian Healing: Faith Tabernacle Congregation in Southern Colonial Ghana, 1918–26." *Journal of African History* 52, no.1 (2011): 63–83.

———, "Missionary Medicine and Akan Therapeutics: Illness, Health and Healing in Southern Ghana's Basel Mission, 1828–1918." *Journal of Religion in Africa* 39, no. 4 (2009): 429–61.

Monrad, H. C. *A Description of the Guinea Coast and Its Inhabitants*. Edited by Selena Axelrod Wisnes. Accra: Sub-Saharan Publishers, 2009.

Moore, Decima, and F. G. Guggisberg, C.M.G.R.E. *We Two in West Africa*. New York: Charles Scribner & Sons, 1909.

Moore, Ronnie, and Stuart McClean, eds. *Folk Healing and Health Care Practices in Britain and Ireland: Stethoscopes, Wands, and Crystals*. New York: Berghahn Books, 2010.

Morton-Williams, Peter, William Bascom, and E. M. McClelland. "Two Studies of Ifa Divination. Introduction: The Mode of Divination."

Africa: Journal of the International African Institute 36, no. 4 (October 1966): 406–31.

Mouser, Bruce L., and Samuel Gamble. *A Slaving Voyage to Africa and Jamaica: The Log of the Sandown, 1793–1794*. Bloomington: Indiana University Press, 2002.

Mshana, N. R., *Traditional Medicine and Pharmacopoeia: Contributions to the revision of Ethnobotanical and Floristic Studies in Ghana*. Accra: Organization of African Unity/Scientific, Technical and Research Commission, 2002.

Mukharji, Projit. "Lokman, Chholeman and Manik Pir: Multiple Frames of Institutionalising Islamic Medicine in Modern Bengal." *Social History of Medicine* 24, no. 3 (2011): 720–38.

Mullings, Leith. *Therapy, Ideology, and Social Change: Mental Healing in Urban Ghana*. London: University of California Press, 1984.

Mumuni, Haji Sulemana. "Islamic Literacy Tradition in Ghana." *Maghreb Review* 28, no. 2/3 (2003): 170–85.

Murray, John. *A System of Materia Medica and Pharmacy*. Edinburgh: W. Laing, et al., 1810.

Nahin, R. L. "Costs of Complementary and Alternative Medicine (CAM) and Frequency of Visits to CAM Practitioners: United States, 2007." *National Health Statistics Reports* 18 (2009).

Nájera, José A., M. González-Silva, and P. L. Alonso. "Some Lessons for the Future from the Global Malaria Eradication Programme (1955–1969)." *PLoS Medicine* 8, no. 1 (2011).

Neequaye, Alfred R., Janet E. Neequaye, and Robert J. Biggar. "Factors That Could Influence the Spread of AIDS in Ghana, West Africa: Knowledge of AIDS, Sexual Behaviour, Prostitution, and Traditional Medical Practices." *JAIDS Journal of Acquired Immune Deficiency Syndromes* 4, no. 9 (September 1991): 914–19.

Neill, Deborah. *Networks in Tropical Medicine: Internationalism, Colonialism, and the Rise of a Medical Specialty, 1890–1930*. Stanford, CA: Stanford University Press, 2012.

Nelson, C., and L. Grossberg, eds. *Marxism and the Interpretation of Culture*. Basingstoke, UK: Macmillan Education, 1988.

Newell, Stephanie. *Literary Culture in Colonial Ghana: "How to Play the Game of Life."* Bloomington: Indiana University Press, 2002.

———. *The Power to Name: A History of Anonymity in Colonial West Africa*. Athens: Ohio University Press, 2013.

Newell, Stephanie, and Audrey Gadzekpo, eds. *Selected Writings of a Pioneer West African Feminist*. Nottingham: Trent, 2004.

Ngalamulume, Kalala. "Keeping the City Clean: Yellow Fever and the Politics of Prevention in Colonial Saint-Louis-du-Senegal, 1854–1914." *Journal of African History* 45 (2004): 183–202.

Niane, D. T. *Sundiata, an Epic of Old Mali*. London, (1965) 2001.

Nketia, J. H. "Changing Traditions of Folk Music in Ghana." *Journal of the International Folk Music Council* 11 (1959): 31–36.

Noret, Joel. "Morgues et prise en charge de la mort au Sud-Benin." *Cahiers d'études africaines* 44, no. 4 (2004): 745–67.

Norregard, Georg. *1658–1850: Danish Settlements in West Africa*. Boston: Boston University Press, 1968.

Norton, Marcy. *Sacred Gifts, Profane Pleasures: A History of Tobacco and Chocolate in the Atlantic World*. Ithaca, NY: Cornell University Press, 2008.

O'Barr, William M. *Culture and the Ad: Exploring Otherness in the World of Advertising*. Boulder, CO: Westview, 1994.

Obermeyer, Carla Makhlouf. "Pluralism and Pragmatism: Knowledge and Practice of Birth in Morocco." *Medical Anthropology Quarterly* 14, no. 2 (June 2000): 180–201.

Odaamtten, S. K. *The Missionary Factor in Ghana's Development (1820–1880)*. Accra: Waterville, 1978.

Odoom, K. O. "A Document on Pioneers of the Muslim Community in Accra." *Institute of African Studies: Research Review* 7, no. 3 (1971): 1–31.

Odotei, Irene. "About the Guinea Coast in General: Draft Translation of F. L. Rømer." Supplement, *Research Review*, no. 8 (1995).

———. "Pre-colonial Economic Activities of Ga." *Research Review* 11 (1995): 60–74.

Officer, Lawrence H., and Samuel H. Williamson. *Cliometric Currency Calculator*. http://measuringworth.com/calculators/uscompare.

Ofori-Adjei, David. "David Ofori-Adjei: Building Bridges for Health Care and Research in Ghana. Interviewed by Julia Royall." *Lancet, Infectious Diseases* 3, no. 4 (2003): 251–54.

Okware, S., J. Kinsman, S. Onyango, A. Opio, and P. Kaggwa. "Revisiting the ABC Strategy: HIV Prevention in Uganda in the Era of Antiretroviral Therapy." *Postgraduate Medical Journal* 81 (2005): 625–28.

Oliver-Bever, Bep. *Medicinal Plants in Tropical West Africa*. Cambridge: Cambridge University Press, 1986.

Oppong, Joseph R. "A Vulnerability Interpretation of the Geography of HIV/AIDS in Ghana, 1986–1995." *Professional Geographer* 50, no. 4 (November 1998): 437–48.

Ordinances of the Gold Coast Colony. London: Stevens & Sons, 1903.

Orlove, Benjamin, ed. *The Allure of the Foreign: Imported Goods in Postcolonial Latin America.* Ann Arbor: University of Michigan Press, 1997.

Ortiz, Fernando. *Cuban Counterpoint: Tobacco and Sugar.* Translated by Harriet de Onís. Durham, NC: Duke University Press, 1995.

Osseo-Asare, Abena Dove. *Bitter Roots: The Search for Healing Plants in Africa.* Chicago: University of Chicago Press, 2014.

Owusu, George, and Samuel Agyei-Mensah. "A Comparative Study of Ethnic Residential Segregation in Ghana's Two Largest Cities, Accra and Kumasi." *Population and Environment* 32 (2011): 332–52.

Owusu-Ansah, David. *Historical Dictionary of Ghana.* Lanham, MD: Rowman & Littlefield, 2014.

———. "Islamic Influence in a Forest Kingdom: The Role of Protective Amulets in Early 19th Century Asante." *Transafrican Journal of History* 12 (1983): 100–133.

Packard, Randall. *The Making of a Tropical Disease: A Short History of Malaria.* Baltimore, MD: Johns Hopkins University Press, 2007.

"Paludrine: A New Anti-malarial Drug," *Nature* 156 (1945): 596–97.

Parker, John. *Making the Town: Ga State and Society in Early Colonial Accra.* Portsmouth, NH: Heinemann, 2000.

———. "Witchcraft, Anti-witchcraft and Trans-regional Ritual Innovation in Early Colonial Ghana: Sakrabundi and Aberewa, 1889–1910." *Journal of African History* 45, no. 3 (2004): 393–420.

Parker, John, and Richard J. Reid. *Oxford Handbook of Modern African History.* Oxford: Oxford University Press, 2016.

Parrinder, Geoffrey. *Religion in an African City.* London: Oxford University Press, 1953.

———. *West African Religion: A Study of the Beliefs and Practices of Akan, Ewe, Yoruba, Ibo, and Kindred Peoples.* New York: Barnes & Noble, 1970.

Patterson, K. David. *Health in Colonial Ghana: Disease, Medicine, and Socio-economic Change, 1900–1955.* Waltham, MA: Crossroads, 1981.

———. "Health in Urban Ghana: The Case of Accra, 1900–1940." *Social Science and Medicine* 13 B, no. 4 (1979): 251–68.

———. "Health in Urban Ghana: The Case of Accra, 1900–1940." Unpublished manuscript, last modified 1978. Held at Northwestern University Library.

———. "The Influenza Epidemic of 1918–19 in the Gold Coast." *Journal of African History* 24, no. 4 (1983): 485–502.

Patton, Adell, Jr. "Dr. John Farrell Easmon: Medical Professionalism and Colonial Racism in the Gold Coast, 1856–1900." *International Journal of African Historical Studies* 22, no. 4 (1989): 601–36.

———. *Physicians, Colonial Racism, and Diaspora in West Africa.* Gainesville: University of Florida Press, 1996.

Pearson, Jessica Lynne. *The Colonial Politics of Global Health: France and the United Nations in Postwar Africa.* Cambridge, MA: Harvard University Press, 2018.

Peel, J. D. Y. *Aladura: A Religious Movement among the Yoruba.* London: Oxford University Press, 1968.

———. "The Pastor and the 'Babalawo': The Interaction of Religions in Nineteenth-Century Yorubaland." *Africa: Journal of the International African Institute* 60, no. 3 (1990): 338–69.

———. *Religious Encounter and the Making of the Yoruba.* Bloomington: Indiana University Press, 2000.

———. "Syncretism and Religious Change." *Comparative Studies in Society and History* 10, no. 2 (1968): 121–41.

Pellow, Deborah. "Cultural Differences and Urban Spatial Forms: Elements of Boundedness in an Accra Community." *American Anthropologist* 103, no. 1 (March 2001): 59–75.

———. "Muslim Segmentation: Cohesion and Divisiveness in Accra." *Journal of Modern African Studies* 23, no. 3 (1985): 419–44.

———. "The Power of Space in the Evolution of an Accra Zongo." *Ethnohistory* 38, no. 4 (Autumn 1991): 414–50.

———. "Research Article: STDs and AIDS in Ghana." *Genitourinary Medicine* 70 (1994): 418–42.

Pesek, Michael. "Foucault Hardly Came to Africa: Some Notes on Colonial and Post-colonial Governmentality." *Comparativ* 21 (2011): 41–59.

Pesewua, George A., Ronald R. Cutlera, and David P. Humbera. "Antibacterial Activity of Plants Used in Traditional Medicines of Ghana with Particular Reference to MRSA." *Journal of Ethnopharmacology* 116, no. 1 (February 28, 2008): 102–11.

Peterson, Derek R., and Darren R. Walhof. *The Invention of Religion: Rethinking Belief in Politics and History.* New Brunswick, NJ: Rutgers University Press, 2002.

Pickstone, John V., Terence Ranger, and Paul Slack. "Dearth, Dirt and Fever Epidemics: Rewriting the History of British 'public health',

1780–1850." In *Epidemics and Ideas*, edited by Terence Ranger and Paul Slack, 125–48. Cambridge: Cambridge University Press, 1992.

Pierre, Jemima. *The Predicament of Blackness: Postcolonial Ghana and the Politics of Race*. Chicago: University of Chicago Press, 2013.

Pietz, William. "The Problem of the Fetish, I." *Res* 9 (Spring 1985): 5–17.

———. "The Problem of the Fetish, II." *Res* 13 (Spring 1987): 23–45.

———. "The Problem of the Fetish, IIIa: Bosman's Guinea and the Enlightenment Theory of Fetishism." *Res* 16 (Autumn 1988): 105–23.

Piot, Charles. *Remotely Global: Village Modernity in West Africa*. Chicago: University of Chicago Press, 1999.

Plageman, Nate. "'Accra Is Changing, Isn't It?': Urban Infrastructure, Independence, and Nation in the Gold Coast's *Daily Graphic*, 1954–57." *International Journal of African Historical Studies* 43, no. 1 (2010): 137–60.

"Plague at Accra." *Lancet*, January 25, 1908, 248.

Polednak, Anthony P. "Albert Schweitzer and International Health." *Journal of Religion and Health* 28, no. 4 (Winter 1989): 323–29.

Pool, Robert. *Dialogue and the Interpretation of Illness: Conversations in a Cameroon Village*. Oxford: Berg, 1994.

Pope, Daniel. *The Making of Modern Advertising*. New York: Basic Books, 1983.

Poplin, Irene Schuessler. "Nursing Uniforms: Roman Idea, Functional Attire, or Instrument of Social Change?" *Nursing History Review* 2 (1993): 153–70.

Porter, Roy, ed. *The Cambridge History of Medicine*. Cambridge: Cambridge University Press, 2006.

———. "The Patient's View: Doing Medical History from Below." *Theory and Society* 14 (1985): 175–98.

———. *Quacks: Fakers and Charlatans in English Medicine*. Charleston, SC: Tempus, 2000.

Poser, C. M., and G. W. Bruyn, eds. *An Illustrated History of Malaria*. New York: Informa Healthcare, 1999.

Postal Domestic Course in Medical Herbalism. Birmingham, UK: National Institute of Medical Herbalists, 1950.

Power, Helen. *Tropical Medicine in the 20th Century*. New York: Routledge, 2016.

Prais, Jinny Kathleen. "Imperial Travelers: The Formation of West African Urban Culture, Identity, and Citizenship in London and Accra, 1925–1935." PhD diss., University of Michigan, 2008.

Pratt, Mary Louise. *Imperial Eyes: Travel Writing and Transculturation*. New York: Routledge, 2008.

Prins, G. "But What Was the Disease? The Present State of Health and Healing in African Studies." *Past & Present*, 1989, 159–79.

Protten, Jacobsen. En nyttig grammaticalsk indledelse til tvende hidindtil ubekiendte Sprog, Fanteisk og acraisk [. . .]. Copenhagen, 1764.

"The Public Health Bill, 1875." *British Medical Journal*, April 3, 1875, 449–51.

Punday, Daniel. "Foucault's Body Tropes." *New Literary History* 31, no. 3 (2000): 509–28.

Quarcoopome, Nii Otokunor. "Thresholds and Thrones: Morphology and Symbolism of Dangme Public Altars." *Journal of Religion in Africa* 24, no. 4 (November 1994): 339–57.

Quarcoopome, Samuel S. "The Impact of Urbanization on the Sociopolitical History of the Ga Mashie of Accra: 1877–1957." PhD diss., Institute of African Studies, University of Ghana, 1993.

Quartey Papafio, A. B. "The Ga Homowo Festival." *Journal of the Royal African Society* 19, no. 74 (January 1920): 126–34.

———. "The Ga Homowo Festival." *Journal of the Royal African Society* 19, no. 75 (April 1920): 227–32.

Quartey, Seth. *Missionary Practices on the Gold Coast, 1832–1895: Discourse, Gaze, and Gender in the Basel Mission in Pre-colonial West Africa.* Youngstown, NY: Cambria, 2007.

Quayesi-Amakye, Joseph. "The Church, Medicine and Healing: The Ghanaian Pentecostal Response." *Ogbomoso Journal of Theology* 18, no. 2 (2013):1–16.

"Quininism." *Lancet*, January 13, 1838, 550–51.

R., B. L. H. "F. V. Nanka-Bruce, O.b.e., M.b., Ch.b." *British Medical Journal* 2, no. 4830 (1953): 289–90.

Ranger, Terence. *Voices from the Rocks: Nature, Culture, and History in the Matopos Hills of Zimbabwe.* Bloomington: Indiana University Press, 1999.

Ranger, Terence, and Paul Slack, eds. *Epidemics and Ideas.* Cambridge: Cambridge University Press, 1992.

Rankin, F. H. *The White Man's Grave: A Visit to Sierra Leone in 1834.* 2 vols. London, 1836.

Ransford, Oliver. *"Bid the Sickness Cease": Disease in the History of Black Africa.* London: J. Murray, 1983.

Rapp, Eugen L. "Review of M. J. Field: *Religion and Medicine.*" *Africa: Journal of the International African Institute* 11, no. 4 (October 1938): 513–14.

Rask, Johannes, and H. C. Monrad. *Two Views from Christiansborg Castle.* Translated by Selena Wisnes. Legon, Accra, Ghana: Sub-Saharan Publishers, 2009.

Rasmussen, Susan. *Healing in Community: Medicine, Contested Terrains, and Cultural Encounters among the Tuareg.* Westport, CT: Bergin & Garvey, 2001.

Rattray, Robert Sutherland. *Religion & Art in Ashanti.* Oxford: Clarendon, 1927.

Reconstructive Surgery Africa. Accessed September 22, 2014. http://www.resurgeafrica.org.

Reindorf, Carl Christian. *The History of the Gold Coast and Asante: Based on Traditions and Historical Facts Comprising a Period of More Than Three Centuries from about 1500 to 1860.* Accra: Ghana Universities Press, 1966.

Reindorf, C. E. "Influence of Fifty Years of Scientific Medicine on Beliefs and Customs in the Gold Coast." *West African Medical Journal* 3, no. 3 (September 1955): 115–19.

———. "The Problem of Venereal Disease on the Gold Coast and the Possibilities of Control." *West African Medical Journal,* 1927, 8–9.

Rekdal, Ole Bjørn. "Cross-cultural Healing in East African Ethnography." *Medical Anthropology Quarterly* 13, no. 4 (December 1999): 458–82.

Rentink, Sonja. "Kpanlogo: Conflict, Identity Crisis and Enjoyment in a Ga Drum Dance." Research paper for the Department of Musicology, University of Amsterdam, 2003. https://www.yumpu.com/en/document/read/8503960/conflict-identity-crisis-and-enjoyment-in-a-ga-drum-dance.

Reynolds, Edward. *Trade and Economic Change on the Gold Coast, 1807–1874.* New York: Longmans, 1974.

Ribbands, C. R. "Effects of Bush Clearance on Flighting of West African Anophelines." *Bulletin of Entomological Research* 37 (1946): 33–41.

———. "Moonlight and House-Haunting Habits of Female Anophelines in West Africa." *Bulletin of Entomological Research* 36 (1945): 395–415.

Richards, Thomas. *The Commodity Culture of Victorian England: Advertising and Spectacle, 1851–1914.* Stanford, CA: Stanford University Press, 1990.

The Rise of Independent Churches in Ghana. Accra: Asempa, 1990.

Risse, Geunter B. *Mending Bodies, Saving Souls: A History of Hospitals.* New York: Oxford University Press, 1999.

Rivett, Geoffrey. *The Development of the London Hospital System, 1823–1982.* Oxford: Oxford University Press, 1986.

Robertson, Claire C. "The Death of Makola and Other Tragedies." *Canadian Journal of African Studies* 17, no. 3 (1983): 469–95.

————. *Sharing the Same Bowl: A Socioeconomic History of Women and Class in Accra, Ghana.* Bloomington: Indiana University Press, 1984.

Robinson, David. *Muslim Societies in Africa.* Cambridge: Cambridge University Press, 2004.

Rocco, Fiametta. *Quinine: Malaria and the Quest for a Cure That Changed the World.* New York: Harper Collins, 2003.

Roller, Heather Flynn. "Colonial Collecting Expeditions and the Pursuit of Opportunities in the Amazonian Sertão, c. 1750–1800." *Americas* 66, no. 4 (April 2010): 435–67.

Rømer, Ludvig Ferdinand. *A Reliable Account of the Coast of Guinea (1760).* Translated by Selena Axelrod Wisnes. Oxford: Oxford University Press, 2001.

Rosen, George. *A History of Public Health.* Baltimore, MD: Johns Hopkins University Press, 1993.

Ross, David. "European Models and West African History: Further Comments on the Recent Historiography of Dahomey." *History in Africa* 10 (1983): 293–305.

Ross, Ivan A. *Medicinal Plants of the World: Chemical Constituents, Traditional and Modern Medicinal Uses.* Totowa, NJ: Humana Press, 1999.

Ross, Ronald. "Letters to Editor: The Inoculation Accident at Mulkowal." *Nature* 75 (March 21, 1907): 486–87.

————. *Malaria Fever: Its Cause, Prevention, and Treatment.* London: Liverpool School of Tropical Medicine, 1902.

Rouch, Jean. *Ciné-ethnography.* Vol. 13 of *Visible Evidence.* Edited and translated by Stephen Feld. Minneapolis: University of Minnesota Press, 2003.

————. "Jean Rouch Talks about His Films to John Marshall and John W. Adams (September 14th and 15th, 1977)." *American Anthropologist* 80 (1978): 1005–20.

————. *Notes on Migration into the Gold Coast: First Report of the Mission Carried Out in the Gold Coast from March to December, 1954.* N.p.: J. Rouch, 1955.

Royal Society. *Reports of the Malaria Committee of the Royal Society.* 10 vols. London, 1900.

Royall, J. "David Ofori-Adjei Building Bridges for Health Care and Research in Ghana." *Lancet Infectious Diseases* 3, no. 4 (April 2003): 251–54.

Russell, Helen. "Experimental Relapsing Fever, Accra, 1931." *West African Medical Journal* 6 (1933): 36–43.

Ryley, J. F. "The Mode of Action of Proguanil and Related Antimalarial Drugs." *British Journal of Pharmacology and Chemotherapy* 8, no. 4 (1953): 424–30.

Sabben-Clare, E. E., David J. Bradley, and Kenneth Kirkwood, eds. *Health in Tropical Africa during the Colonial Period.* Oxford: Clarendon, 1980.

Salm, Steven J., and Toyin Falola. *Culture and Customs of Ghana.* Westport, CT: Greenwood, 2002.

Sama, Martyn, and Vinh-Kim Nguyen. *Governing Health Systems in Africa.* Dakar, Senegal: Council for the Development of Social Science Research in Africa, 2008.

Sampson, Magnus J. *Gold Coast Men of Affairs (Past and Present).* London: Dawsons, 1969.

Sandosham, A. A., and Vijayamma Thomas. *Malariology: With Special Reference to Malaya.* Singapore: National University of Singapore Press, 1983.

Sanjek, Roger. "The Ethnographic Present." *Man* 26, no. 4 (1991): 609–28.

Sanneh, L. *Translating the Message: Missionary Impact on Culture.* Maryknoll, NY: Orbis, 1991.

Saunders, C. C., H. Phillips, and H. E. Van. *Studies in the History of Cape Town.* Vol. 4. Cape Town: University of Cape Town, Dept. of History, 1984. In association with Centre for African Studies.

Scenes and Services in South Africa: The Story of Robert Moffat's Half-Century of Missionary Labours. London: J. Snow, 1876.

Schoenbrun, David Lee. "Conjuring the Modern in Africa: Durability and Rupture in Histories of Public Healing between the Great Lakes of East Africa." *American Historical Review* 111, no. 3 (December 2006): 1403–39.

———. *A Green Place, a Good Place: Agrarian Change, Gender, and Social Identity in the Great Lakes Region to the 15th Century.* Portsmouth, NH: Heinemann, 1998.

Schoffeleers, Matthew. "Folk Christology in Africa: The Dialectics of the Nganga Paradigm." *Journal of Religion in Africa* 19, no. 2 (June 1989): 157–83.

———. "Ritual Healing and Political Acquiescence: The Case of the Zionist Churches in Southern Africa." *Africa* 61, no. 1 (1991): 1–25.

Schumaker, Lyn, Diana Jeater, and Tracy Luedke. "Introduction: Histories of Healing; Past and Present Medical Practices in Africa and the Diaspora." *Journal of Southern African Studies* 33, no. 4 (December 2007): 707–14

Scott, David. *Epidemic Disease in Ghana, 1901–1960.* London: Oxford University Press, 1965.

Sederberg, Peter C. "The Gold Coast under Colonial Rule: An Expenditure Analysis." *African Studies Review* 14, no. 2 (September 1971): 179–204.

Selin, Helaine, and Hugh Shapiro. *Medicine across Cultures: History and Practice of Medicine in Non-Western Cultures*. Dordrecht: Kluwer Academic Publishers, 2003.

Selwyn-Clarke, Percy, G. E. H Le Fanu, and A. Ingram. "Relapsing Fever in the Gold Coast." *Annals of Tropical Medicine and Parasitology* 17, no. 3 (1923): 389–426.

Semley, Lorelle. "Public Motherhood in West Africa as Theory and Practice." *Gender & History* 24, no. 3 (2012): 600–16.

Senah, Kodjo Amedjorteh. *Money Be Man: The Popularity of Medicines in a Rural Ghanaian Community*. Amsterdam: Het Spinhuis, 1997.

Shaw, Rosalind. *Memories of the Slave Trade: Ritual and the Historical Imagination in Sierra Leone*. Chicago: University of Chicago, 2002.

Sheridan, Richard B. *Doctors and Slaves: A Medical and Demographic History of Slavery in the British West Indies, 1680–1834*. Cambridge: Cambridge University Press, 1985.

———. "The Guinea Surgeons on the Middle Passage: The Provision of Medical Services in the British Slave Trade." *International Journal of African Historical Studies* 14, no. 4 (1981): 601–25.

Silver, John B. *Mosquito Ecology: Field Sampling Methods*. 3rd ed. Dordrecht, Netherlands: Springer, 2008.

Silverman, Raymond A., and David Owusu-Ansah. "The Presence of Islam among the Akan of Ghana: A Bibliographic Essay." *History in Africa* 16 (1989): 325–39.

Simpson, William John Ritchie. *Report on Plague in the Gold Coast, 1908*. London: J & A Churchill, 1909.

———. "Statement on the Outbreak of Plague in the Gold Coast Colony." In *Government Gazette*. Accra, Gold Coast, West Africa, 1908.

———. *A Treatise on Plague: Dealing with the Historical, Epidemiological, Clinical, Therapeutic, and Preventative Aspects of the Disease*. Cambridge: Cambridge University Press, 1905.

Skinner, David E. "Mande Settlement and the Development of Islamic Institutions in Sierra Leone." *International Journal of African Historical Studies* 11, no. 1 (1978): 32–62.

Slater, Ransford. "Changing Problems of the Gold Coast." *Journal of the Royal African Society* 29, no. 117 (October 1930): 461–66.

Smith, Noel. *The Presbyterian Church of Ghana, 1835–1960*. Accra: Ghana Universities Press, 1966.

Smith, Philippa Mein. "King, Sir (Frederic) Truby (1858–1938)." In *Oxford Dictionary of National Biography*. Oxford: Oxford University Press, 2004. http://www.oxforddnb.com/view/article/34320.

Sneader, Walter. *Drug Discovery: A History*. West Sussex, UK: John Wiley & Sons, 2005.

Songsore, J., and G. McGranahan. "Environment, Wealth and Health: Towards an Analysis of Intra-urban Differentials within the Greater Accra Metropolitan Area, Ghana." *Environment and Urbanization* 5, no. 2 (1993): 10–34.

Sparks, Randy J. *Where the Negroes Are Masters: An African Port in the Era of the Slave Trade*. Cambridge, MA: Harvard University Press, 2014.

Spitzer, Leo. "The Mosquito and Segregation in Sierra Leone." *Canadian Journal of African Studies / Revue Canadienne des Études Africaines* 2, no. 1 (Spring 1968): 49–61.

Stanley, Henry M., and Melton Prior. *Coomassie and Magdala: The Story of Two British Campaigns in Africa*. London: Sampson Low, Marston, Low & Searle, 1874.

Stanton, J. "Listening to the Ga: Cicely Williams' Discovery of kwashiorkor on the Gold Coast." *Clio Medica* 61 (2001): 149–71.

Stearns, Peter N., and William Leonard Langer. *The Encyclopedia of World History: Ancient, Medieval, and Modern*. New York: Houghton Mifflin Harcourt, 2001.

Steiner, Rudolf. *Fundamentals of Anthroposophical Medicine: Four Lectures Given to Doctors*. Stuttgart, 1922. Published online through the Mercury Press. http://wn.rsarchive.org/Lectures/GA314/English/MP1986/FunAnt_index.html.

Stepan, Nancy. *Eradication: Ridding the World of Disease*. London: Reaktion, 2011.

Stephens, Rhiannon. *A History of African Motherhood: The Case of Uganda, 700–1900*. Cambridge: Cambridge University Press, 2015.

Stewart, Charles, and Rosalind Shaw, eds. *Syncretism/Anti-syncretism: The Politics of Religious Synthesis*. New York: Routledge, 1994.

Stock, R. "Traditional Healers in Rural Hausaland." *Geojournal* 5, no. 4 (July 1981): 363–68.

Stoller, Paul. *The Cinematic Griot: The Ethnography of Jean Rouch*. Chicago: University of Chicago Press, 1992.

Stuart, David C. *Dangerous Garden: The Quest for Plants to Change Our Lives*. Cambridge, MA: Harvard University Press, 2004.

Sundkler, Bengt. *Bantu Prophets in South Africa*. 2nd ed. London: Oxford University Press, 1961.

Svalesen, Leif. *The Slave Ship* Fredensborg. Bloomington: Indiana University Press, 2000.

Swanson, Maynard. "The Sanitation Syndrome: Bubonic Plague and Urban Native Policy in the Cape Colony, 1900–1909." *Journal of African History* 18, no. 3 (1977): 387–410.

Swinson, Arthur. *The History of Public Health*. Exeter: A. E. Wheaton, 1965.

Tanabe, Makoto, Peter van den Besselaar, and Toru Ishida, eds. *Digital Cities*. Vol. 2. Berlin: Springer, 2002.

Tanner, Thomas Hawkes. *An Index of Diseases and Their Treatment*. 3rd ed. London: Henry Renshaw, 1883.

———. *A Manual of the Practice of Medicine*. London: Lindsay & Blakiston, 1858.

Taylor, W. R. "An Arabic Amulet." *Muslim World* 25, no. 2 (1935): 161–65.

Teixiera da Mota, A., and P. E. H. Hair. *East of Mina: Afro-European Relations on the Gold Coast in the 1550s and the 1560s*. Madison: African Studies Program, University of Wisconsin-Madison, 1988.

Thomas, Hugh. *The Slave Trade: The Story of the Atlantic Slave Trade: 1440–1870*. New York: Simon & Schuster, 1997.

Thomas, Keith. *Religion and the Decline of Magic*. Harmondsworth: Penguin Books, 1973.

Thompson, E. P. "The Moral Economy of the English Crowd in the Eighteenth Century." *Past & Present* 50 (February 1971): 76–136.

Thompson, John D., and Grace Goldin. *The Hospital: A Social and Architectural History*. New Haven, CT: Yale University Press, 1975.

Thornton, John. *Africa and Africans in the Making of the Atlantic World, 1400–1680*. Cambridge: Cambridge University Press, 1992.

Tonelli, M. R., and T. C. Callahan. "Why Alternative Medicine Cannot Be Evidence-Based." *Academic Medicine: Journal of the Association of American Medical Colleges* 76, no. 12 (2001): 1213–20.

The Trans-Atlantic Slave Trade Database. http://www.slavevoyages.com.

Trape, J. F. "The Public Health Impact of Chloroquine Resistance in Africa." *American Journal of Tropical Medicine and Hygiene* 64, no. 1 (January 2001). http://www.ncbi.nlm.nih.gov/books/NBK2616/.

Tudhope, W. T. D. "The Development of the Cocoa Industry in the Gold Coast and Ashanti." *Journal of the Royal African Society* 9, no. 33 (October 1909): 34–45.

Turino, Thomas. *Nationalists, Cosmopolitans, and Popular Music in Zimbabwe*. Chicago: University of Chicago Press, 2000.

Tutu, John Kwadwo Osei. "The Asafoi (Socio-military Groups) in the History of Politics of Accra (Ghana) from the 17th to the Mid-20th

Century." PhD diss., Norwegian University of Science and Technology, 2000.

Twumasi, Patrick A. "Colonialism and International Health: A Study in Social Change in Ghana." *Social Science & Medicine* 15 B (1981): 147–51.

———. *Medical Systems in Ghana*. Accra: Ghana Publishing Corporation, 2005.

———. "A Social History of the Ghanaian Pluralistic Medical System." *Social Science & Medicine, Part B: Medical Anthropology* 13, no. 4 (1979): 349–56.

UNESCO. *Visual Aids in Fundamental Education*. N.p.: UNESCO, 1952.

UNICEF. *Malaria: A Major Cause of Child Death and Poverty in Africa*. N.p.: UNICEF, 2004.

US Supreme Court. *Manhattan Medicine Co. v. Wood*, 108 U.S. 218 (1883).

van Binsbergen, Wim, and Peter Geschiere. *Commodification: Things, Agency, and Identities (The Social Life of Things Revisited)*. Vol. 8. Munster: Lit, 2005.

van Dantzig, Albert. *Forts and Castles of Ghana*. Accra: Sedco, 1999.

van den Bersselaar, Dmitri. *The King of Drinks: Schnapps Gin from Modernity to Tradition*. Leiden: Brill, 2007.

van der Geest, Sjaak. "Marketplace Conversations in Cameroon: How and Why Popular Medical Knowledge Comes Into Being." *Culture, Medicine and Psychiatry* 15, no. 1 (1991): 69–90.

van der Geest, Sjaak, and Susan Reynolds Whyte. "The Charm of Medicines: Metaphors and Metonyms." *Medical Anthropology Quarterly*, n.s., 3, no. 4 (December 1989): 348–50.

van Dijk, Rijk. "Contesting Silence: The Ban on Drumming and the Musical Politics of Pentecostalism in Ghana." *Ghana Studies* 4 (2001): 31–64.

———. "From Camp to Encompassment: Discourses of Transsubjectivity in the Ghanaian Pentecostal Diaspora." *Journal of Religion in Africa* 27, fasc. 2 (May 1997): 135–59.

———. "Localisation, Ghanaian Pentecostalism and the Stranger's Beauty in Botswana." *Africa: Journal of the International African Institute* 73, no. 4 (2003): 560–83.

van Dijk, Rijk, Ria Reis, and Marja Speirenburg. *The Quest for Fruition through Ngoma*. Oxford: James Currey, 2000.

Van Heyningen, Elizabeth. "Cape Town and the Plague of 1901." In *Studies in the History of Cape Town*, vol. 4. Cape Town: University of Cape Town, Centre for African Studies, 1981, 72.van Kessel, I., ed. *Merchants, Missionaries & Migrants: 300 Years of Dutch-Ghanaian Relations*. Amsterdam: KIT Publishers, 2002.

Vansina, Jan. *Oral Tradition as History*. Madison: University of Wisconsin Press, 1985.

———. *Paths in the Rainforests: Toward a History of Political Tradition in Equatorial Africa*. Madison: University of Wisconsin Press, 1990.

Vartanian, Aram. *Science and Humanism in the French Enlightenment*. Charlottesville, VA: Rookwood, 1999.

Vaughan, Megan. *Curing Their Ills: Colonial Power and African Illness*. Stanford, CA: Stanford University Press, 1991.

Ventevogel, Peter. *Whiteman's Things: Training and Detraining Healers in Ghana*. Amsterdam: Het Spinhuis, 1996.

Vermeer, Donald E. "Geophagy among the Ewe of Ghana." *Ethnology* 10, no. 1 (January 1971): 56–72.

Villault, Nicholas. *Relation des Costes d'Afrique Appelees Guinee*. Paris, 1669.

"Vogeler's Curative Compound." *Meyer Brothers Druggist* 26, no. 10 (1905): 113.

Von Brazi, Calus. "Controversy Unlimited: The Nigerian 'Re-invasion' of Ghana." *Ghana Web News*, September 13, 2009. http://www.ghanaweb.com/GhanaHomePage/NewsArchive/artikel.php?ID=168530.

Waddington, C. J., and K. A. Enyimayew. "A Price to Pay: The Impact of User Charges in Ashanti-Akim District, Ghana." *International Journal of Health Planning and Management* 4, no. 1 (January/March 2006): 17–47.

Waite, Gloria. *A History of Traditional Medicine and Health Care in Precolonial East-Central Africa*. Lewiston, NY: Mellen, 1992.

Wall, L. Lewis. *Hausa Medicine*. Durham, NC: Duke University Press, 1988.

Wangensteen, Owen H., and Sarah D. Wangensteen. *The Rise of Surgery: From Empiric Craft to Scientific Discipline*. Minneapolis: University of Minnesota Press, 1978.

Weinberg, S. Kirson. "'Mental Healing' and Social Change in West Africa." *Social Problems* 11, no. 3 (Winter 1964): 257–69.

Weiss, Holger. *Social Welfare in Muslim Societies in Accra*. Uppsala: Nordic Africa Institute, 2002.

Wellman, Barry, and Keith Hampton. "Living Networked On and Offline." *Contemporary Sociology* 28, no. 6 (November 1999): 648–54.

Welman, C. W. "James Fort, Accra, and the Oyeni Fetish." *Gold Coast Review* 3 (1927): 78.

Wesseling, H. L. *Expansion and Reaction: Essays on European Expansion and Reaction in Asia and Africa*. Leiden: Leiden University Press, 1978.

Westermann, Diedrich. *Evefiala or Ewe-English Dictionary*. Berlin: Kraus, 1973.

White, Hayden V. *The Content of the Form: Narrative Discourse and Historical Representation.* Baltimore, MD: Johns Hopkins University Press, 1987.

White, Luise. *Speaking with Vampires: Rumour and History in Colonial Africa.* Los Angeles: University of California Press, 2000.

Whyte, Susan Reynolds. "Pharmaceuticals as Folk Medicine: Transformations in the Social Relations of Health Care in Uganda." *Culture, Medicine and Psychiatry* 16, no. 2 (June 1992): 163–86.

———. *Questioning Misfortune: The Pragmatics of Uncertainty in Eastern Uganda.* Cambridge Studies in Medical Anthropology 4. Cambridge: Cambridge University Press, 1997.

Wilcocks, Charles. *Aspects of Medical Investigation in Africa.* London: Oxford University Press, 1962.

Wilks, Ivor. "Akwamu and Otublohum: An Eighteenth-Century Akan Marriage Arrangement." *Africa: Journal of the International African Institute* 29, no. 4 (October 1959): 391–404.

———. *Asante in the Nineteenth Century: The Structure and Evolution of a Political Order.* London: Cambridge University Press, 1975.

———. "The Rise of the Akwamu Empire, 1650–1710." *Transactions of the Historical Society of Ghana* 3 (1957): 99–136.

Willcox, R. E. "Obituary George Marshall Findlay, 6th January 1893–14th March 1952." *Journal of Pathology and Bacteriology* 65, no. 2 (April 1953): 621–25.

Willcox, R. R. "Venereal Disease in British West Africa." *Nature* 157 (1946): 416–19.

Williams, Cicely. "Child Health in the Gold Coast." *Lancet,* January 8, 1938, 97–102.

———. "Malnutrition." *Lancet,* August 18, 1962, 342–44.

———. "A Nutritional Disease of Childhood Associated with a Maize Diet." *Archives of Disease in Childhood* 8 (1933): 423–33.

———. "Witchdoctors." *Pediatrics* 46, no. 3 (September 1970): 448–55.

Williams, David A., and Thomas L. Lemke. *Foye's Principles of Medicinal Chemistry.* 5th ed. Baltimore: Lippincot William & Wilkins, 2002.

Williams, T. David. "Sir Gordon Guggisberg and Educational Reform in the Gold Coast, 1919–1927." *Comparative Education Review* 8, no. 3 (December 1964): 290–306.

Winters, Robert W. *Accidental Medical Discoveries: How Tenacity and Pure Dumb Luck Changed the World.* New York: Skyhorse, 2016.

Wiredu, Kwasi. *Philosophy and an African Culture.* Cambridge: Cambridge University Press, 1980.

Wiredu, Kwasi, and Kwame Gyekye. *Person and Community: Ghanaian Philosophical Studies I.* Washington, DC: Council for Research in Values and Philosophy, 1992.

Wisnes, Selena Axelrod. *Letters on West Africa and the Slave Trade: Paul Erdmann Isert's Journey to Guinea and the Caribbean Islands in Columbia (1788).* Oxford: Oxford University Press, 1992.

Wood, Gloria, and Paul Thompson. *The Nineties: Personal Recollections of the 20th Century.* London: BBC Books, 1993.

Woodham, Jonathan. "Images of Africa and Design at the British Empire Exhibitions between the Wars." *Journal of Design History* 2, no. 1 (1989): 15–33.

Wraith, R. E. *Guggisberg.* London: Oxford University Press, 1967.

Wright, Gwendolyn. *The Politics of Design in French Colonial Urbanism.* Chicago: University of Chicago Press, 1991.

Wulff, Wulff Joseph, and Selena Axelrod Wisnes. *A Danish Jew in West Africa: Wulff Joseph Wulff; Biography and Letters 1836–1842.* Legon-Accra, Ghana: Sub-Saharan Publishers, 2013.

Xulu, Sheikh Aazam. "Description Money Spell." Accessed March 10, 2018. https://www.myjoymarket.com/ads/view/74192.

Yerxa, Donald A. *Recent Themes in the History of Africa and the Atlantic World: Historians in Conversation.* Columbia: University of South Carolina Press, 2008.

Young, Crawford. *The African Colonial State in Comparative Perspective.* New Haven, CT: Yale University Press, 1994.

Zimmerman, Johannes. *Grammatical Sketch of the Akra or Ga Language, Including a Vocabulary of the Akra or Ga Language with an Adangme Appendix.* Stuttgart, 1858.

INDEX

Figure numbers in *italics* indicate illustrations.

392 INDEX

JONATHAN ROBERTS is Associate Professor of History at Mount Saint Vincent University in Halifax.

Printed and bound by CPI Group (UK) Ltd, Croydon, CR0 4YY

27/10/2024

14580189-0002